Addiction
Therapy and Treatment

Addiction Therapy and Treatment

A Systems Approach

LARRY FRITZLAN, LMFT,
with AVIS RUMNEY, LMFT

Foreword by Brad Reedy, Ph.D.

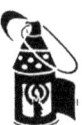

McFarland & Company, Inc., Publishers
Jefferson, North Carolina

ALSO OF INTEREST
AND FROM MCFARLAND

Dying to Please: Anorexia, Treatment and Recovery,
2d ed., by Avis Rumney (2009)

"Requiem: My Mother's Unspeakable Illness" by Cynthia Gorey (Appendix I) is reprinted with the permission of the author.

The Ten Principles of Successful Addiction Treatment by Kevin McCauley, MD (Appendix D) is reprinted with the permission of the author.

The excerpts from *Alcoholics Anonymous,* the Big Book and pamphlets "Is A.A. For You?" and "If You Are a Professional, A.A. Wants to Work with You" are reprinted with the permission of Alcoholics Anonymous World Services, Inc. ("A.A.W.S."). Permission to reprint these excerpts does not mean that A.A.W.S. has reviewed or approved the contents of this publication, or that A.A. necessarily agrees with the views expressed herein.

The 10-page excerpt from Chapter 8, "Transgenerational Models," is taken from Goldenberg/Stanton/Goldenberg, *Family Therapy,* 9E, © 2017 Delmar Learning, part of Cengage, Inc., and is reproduced by permission.

ASAM's short and long definitions of addiction are reprinted by permission from ASAM.

LIBRARY OF CONGRESS CATALOGUING-IN-PUBLICATION DATA

Names: Fritzlan, Larry, author. | Rumney, Avis, author. | Reedy, Brad M., author of foreword.
Title: Addiction therapy and treatment : a systems approach / Larry Fritzlan, LMFT, with Avis Rumney, LMFT ; foreword by Brad Reedy, Ph.D.
Description: Jefferson, North Carolina : McFarland & Company, Inc., Publishers, 2023 | Includes bibliographical references and index.
Identifiers: LCCN 2022039605 | ISBN 9781476688145 (paperback : acid free paper) ∞
ISBN 9781476647289 (ebook)
Subjects: LCSH: Substance abuse—Treatment. | Substance abuse—Patients—Family relationships. | Substance abuse—Treatment—Case studies. | Substance abuse—Patients—Counseling of. | BISAC: PSYCHOLOGY / Psychopathology / Addiction
Classification: LCC RC564 .F753 2022 | DDC 362.29—dc23/eng/20220929
LC record available at https://lccn.loc.gov/2022039605

BRITISH LIBRARY CATALOGUING DATA ARE AVAILABLE

ISBN (print) 978-1-4766-8814-5
ISBN (ebook) 978-1-4766-4728-9

© 2023 Larry Fritzlan and Avis Rumney. All rights reserved

No part of this book may be reproduced or transmitted in any form or by any means, electronic or mechanical, including photocopying or recording, or by any information storage and retrieval system, without permission in writing from the publisher.

Front cover images and design by Alan Hebel

Printed in the United States of America

McFarland & Company, Inc., Publishers
Box 611, Jefferson, North Carolina 28640
www.mcfarlandpub.com

*To all those affected by addiction and codependency,
and to the courageous practitioners dedicated to helping them,
that our society may begin to heal and recover
from the damage wrought by addiction.*

Table of Contents

Acknowledgments	ix
Foreword	1
Introduction	7

PART ONE. THEORY AND PRINCIPLES

Chapter 1—Addiction Treatment: Introducing a New Paradigm	11
Chapter 2—The Fourteen Principles of Family Recovery Therapy	34
Chapter 3—What Is Addiction?	67
Chapter 4—Effective Treatment—FRT's Fourteen Principles and the Federal Guidelines for Addiction Treatment	88
Chapter 5—Bowen's Theory of Family Systems	107

PART TWO. PRACTICE

Chapter 6—Introduction to Case Studies	131
Chapter 7—Case Study—Young Adult	137
Chapter 8—Case Study—Spouse	159
Chapter 9—Case Study—Parent	184
Chapter 10—Case Study—Adolescent	207
Chapter 11—Stephanie Brown's Developmental Model of Family Recovery and FRT	216

PART THREE. USING ADJUNCTIVE RESOURCES

Chapter 12—Working with Other Treatment Providers	233
Chapter 13—Social Support and Mutual Aid Groups	251
Chapter 14—Drug Testing	281
Conclusion	289
Appendix A. Erik Erikson's Eight Stages of Psycho-Social Development	293
Appendix B. The Fourteen Principles of Family Recovery Therapy	297

Appendix C. How AA Works with Professionals   299

Appendix D. Dr. Kevin McCauley's Ten Principles of Successful Addiction Treatment   302

Appendix E. Addiction/Codependency Family Treatment Agreement   305

Appendix F. Additional Resources   307

Appendix G. Testing Instruments   308

Appendix H. The Cost of Addiction Treatment   311

Appendix I. "REQUIEM: My Mother's Unspeakable Illness" by Cynthia Gorney   313

Appendix J. From Addiction to Healthy Self   316

Appendix K. How to Find Social Support Groups   318

Appendix L. Spiritual Experience   319

References   321

Index   327

Acknowledgments

It is humbling to imagine who and where I would be today without the inspiration and support of many other people.

Addiction is a disease that tells us that we don't have a disease. We owe a large debt to the pioneers, particularly to the doctor and the stockbroker who, in the 1930s, discovered a simple solution to the paradox of addiction, and founded Alcoholics Anonymous. The millions who have found sobriety, by various paths, have paved the way for others to follow.

There are many people I would like to thank for helping me on my recovery path—too many to acknowledge here individually—but three stand out: T.K., Jack C, and Todd J. These men took me into their homes and their hearts and spent countless hours in numerous venues, guiding me towards sanity.

Three professors, Steven Bosky, Ph.D., Brant Cortright, Ph.D., and Michael Kahn, Ph.D., profoundly inspired in me a fierce wind to blow open doors I did not even know existed.

Stephanie Brown, Ph.D., from my first meeting with her in 1997, has been a beacon of light, helping to clarify our understanding of the impact of addiction on individuals and families. Her wisdom and perspective on addiction, codependency, and treatment have slowly coalesced into the basic tenets of the Family Recovery Therapy model. Her availability, her warmth, and her messages have been foundational to the development of my own work.

I am very grateful to Timmen Cermak, M.D. His generosity and unvarnished responses to my questions have often put me back on my heels, in a good way. He has repeatedly corrected my thinking with a wise clarity that has provoked me to reconsider my conclusions and revise this treatment model accordingly.

Over the last twenty years, Brad Reedy, Ph.D., and the rest of the team at Evoke Therapy have helped hone my belief in the efficacy of a family systems treatment model through their creation of a successful residential family systems treatment program. The collaboration and integration of our two models, and the positive outcomes that have been achieved, give me hope for the future of addiction treatment and the adoption of the FRT therapy model. Effective systems-based treatment can encourage a stable individual to differentiate from the enmeshed codependency inherent in the family system of addiction.

Acknowledgments

My wife, Avis Rumney, therapist and author, is on the cover because, well, she has touched every page, edited, corrected, and often challenged my work. She has taught me that it is possible to fall in love and also have a fierce, separate self. She has shown me what a healthy, functioning, growing bond of love can really be.

I am indebted to Katy Butler, journalist and author, whose wordsmith skills introduced my treatment model to the families and the clinicians in my community and started the ball rolling on this project; to Brant Cortright, Ph.D., whose wise guidance has informed this project over the last 30 years; to Leslie Keenan, the book muse, the gal who gets books published, and her endlessly calm voice that keeps reminding me that this book is only a day at a time, a page at a time, and it will all work out; to Stephanie Daigre, LMFT, who somehow can find myriad references and contort them into appropriate APA-style citations; to Julia McNeal, who can edit a whole book and make the meaning clearer with thousands of small—and sometimes large—suggestions; to Mariah Parker, graphics whiz whose ability to take my ideas and put them in visual form has greatly enhanced this book.

To these wise and giving individuals, I say thank you. And to Jon, you know all of this, since it is you, since 1991, fifty minutes a week, sometimes with me kicking and screaming, who have helped disconfirm the beliefs I learned growing up in an alcoholic and codependent family, to replace the programming installed in me during my childhood and led me to a new view of reality. You have shown me that love and the wisdom of now are all that really matter.

I need to acknowledge whatever power in the universe has given me a relentless desire to grow. My drinking years were full of dangerous, self-willed adventures, but my addiction predictably led me to a desperate, suicidal hell. In the early months of waking up from addiction, I discovered not only that were there others I could trust, but that I also desperately needed to listen to them and follow their guidance. This was a start. I regularly turned my will and my life over to wise others who helped me wake up and slowly discover the wonder of life, love, and the real world.

Foreword

by Brad Reedy, Ph.D.

The air was hot and heavy in the Ochoco mountains of Oregon as I sat outside, facing a group of young adults who were enrolled in the wilderness program run by my company, Evoke Therapy. The young people, ranging in age from 17 to 24, were arrayed loosely along the side of a small ravine. One young man, arms folded, barely looked up as I began to address the group.

"I want to talk to you about your parents. I want you to know that I know they are crazy." This opening tends to get the attention of the "identified patients"—the young adults in treatment—and it was having its effect here. I went on to talk about how families are organized in such a way that one member of the family often bears the burden of the family's pathology. I explained the term "identified patient" and gave a short lesson on the history of a scapegoat from the Jewish tradition. The longer I talked, the more the eyes of the young people met mine.

One young man, the one whose arms were folded and whose eyes were conspicuously looking away from me when I began talking, met my gaze as I paused. "I'm listening," he said.

That was enough to make my trip to talk with these young adults worth it.

I returned my focus to the young people gathered in front of me. "You cannot fix your parents. Some of them might never change. They may never have the courage to look at themselves closely enough to recognize their contribution to your family's patterns. You may have to go it alone. We haven't given up on them, but I think you should consider the reality that many families like yours don't do the work to heal. We have support meetings, assignments, tools, and resources for them. And while they have dented you, the dents are now yours."

As I continued to speak, one young man interrupted, "I am having the weirdest feeling. It feels like I'm high. It seems like you're high. Maybe we are both high? Logically I know it's not true, but that's the way it feels...."

"As far as you know," I joked. "Seriously, do you know why you feel that way? That is what it feels like when you feel seen and understood—when someone is connecting with you. Your brain is releasing chemicals that communicate a sense of well-being. It's no wonder," I swept my hand around, briefly gesturing toward each of them, "that you are self-medicating with drugs or other addictive substances or behaviors. You are seeking this feeling."

The work we do at Evoke Therapy that is so effective at reaching these young people is based entirely in Family Systems theory. It goes counter to the "identified patient" mode typical of most residential treatment programs in which the staff and family just want the "problem person" to get better, but the enabling family system remains unchanged. A Family Systems approach views the family as a whole, and acknowledges the effect every person in the family (or any system) has on the others—just as touching one part of a mobile hanging over a baby's crib causes the other parts to move.

As this book describes, Family Recovery Therapy (FRT) codifies the work of Family Systems theory, working with families struggling with addiction and helping the family heal, beginning with the initial phone call and extending through the first year of sustained recovery. It sees the client as the *entire family system*.

I was attracted to Family Systems and Family Therapy by my own experience of growing up in a family where I was deemed the problem. When my parents divorced, I was raised by my single mother, who was depressed. With the legacy of alcoholism on both my mother's and my father's sides of the family, I played the role of the identified patient. I was angry, searching for answers, meaning, and belonging. Therapists, teachers, and other adults had told me my whole life that my anger was the problem. It took me well into adulthood before I realized that my anger was in fact a *healthy* response to an *unhealthy* system.

When I finished my course work for my Ph.D. in Marriage and Family Therapy, I took a job treating adolescents at an experientially-based program. Our clients suffered from mental health issues including anxiety and mood disorders, depression and suicidality, and addiction. I was excited to enter the work force armed with the information from all my Family Systems classes where professors had promised that the systems revolution was well underway and in full force. Yet, days into my job, when I suggested that we offer more time and resources to the parents of the still-developmentally-malleable teens, I was told in clear terms, "You are wasting your time. The parents didn't send their kids here to have the focus of the work turned on them. Just do your work with the child and send them on to another school or program for longer term care. Leave the parents alone."

My enthusiasm for my chosen field was shattered. I thought the Family Systems revolution was in full swing, but I ran into the same wall that I'd been told had been toppled in the 1970s and 80s—the *identified patient model*. Surely everyone can understand the power of a system to regulate itself using homeostatic processes that move the family dynamics back towards the previous status quo. As Harriet Lerner wisely describes in her book on boundaries, *The Dance of Anger*, when we change our behavior, we are prudent to expect "change back" energy from the others in our system. On a lighter note, I love a quote from Alistair Moses that I saw recently. He said, "If you aren't an asshole in someone's story, you haven't been setting healthy boundaries." While family members may not wish to acknowledge their contribution to the status quo, professionals owe it to the addict, and to those who love them, to explain these dynamics.

I went on to found Evoke Therapy and brought systems theory to the residential treatment programs I run (in-patient). Larry Fritzlan has developed out-patient programs for families grappling with addiction using a Family Systems approach. He found a way to address head-on the elephant in the room, the fact that many treatment centers are not treating the whole disease, but only one small part—the addict—making relapse much more likely.

Larry Fritzlan's Family Recovery Therapy (FRT) approach has become well known to Evoke Therapy's residential wilderness staff. Over the last 20 years, we have collaborated in treating perhaps 30 families. It is refreshing, albeit rare, to have a referent who understands Family Systems theory and treatment. We know that when Fritzlan refers a family to our residential wilderness program, the family is *already in treatment* with a systems therapist. The reality is that in Fritzlan's approach, in which the family receives comprehensive treatment through the *first year of continuous sobriety*, our wilderness program is just one component of his intensive outpatient program (IOP) treatment model.

In our Family Systems–based wilderness program, the parents are assigned homework from day one. The parents meet weekly on a phone call with their child's field therapist, and Larry Fritzlan is on this call as well. Larry has a second session each week in his office with just the parents during which he helps them integrate both what they are learning from us and what they are discovering from the outside support groups they are attending.

Evoke Therapy's approach has always been based on treating the family system. Fritzlan's FRT model and Evoke Therapy both acknowledge that the solution to the presenting problem may be deeply entrenched in long-standing family patterns, and that recovery requires an integrated and comprehensive "reboot" of the family system's dynamics. While Evoke attends to the family's young adults on a 24/7 basis over their 7-to-10-week residential stay, Fritzlan guides the parents back at home through a parallel process to get underneath some of the presenting issues and to fundamentally shift the homeostasis, including modifying relationships among individuals in the family.

It has been gratifying to see this play out over the years, to witness long-term change unfold as families recover from addiction and codependency, heal, and develop new, more functional relationship patterns. In one case, a young man suffering from a serious addiction problem whom Fritzlan referred to Evoke was able, over the course of a number of years, to get and stay sober, grow and develop, become a licensed psychotherapist, and then return to Evoke Therapy as a field psychotherapist treating young adults.

The role of the family in addiction and in recovery is pivotal. Those recovering from addiction know the disease only from their own perspective. They don't know what it is like to suffer as a parent, spouse, or sibling of someone who is killing themselves to attempt to feel better or numb their pain. They have little insight into the dynamics of the system and rarely grasp that each family member acts like one part of a mobile, springing back into place without changing.

To illustrate this point, I mention an experience I had some time ago with a friend who had several years of recovery from substance use disorder. He shared with me his dilemma regarding his engagement to his fiancée. He confessed, "I don't want to get married. I never really agreed to it, but the plans seem to be marching towards that end. I don't know how to tell my fiancée."

"Have you ever thought of going to a Co-dependents Anonymous meeting?" I asked.

"Why would you say that?" was his reply.

"Well, if you are getting married to someone because you don't know how to express your honest truth—to set a very simple and profound boundary—you might have some issues with codependency." It is not inconsequential to note that this friend was the director of a reputable treatment program for addiction. Yet he had little to no idea about the dynamics that characterize *families* that suffer from addiction. He was charismatic and could retell story after story of his success at reaching stubborn and resistant alcoholics and addicts, but he couldn't relate to the *family members of his clients* in a way that spoke to *their* disease, to *their* participation in the dance.

So yes, FRT is still a revolutionary idea. And I am sure the reason that working with a family is still a novel idea—long after the Family Systems people deemed that the identified patient model is dead—is that the FRT approach asks each member of the family system to heroically look at themselves. In 2015 I wrote a book, *The Journey of the Heroic Parent*, and I am often asked about the meaning of the title. I have learned to distill it down to one simple idea: looking at yourself and your contribution to the problem in your family takes courage and is so rare that it can be considered *heroic*.

FRT is a comprehensive approach in which the treatment team is coordinated by a licensed professional therapist who has the training and perspective to offer healing for the entire family and each of its members. As Johan Hair suggested in his profound TedTalk, *Everything We Think We Know About Addiction Is Wrong*, "The opposite of addiction isn't abstinence. It's connection." Establishing authentic connection among family members, as well as for each family member with their support system, is key to the healing process.

We are wounded in relationships, and we heal in relationships. We know the impact on an individual's healing of addressing the entire family system, and we recognize that this is the most consequential tool at our disposal. Beyond the reward of having a loved one move from active addiction into healing and recovery is the gift of having each member of the system increase their joy, awareness, and empowerment in extricating themselves from addictive patterns. FRT offers a template for this work and provides the answer to the question frequently asked by desperate parents, spouses, siblings, and other concerned family members of an addict, "What should I do?"

Brad Reedy, Ph.D., *is a co-owner and the clinical director of Evoke Therapy Programs, providing outdoor-based therapy for adolescents, young adults, and families. Previously, Reedy served as a Primary Therapist, Executive Director and Director of Clinical Services at Second Nature. He has served on the board of the Utah Department of Child and Family Services and the board of the National Association of Therapeutic Schools and Programs. He is the author of the books* The Journey of the Heroic Parent: Your Child's Struggle & the Road Home *and* The Audacity to Be You: Learning to Love Your Horrible, Rotten Self. *Reedy is host of the podcast* Finding You: An Evoke Therapy Podcast. *He lives in Salt Lake City, Utah, with his family.*

Introduction

Addiction is a national mental health crisis, responsible for untold costs to our society and immense suffering for innumerable people. As I write this book, addiction treatment providers are failing to reach the vast majority of those who suffer from addiction. The stark reality is that 50 percent of those who receive addiction treatment fail to sustain recovery after treatment. This statistic has not improved throughout many decades of treating this problem (National Institute on Drug Abuse, 2020). Providers are also failing to address the collateral damage created by addiction. *Facing Addiction in America: The Surgeon General's Report on Alcohol, Drugs, and Health* found that only 10 percent of addicts receive any treatment at all, and the number of addicts continues to increase as new, readily available, addictive substances and behaviors proliferate (Office of the Surgeon General, 2016).

I believe that a new and different approach is essential. And, after 25 years of successfully treating addicted families, by which I mean that most addicts and their families sustain their recovery after treatment, I know for a fact that this approach works significantly better than the addiction treatment model that is currently generally accepted and widely practiced.

In this book, I propose a radically different approach to the current addiction treatment paradigm. Specifically, I suggest organizing treatment around a single professional—a state-licensed, mental or medical health professional trained in Family Recovery Therapy (FRT)—who acts as a Treatment Team Manager and coordinates, case manages, oversees, and treats the members of the addicted/codependent system in an integrated continuum of care, from the first phone call through at least the first year of continuous sobriety. The FRT therapist, who is both case manager and primary treating clinician, bridges and integrates the benefits of evidence-based, medically assisted treatment with that of the widely available—and free—social support and mutual aid groups. This model stands in stark contrast to the traditional, unregulated, fragmented approach that treats the addict in the short term and does not directly address those who *enable* the addict.

Addiction has been with us since the beginning of humanity. And now, smartphones, TV, and other technology-based innovations offer us additional ways to trigger our brains' neurotransmitters, often resulting in out-of-control, compulsive, and life-threatening behaviors that are now being categorized as addictions.

My hope is that you, the practitioner who is interested in studying and treating addiction, will find that adopting this new model can help you achieve more successful outcomes with your clients. My hope is that families contending with addiction will find a clear road map with this approach to help them navigate the dizzying array of treatments and interventions offered in the largely unregulated American addiction treatment industry.

And my hope is that you, the family member who is concerned about an addicted loved one, will find solace in the knowledge that there is a path toward sustained recovery for you and your family, and that there are now practitioners who can help to guide you in that process.

Of course, private practitioners will encounter only a portion of the addicts who need treatment. This book is primarily addressed to those working with clients who have access to medical care. For this new method to succeed with the entire population, including with those who are dependent on government funding, it will need to be adopted by social service agencies, many of which have unwittingly enabled addiction by providing untreated addicts with money that they then use to buy alcohol and drugs. By making this model available to all, it is my hope that it will begin to be adopted by those who serve the populations I am not able to reach.

The goal of Family Recovery Therapy is to restore the addict, each family member, and the family system as a whole to healthy development. As illustrated by Erik Erikson's Eight Stages of Psycho-Social Development (see Appendix A), human beings go through predictable stages of growth, and the tasks of each stage optimally should be mastered before proceeding to the next stage. Effective treatment reestablishes the normal life progression that would have been achieved had addiction not derailed the process. Since recovery, just like development, is an ongoing process, it is customary to use the terms "in recovery" or "recovering" rather than "recovered" to describe the trajectory of growth and healing attained through treatment. Although in the ideal world, and particularly in families where addiction has wreaked havoc, it might be a relief to think that an addict "has recovered" or attained "full recovery," the nature of addiction, and also of human development, is such that recovery does not reach an end point.

It is finally time to move addiction treatment into the modern era. It is time to integrate modern mental and medical health treatment with the long-established residential rehab movement. It is time to acknowledge that addiction is almost always enabled by well-meaning individuals who need their own support. It is time to understand the need for addiction treatment to comprehensively treat the addict through at least the first year of continuous sobriety. This book, *Addiction Therapy and Treatment: A Systems Approach*, describes exactly how this will work. Individuals seeking treatment for addiction should start with a therapist certified in Family Recovery Therapy (FRT). And rehabs seeking interventionists are best served by referring to certified FRT therapists who will work with the addict and the family—the family system—hands on, before and after a residential stay and throughout the initial year of continuous sobriety.

Part One

Theory and Principles

Chapter 1

Addiction Treatment: Introducing a New Paradigm

We are finally getting a more complete, more accurate picture of the complex biological, psychological, social, and spiritual nature of addiction. We are beginning to fully understand the brain physiology of addiction and the social components that often support addiction, and we are developing new treatment modalities that can effectively address this medical and mental disorder.

To be clear, not all substance abuse is "addiction." Nor do all compulsive behaviors, like compulsive gambling or computer gaming, meet the criteria for addiction. This book, and Family Recovery Therapy (FRT), address the kind of "addiction" clearly spelled out in the "Long Definition of Addiction" of the American Society of Addiction Medicine (ASAM [2011]) which is reprinted with permission in Chapter 3.

ASAM describes an addicted brain as diseased and disordered. The underlying neurological changes associated with long-term addiction render an addict literally *incapable of refraining from ongoing usage without external support.* This reality speaks to a critical distinction between simple abuse—overuse of a substance or behavior—and medically defined addiction. And yet, before or during treatment, it is often difficult to differentiate between an addict and others who may not be addicts, but who exhibit symptoms of addiction. As with all medical disorders, diagnostic due diligence is necessary in order to identify or rule out a disease, as well as to modify treatment as new evidence emerges. And yes, there are a few who go through addiction treatment who were misdiagnosed and can actually control their behavior, but it is a very small minority.

Addiction in one form or another directly affects nearly half of all families (Gramlich, 2017). Family members, concerned about their addict, are drawn into the addict's drama, becoming interdependent (codependent) in ways that can profoundly disrupt their lives and their healthy development. While advances in addiction treatment continue to evolve, we still have to face the reality that approximately half of those who enter some sort of addiction treatment program relapse within a year and resume their addiction, resulting in costly, and potentially deadly, outcomes. This happens in part because, in the current, fragmented treatment model, a split exists between the abstinence-only social support group approach (such as Alcoholics Anonymous) and the equally useful "medically assisted treatment" (M.A.T.). Each approach often fails to fully benefit from what the other offers.

This book proposes a plan to fundamentally alter the predominant, existing approach and set the stage for a new paradigm in treatment—one that integrates processes that are currently fragmented and ineffective into a model that can produce significantly better outcomes. This new paradigm is based on science, evidence, and research, and is supported by the findings in *Facing Addiction in America: The Surgeon General's Report on Alcohol, Drugs, and Health* (Office of the Surgeon General, 2016). I propose that treatment programs, government agencies, drug counselors, and all others involved in addiction treatment start to "row in the same direction," and that they all employ the Family Recovery Therapy (FRT) treatment model. According to this model, an addiction-trained, licensed mental health professional, an "FRT therapist," coordinates a treatment team that treats all aspects of the addictive/codependent family system from the very beginning—from the first phone call—through at least the initial year of sobriety.

Social support and mutual aid groups are central to the rehabilitation of addicts and are used in nearly all addiction treatment programs. The most widespread of these is Alcoholics Anonymous (AA). Others include LifeRing Secular Recovery (LifeRing), SMART Recovery®, and Women for Sobriety. The AA groups began in the 1930s, when several alcoholics met together to help each other not drink for that one day—and met again the next day to help each other not drink that day, and again the day after that—one day at a time. Today, nearly every approach to addiction treatment includes some kind of group support in which recovering individuals talk about what they are thinking and feeling, share their pain and their problems, and get support from each other—an authentic support that is absent elsewhere in the lives of most addicts.

I understand that AA meetings and other 12-Step fellowships comprise by far the majority—perhaps over 90 percent—of free social support and mutual aid groups for addicts. While 12-Step programs are not for everyone, they do dominate the recovery field. A professor in my graduate program once called 12-Step programs "the world's fastest-growing spiritual movement," and that is not hyperbole. The book *Alcoholics Anonymous* has sold more than 40 million copies (in English editions alone) (Alcoholics Anonymous®, n.d.-c). and has been translated into 72 other languages (Alcoholics Anonymous®, n.d.-a) (and counting) since it was first published in English in 1939. *Time* magazine, in 2011, placed the book on its list of the "100 best and most influential books written in English" (Sun, 2011). The Library of Congress designated it "one of the 88 books that shaped America" (Library of Congress, 2012).

The 12-Step approach for alcoholics has spawned dozens of offshoots, such as Narcotics Anonymous, Overeaters Anonymous, Sex and Love Addicts Anonymous, Gamers Anonymous, Gamblers Anonymous, and Debtors Anonymous. These programs offer a practical, step-by-step solution to suffering addicts, whose disordered midbrains have hijacked their thinking prefrontal cortices, rendering them susceptible to compulsive and self-harming behavior (see Figures 3.1, 3.2, and 3.3 in Chapter 3).

The 12-Step approach has many detractors, but the fact that its principles are based on anonymity makes it both an underappreciated gem and a defenseless target when it comes to documenting its successes and failures. Millions of its members, many of them famous, remain silent about their 12-Step involvement and their successful remission from this chronic disorder using the support of these free and readily available programs. And, as mentioned, there are other social support groups for addicts that may be a better fit for some individuals.

In considering treatment and addiction, it is critical to differentiate "true addicts" from those who engage in addictive behaviors but do not suffer from the brain disorder of addiction. The American Society of Addiction Medicine (ASAM) is unambivalent: substance addiction is fundamentally a neurological disorder, a disease of the brain (2011). For many years, neuroscientists, using a variety of complex imaging technologies, have delved deeply into the mysteries of how the brain works, and they have substantiated what the American Medical Association (AMA) pronounced in 1956, that addiction is a medical illness. Harm reduction approaches, such as psychodynamic therapy and cognitive behavioral therapy, are appropriate for treating individuals who exhibit obsessive and compulsive "addictive-like" thinking and behavior. Many afflicted individuals are successfully treated using these and similar approaches—but only if they are not "true" addicts who suffer from the neurological disorder of addiction.

How can we know if someone is a true addict? Often the answer comes from looking in a rearview mirror. In his book, *Harm Reduction Psychotherapy*, Andrew Tatarsky acknowledges the necessity of referral of "certain cases" to AA where abstinence, not harm reduction, is indicated (2002). Lance Dodes, author of *The Heart of Addiction* (2002), who advocates addressing the psychological issues underlying addictive behaviors, would welcome a client finding the help they needed in AA or another support group, if they fail to recover with the assistance of his psychodynamic approach. We clinicians may try a number of approaches to help relieve our clients' suffering, until hopefully we are able to guide an individual to remission. Like turtles and dolphins getting caught inadvertently in fishing nets, some individuals are referred to addiction treatment and then discover later, once their substance use has stopped and other issues have been addressed, that, in fact, they are not addicts, and they can use and control mood-altering substances, including alcohol, without developing a harmful dependency.

It is impossible to know 100 percent of the time if a new client is a true addict. Clinically speaking, it is appropriate to rapidly escalate treatment when clients are engaging in dangerous behavior. Of course, we continue to assess presenting issues and modify our approach as needed.

To be clear, this book and the 14 Principles described in it are intended to guide clinicians working with *addicts*—those who have the brain disease of addiction as defined by ASAM. (See Chapter 3 for more detail.)

Currently, two primary approaches dominate the addiction treatment field. One is the abstinence approach, which is espoused by the social support groups such as AA, and the other is medically assisted treatment (M.A.T.), which is advocated by medical doctors and is increasingly supported by the government. Both have strong evidence supporting their efficacy, but neither comes even close to offering a fully integrated, comprehensive, and unified treatment method. Hence each approach has less than optimal long-term success rates.

Psychiatrists who espouse using M.A.T. focus on possible organic deficits that will benefit from different kinds of medication. There are many recovering addicts with long-term "sobriety" who are taking any number of medications to help stabilize their nervous systems. The benefits of Suboxone (buprenorphine) are well established. Suboxone can get the user "high," but used correctly and under a doctor's care, it can allow an opiate addict to stabilize and stop using heroin and other opiates. Methadone has been used for many years to help keep opiate addicts from returning to dangerous street drugs. Naltrexone and Vivitrol will block the high from opiates and can assist opiate addicts resist relapse. Many other medications, such as antidepressants, can help addicts turn away from their addictive drug of choice and get their lives back on track.

Some AA members, especially "old-timers" who have been with the program for many decades, discourage the use of medication because they believe that only abstinence from all psychoactive drugs constitutes real sobriety. In fact, AA does not have an opinion—neither for nor against medication. Today we know that many addicts benefit from medical support, and others cannot thrive without it. The concern voiced by most proponents of the traditional, abstinence-based approaches is that M.A.T. fails to incorporate the use of social support and mutual aid groups. These groups provide a vital component of recovery—helping recovering individuals to connect with each other on a daily basis, to get and give mutual support, to be inspired by those with longer recovery, and to find a healthy community. Addicts in the throes of addiction have rarely experienced in any other context the kind of vital support these groups have offered for over 80 years.

Comprehensive treatment must utilize aspects of *both* medical and psychological best practices *and* abstinence-based social support and mutual aid groups. An important component of FRT is the reliance of recovering addicts and family members on community-based, free, social support groups. Chapter 13 is devoted to a discussion of these groups, which together constitute the world's most successful "mental health program" for the treatment of addiction.

Twelve-Step programs, for many, have certainly proven to be a simple and effective way to put many kinds of addiction into remission. However, nearly 40 percent of newly recovering addicts also suffer from dual or multiple mental illnesses, among them, depression, anxiety, bipolar disorder, post-traumatic stress disorder, or personality disorders (National Institute of Mental Health, 2016), and, further, have myriad other problems related to financial, legal, employment, housing, or relationship issues. Various kinds of treatment to address these issues can be essential to recovery, which is why the FRT therapist, who can integrate and coordinate psychiatric, medical, therapeutic, and any other required professional services, plays a vital role in ensuring a continuum of care.

During the years he spent working as staff physician in a clinic on Vancouver's skid row, medical doctor Gabor Maté, author of *In the Realm of Hungry Ghosts* (2010), observed that people with severe substance abuse disorders had invariably suffered traumatic developmental deficits. He cites one of the most comprehensive and prominent studies on the long-term impacts of childhood abuse and neglect: the Adverse Childhood Experiences (ACE) study conducted by the Centers for Disease Control and Prevention in conjunction with Kaiser Permanente. The ACE findings amply demonstrate the crucial role adverse childhood experiences play in predisposing an individual to substance abuse disorders (Felitti, et al., 1998). Childhood trauma and the failure to form secure attachments with loving others early in life make an individual much more likely to fall prey to addiction, and the more severe the deficits in early care, the more likely someone will develop addiction.

For Maté, addiction is essentially a disorder of disconnection. When a child lacks a sense of safety and belonging, this deficit can impair healthy development of the neural pathways that facilitate their ability to feel at home in the world, to live, and love, and prosper in connection with others. We are an affiliative species. If we cannot achieve genuine connection, we seek other ways to repair the breach. Addicts bond with a substance or activity that simulates some of the feelings and sensations associated with healthy human relationships. Tragically, bonding with their drug or compulsive behaviors of choice further impairs the addict's ability to connect with people and to find a home in the human community.

Addicts and alcoholics in recovery from long-term addiction can be especially supportive in helping the practicing addict begin to feel less alone. They've been where the newcomer is and can empathize with his or her plight. The authentic connections that happen in social support and mutual aid groups are healing in and of themselves. Regularly meeting with a committed group of sincere, loving, caring people helps heal the disconnected, alienated soul, and helps ward off the pain of isolation. The significance of human connection in recovery is one of the reasons for the wide success of the many social support groups.

All social support groups provide both affiliation and specific recovery tools. SMART Recovery®, LifeRing, and other non–12-Step groups offer the opportunity for connection and interaction with others in recovery as well as substantial cognitive behavioral tools. Participants in these groups learn to address myriad aspects of recovery that foster healthy development—including preventing relapse, handling emotions, and learning effective and appropriate communication and relationship skills.

Twelve-Step programs offer both the fellowship of community members and the 12 steps, which the newly recovering addict is invited to "work" to recover from the damage done by perhaps years of addiction. It is within the fellowship that addicts find the kind of understanding "others" that most of us need in our lives in order to feel safe and loved. And in "working" the steps, one at a time, with a "sponsor," the addict receives many benefits beyond remission from addiction. These benefits—self-exploration, self-responsibility, awareness of emotions, living with integrity, accepting reality, repairing relationships, embracing spirituality, relating to and helping others—address and ameliorate many mental health and relationship issues.

The Family Recovery Therapy model inserts a mental health professional, the FRT therapist, into a comprehensive treatment process that coordinates both M.A.T. and social support programs. This therapist can monitor and attend to an addict or a family member's co-occurring issues, and guide the addict and the afflicted family members in a timely way to the resources necessary to attain wellness. Through the Family Recovery Therapy process, addicts and codependents achieve recovery and health, and are therefore able to stop the addiction cycle, and to impart to the next generation freedom from a distorted and impoverished development and from the legacy of a poorly differentiated family.

Let's step back and review how we got to where we are now in addiction treatment. In the 1800s and early 1900s, addiction was generally seen as a moral failing or as a form of insanity or demonic possession. Of course, attempts at religious conversion or exorcism were almost always futile. Slowly, over the last hundred years, we have grown in our understanding of addiction and its impact on all of us.

In the early 1900s, Freud and others contributed the concept of the unconscious to our understanding of human behavior. This was important not only for understanding the psychology of the individual, but also for illuminating the underlying unconscious dynamics of family systems and of the larger society. In his book, *Can Love Last?* (2002, p. 22), Stephen Mitchell wrote of Sigmund Freud's work: "Our conscious experience is merely the tip of an immense iceberg of unconscious mental processes that really shape, unbeknownst to us, silently, impenetrably, and inexorably, our motives, our values, our actions."

Freud's contribution to our evolving understanding of addiction is profound, because he helped us to understand that the psychological underpinnings of addiction—on both an individual and a systemic level—are largely unconscious. But in practical terms, psychoanalysis did little to alleviate the suffering of addicts. Psychotherapy alone seldom resolved addiction.

In the 1930s, Bill Wilson and Dr. Bob Smith demonstrated that individuals who were addicted to alcohol could stop drinking simply by gathering together on a regular basis and supporting each other's sobriety—for just that day—one day at a time. Based on this principle, they founded Alcoholics Anonymous. Since then, millions of addicts have managed to achieve in AA what they could not with decades of psychotherapy alone—long-term sobriety and freedom from the ravages of ongoing addiction and relapse (Erikson, M., 2020).

The 1940s saw the beginning of residential treatment programs based on the principles of AA. The programs typically were run by recovering alcoholics who helped alcoholics get sober and get their feet back on the ground.

In the 1950s, Lois Wilson, Bill Wilson's wife, co-founded an organization modeled after AA, called Al-Anon, which offered support for the family members affected by their loved one's addiction. The need for Al-Anon spoke to a central issue in addiction: addiction can legitimately be called a "family disease," since the addict's presence profoundly disrupts family functioning and impedes healthy psychosocial development for all family members, and can lead to codependency. In that same decade, the first residential treatment centers for codependents opened.

Also in the 1950s, the American Medical Association (AMA) recognized that addiction has a biological basis, that it is a disease of an organ—the brain. In 1956, the AMA declared that "alcoholism is a medical illness" (Bettinardi-Angres & Angres, 2010). This acknowledgment began to help remove some of the stigma of alcoholism. In addition, in the 1950s, medical doctors who specialized in addiction medicine began to organize, and eventually formed the American Society of Addiction Medicine (ASAM) to advance both the understanding and the treatment of addiction.

In the 1960s and 1970s, Vernon Johnson, an Episcopal priest, developed the concept of an "intervention" (Johnson, 1990). His idea was to bring together family members—and others significant in an addict's life—in an attempt to motivate the addict to enter treatment. This model is now called the Johnson or "surprise model" of intervention. During the 1960s as well, the psychiatrist Murray Bowen developed a comprehensive psychological theory of family systems that embraced Freud's understanding of the role that the unconscious plays in our actions—in this case, the role of the unconscious in interpersonal relationships among family members (Bowen, 1978). Understanding the role of unconscious actions in a family system is central to the FRT model.

During the 1970s and 1980s, codependency came to be viewed as a psychological and relationship "disorder" (Lancer, 2017). It became clearer not only that codependents experience significant distress, but that unhealthy codependency exacts a severe toll on relationships.

In the 1970s, Dr. Stephanie Brown began her study of addiction. She studied the process of recovery for individuals who belong to Alcoholics Anonymous and published this work in her book, *Treating the Alcoholic: A Developmental Model of Recovery* (1985). In the 1970s and 1980s, she examined the impact on children and on adult children of alcoholics. Dr. Brown partnered with Dr. Virginia Lewis in 1990 to study the process of recovery for the addicted family as a system. Their research demonstrated how family members' pursuit of their own recoveries can contribute to the development of a new, healthy family system over time in recovery. They described their findings about families in recovery in their book *The Alcoholic Family in Recovery: A Developmental Model,* published in 1999.

In the mid-1990s, interventionists and family therapists who understood the dysfunctional roles of family members in addiction and codependency, as well as in recovery, introduced the concept of "systemic" interventions, in contrast to the formerly popular "Johnson" or "surprise" interventions, which can be shame-inducing and often ineffective (Office of the Surgeon General, 2016). This approach acknowledged the crucial role that family dynamics play in the "addictive/codependent system." Systemic interventionists understand the complex codependent enabling forces involved in addiction, and rather than focusing the intervention solely on the addict, offer treatment recommendations to all family members.

Additionally, beginning in the 1990s, scientists and neurophysiologists discovered the disordered structures and chemical reactivity of the addicted brain—features which helped explain why an addict, relying on their own brain, is typically incapable of stopping addictive behavior. The scientific research corroborated what AA had explained decades before—and what every addict self-reports—that willpower alone cannot overcome addiction.

Using modern imaging techniques, addiction researchers discovered that something very peculiar was going on in the brains of addicts who were caught in the throes of active craving (Goldstein & Volkow, 2002). While there was plenty of activity in their midbrain, the prefrontal cortex (that part of the brain responsible for executive functioning) was practically offline. Processes in the midbrain—that portion of the brain shared by all mammals and crucially important in fight-or-flight responses, emotional reactivity, and effective bonding—overwhelm the addict's thinking, reasoning, and decision-making, and drive the addict to repeat addictive behavior to reduce pain and/or to seek temporary euphoria. No amount of moralizing or reasoning can sway a person bereft of executive functioning. The addict is powerless to stop their addiction without external help.

That brings us up to date with where we are today.

Following (pages 19–22) is a graphic representation of the history of addiction treatment.

We have clearly learned a great deal about the disease of addiction and have developed and modified treatment models as new discoveries in biology, psychology, and social interactions have informed our treatment approaches. And yet, despite these advances, we are still stuck with the inconvenient fact that somewhere around fifty percent of those who seek treatment will return to their addiction. Even after attending a number of residential treatment programs, they still fail to maintain sobriety.

I'd like to use the "glass half full/glass half empty" analogy to offer a bird's-eye perspective on the current state of addiction treatment as practiced by medical doctors, mental health professionals, and addiction treatment programs.

Glass Half Full:

- Medical Doctors have deepened their understanding of addiction. A number of medicines have been developed which doctors can prescribe to

Chapter 1. Addiction Treatment: Introducing a New Paradigm

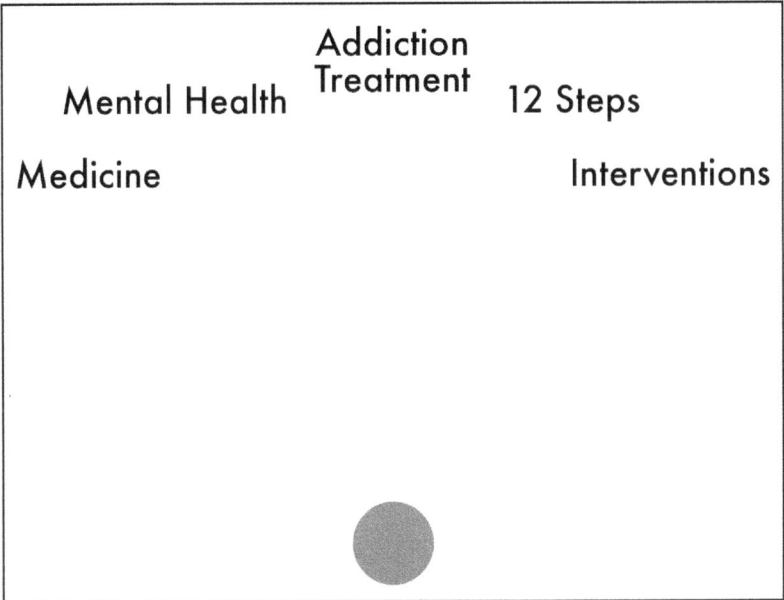

Figure 1.1 *The Year 1900.* At the start of the 20th century, no acceptable treatment for addiction existed.

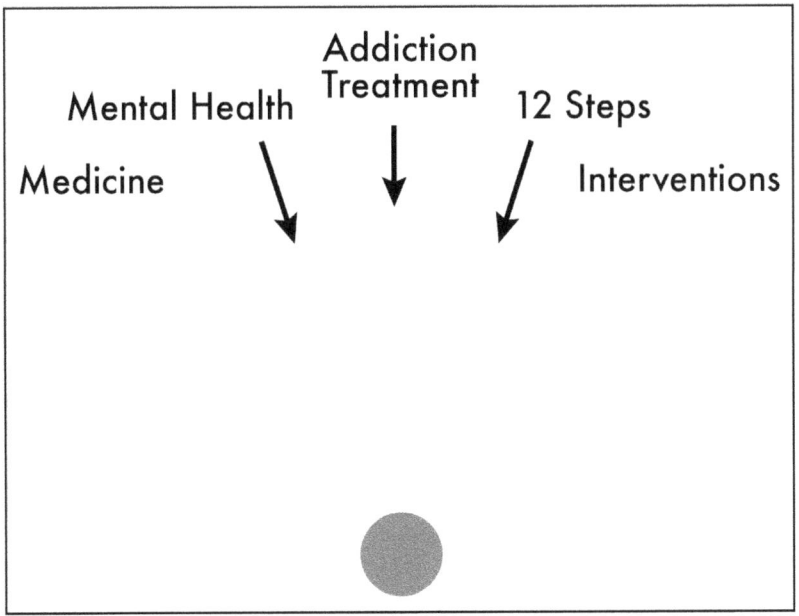

Figure 1.2 *1940s.* Freud, in the early 20th century, described the role of the unconscious in human behavior, and there was a growing awareness that psychological factors influence human thought and action. In the 1930s, AA was founded and began helping addicts get and stay sober, one day at a time. As each year passed, AA membership grew. In the 1940s, with the recognition of the need for addiction treatment, 12-Step-based residential treatment programs were founded.

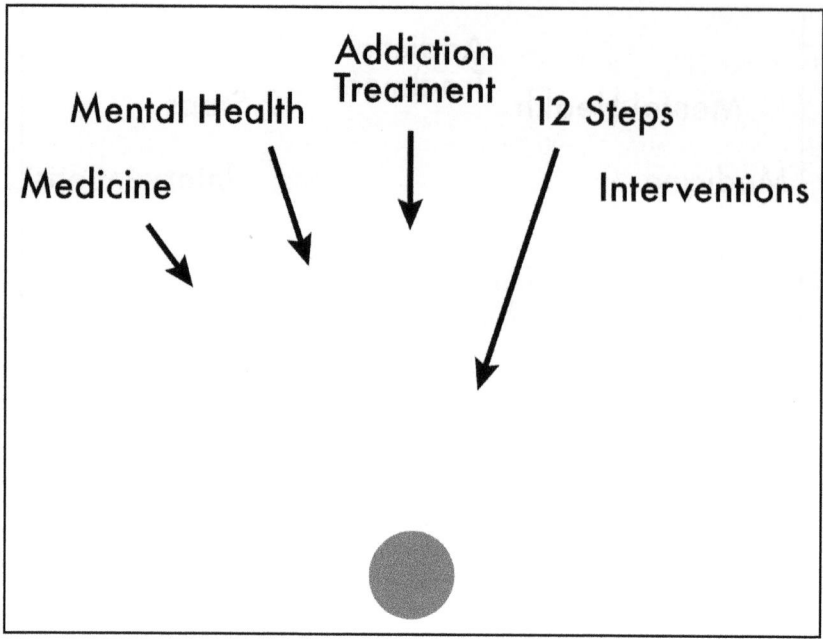

Figure 1.3 *1950s*. The American Medical Association (AMA) acknowledged that addiction is a medical illness. The American Society of Addiction Medicine (ASAM) was established as a forum for doctors to share their knowledge about addiction. The 12-Step program Al-Anon was founded to offer support to family members impacted by addiction. Residential treatment programs for codependents opened.

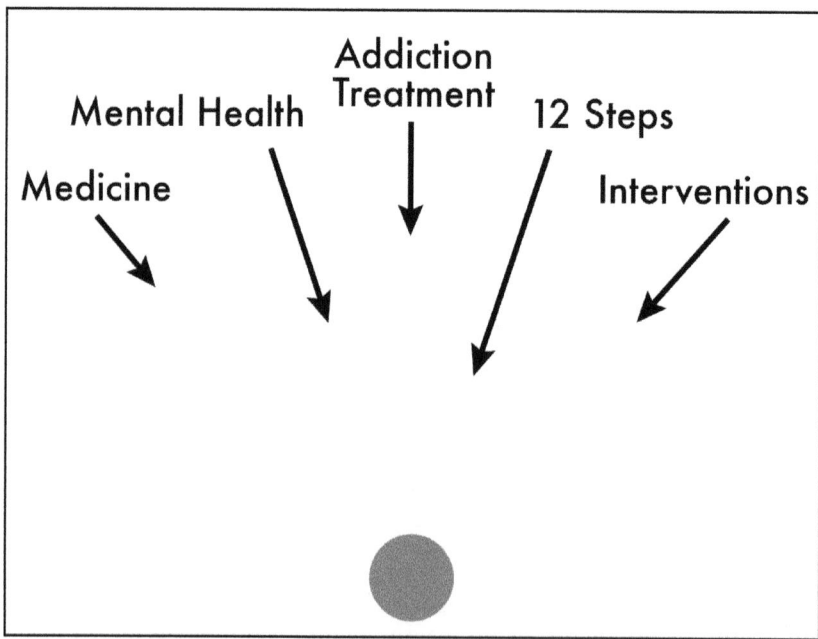

Figure 1.4 *1960s and 1970s*. Murray Bowen described the role that the unconscious plays in family dynamics. Vernon Johnson introduced the "Surprise Model" of intervention.

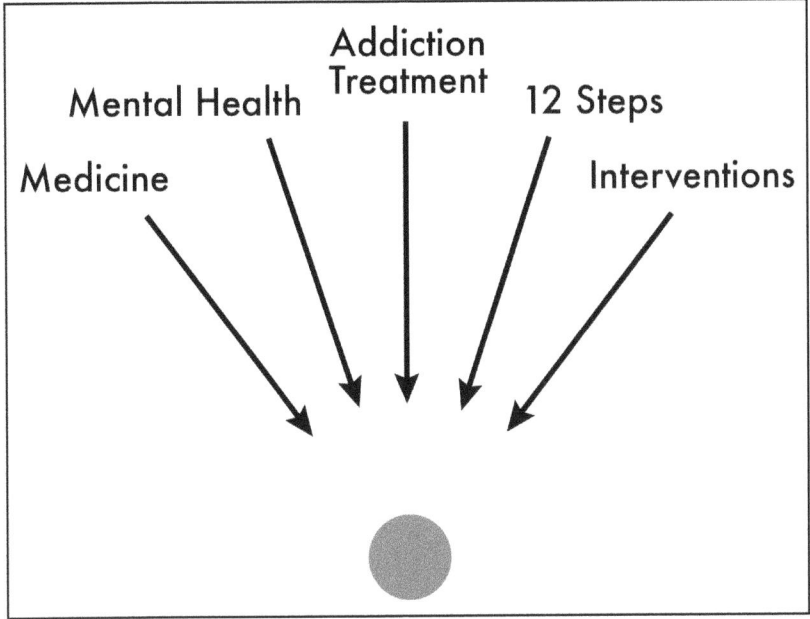

Figure 1.5 *1980s and 1990s.* Brain imaging techniques were developed that could demonstrate differences between brains of addicts and brains of non-addicts. The "Systemic Intervention" was developed, which acknowledged the role of the family system in addiction and recovery. Brown and Lewis published their work on alcoholic families and the developmental model of addiction and recovery.

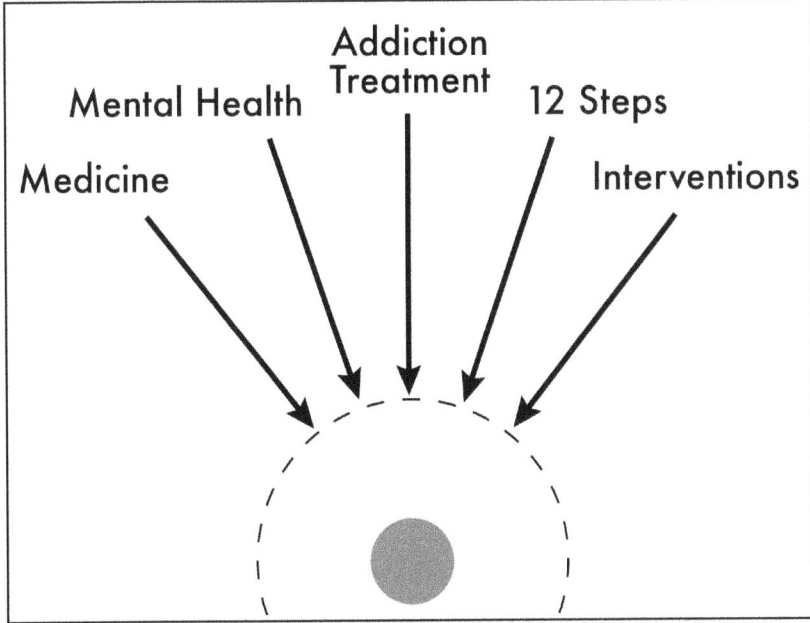

Figure 1.6 *Present Day.* Knowledge about the medical and mental health aspects of addiction has grown, 12-Step programs are thriving, and addiction treatment has improved from where it was decades earlier. However, there is still a 50 percent failure rate of addiction treatment.

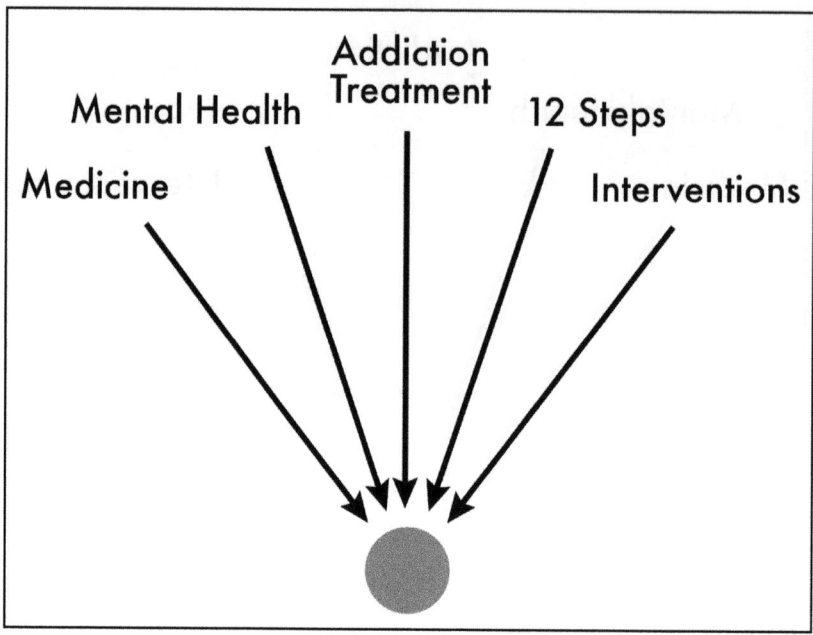

Figure 1.7 *The New Paradigm—Family Recovery Therapy.* In Family Recovery Therapy, the FRT therapist coordinates the treatment of the addictive/codependent family system, facilitating and integrating medicine, social support groups and all adjunctive therapeutic services. Using the FRT model, we can move towards a time when active addiction is rare and, when present, is diagnosed and treated at an early stage, just like any other chronic medical disease.

help the addict go through withdrawal without serious discomfort. Doctors are now able to prescribe legal and readily available medicines that can allow, for instance, opioid addicts to offset their drug cravings. They offer medical treatments for many of the co-occurring physical and psychological disorders that afflict addicts. Doctors are an essential part of an integrated approach to addiction treatment.
- Mental health professionals are highly trained to help relieve the pain of mental disorders. Nearly all addicts entering addiction treatment suffer from mental disorders, which are exacerbated by their addiction-based lifestyle.
- Addiction treatment programs have, for decades, taken in the addict, detoxed and stabilized them, educated them, and given them common sense recommendations upon discharge.

Glass Half Empty:

- Medical doctors get very little training in recognizing addictive disorders, and often treat the *symptoms* of addiction, failing to diagnose the underlying disorder. When they do treat addiction as a medical disorder, they often fail to understand the complex addictive/codependent family system and the social systems surrounding and supporting the addict's malady. They often

do not think to refer the family members for treatment. They often fail to recognize that regular, long-term, attendance in support groups (rather than the brief exposure they may get to such groups during residential treatment) is essential to keeping this chronic brain disorder in remission.
- Mental health professionals are trained to help those suffering from psychological problems to "get a grip" on their problem in order to reestablish mental health and a sense of wellbeing. However, often these professionals have little training in addiction and fail to understand that addiction, by definition, is a disorder characterized by a brain that is *incapable* of control: addicts can control neither their craving nor their subsequent drug-seeking and drug-using behavior. The addicted mind, by definition, will not respond to those who try to strengthen the ego or willpower—something the addict is incapable of benefiting from. Mental health professionals are trying to instruct a brain that has been hijacked to *choose* not to be hijacked. This is demoralizing for the addict who has repeatedly tried and failed to control their behavior.
- Addiction treatment programs, in nearly all cases, fail to address and treat the systemic dynamics underlying, impacting, influencing and enabling the addictive/codependent family system. They acknowledge that the family has a role, but their focus on the addict colludes with the family's denial that family members have a role in the problem. The treatment programs, as well as most family members, continue to believe that the addict "is the problem." Hence, the codependent enablers' "treatment" typically consists of brief education about addiction, and perhaps one meeting with a counselor. But a treatment program's "family program" generally neither engages the codependent family members in long-term treatment, nor addresses the perhaps decades-long, multi-generational, entrenched codependency and lack of differentiation that support the homeostasis of the addictive/codependent system. Differentiation is discussed more fully in the chapters ahead. It is the ability of a person to individuate especially in relation to their family of origin.
- Additionally, treatment for the addict is typically 30, 60, or 90 days in duration. This length of time is simply insufficient to address a long-standing, even decades-long disorder. In some cases, it can take many years for a person to make the substantive changes needed to create a foundation for resuming healthy development. In the current paradigm, everyone crosses their fingers and hopes the patient is "cured," when in fact the work, in most cases, has barely begun.

There is a better way. One that makes the "glass half full/glass half empty" metaphor no longer relevant. This is where we are now.

The current state of addiction treatment brings to mind the parable of the four blind men describing an elephant. One man, holding the trunk, says, "An elephant is like a snake." Another, holding the tail, says, "No, an elephant is like a rope." A third, his arms encircling a leg, says, "No, an elephant is like a tree." And the fourth, grasping an ear, says, "No, an elephant is like a large leaf."

The parable is an apropos analogy. Different phases of treatment are not coordinated into a cohesive whole. I suggest that those in the addiction treatment field step away from the dominant paradigm, and look at the larger picture from a bird's-eye perspective that includes not only the addict, but the family members, as well as the addictive/codependent family and peer system. The blind men above were all correct in their description of the elephant, but they could not see that the part they held was only one portion of a larger whole.

I propose nothing less than a systemic intervention on the addiction treatment field itself. I believe that the addiction treatment industry is addicted to a failed approach and needs an intervention—not unlike an addictive/codependent family system. Such an intervention will give way to a new addiction treatment model—in the same way that an interventionist working with a family recommends new behavior for the codependents and the addict that will create radically different and healthier family dynamics.

This new treatment model is based on current research and evidence-based outcome studies that underpin the guidelines for "best practices" that we know are effective. Unfortunately, the current addiction treatment industry is, like the four blind men, unable to see some key elements, and also not yet equipped to implement them.

Residential treatment programs, drug counselors, family therapists, interventionists, doctors, outpatient programs, government agencies, and others treating addiction are mostly doing their jobs with conviction and dedication—just like the man holding the tail of an elephant would accurately say it was "like a rope."

We are now poised to take the next step in the long evolution from Freud, and AA's founding in the 1930s, incorporating all of the advances in medicine, psychology, clinical practice, and our understanding of family dynamics. It's time to ask the question, "What would it take to put 100% of addicts and their enabling codependent family systems into a treatment process that *effectively* stops this systemic disease in this generation and doesn't pass it on to the next?"

I can imagine a future where teams of doctors, psychologists, drug counselors, treatment programs, and government agencies, working together, put addiction into the category of diseases—like smallpox—that are diagnosed early, treated, and arrested when the first symptoms appear, and even eventually eradicated.

I believe we are ready to adopt a new paradigm. Paradigm shifts are no small thing. Let's take a deeper look at the concept of paradigms, paradigm shifts, and how they relate to addiction treatment. Thomas Kuhn, in his seminal book, *The Structure of Scientific Revolutions* (1962), discusses the stages that science progresses through as it evolves over time. He conceives of the process as traversing four phases. Kuhn suggests that significant change in our perspective and understanding of science occurs not through a linear accumulation of new data, but through revolutionary transformations, which he later termed "paradigm shifts." I think the metaphor is a useful one. Let's explore further.

In Kuhn's view of the evolution of science, during Phase One, or "pre-science," there exist several discordant theories to explain a particular phenomenon. In Phase Two, which Kuhn terms "normal science," a dominant paradigm evolves from the disparate theories, and inconsistencies are resolved within that framework. During Phase Three, anomalies arise that cannot be explained by the dominant paradigm. And finally, in Phase Four, a "scientific revolution" occurs, and a new paradigm emerges which allows for the resolution of previous anomalies.

When the evolution of addiction treatment is viewed through the lens of Kuhn's theory of change, Phase One, the era of pre-science, is comparable to the state of addiction treatment prior to 1956—the point at which the American Medical Association recognized addiction as a medical illness. Before this time, there was no consensus about the nature of addiction or how to treat it. Addiction was viewed variously as evidence of mental illness, lack of willpower, Satanism, or a moral failing. Neither religion nor medicine had been able to effectively offer a "treatment" for addiction.

However, there were a few attempts at treatment as early as 1784, Dr. Benjamin Rush, a civic leader in Philadelphia and signer of the U.S. *Declaration of Independence*, argued that alcoholism was a medical disease that rendered its victims incapable of choosing sobriety. Alcohol, he believed, was the causative agent, not the alcoholic. The alcoholic, Rush contended, should be treated with compassion and weaned from his addiction by the administration of less potent medications (White, 1998).

Decades before Rush, some Native Americans had already begun establishing mutual aid circles and using traditional healing practices (White, 1998) to contend with the terrific toll alcohol abuse and addiction had wrought on an oppressed population living under colonial rule. They were visionaries, but their insights and understanding were lost. Only later would the mainstream scientific community and American society come to similar realizations about the value of peer support in addiction recovery.

Alcoholics Anonymous, founded in the 1930s, offered a glimmer of hope for some addicts, but it was unknown to most people, not widely accepted by medicine, and viewed by many as "religious."

In 1956, Phase Two, the "normal science" stage of addiction treatment, began, and continued through the early 2000s. In this second phase, puzzles are solved within the context of the dominant paradigm. As noted above, doctors began to treat addiction as a *chronic* medical illness that required ongoing, possibly lifelong, monitoring. AA and other social support groups grew, and residential treatment programs emerged as resources to help stabilize addicts.

Murray Bowen and other family systems researchers and practitioners deepened our understanding of the unconscious dynamics that maintain dysfunctional homeostasis in families across generations. Stephanie Brown and her colleagues used this knowledge to delineate these dynamics in families with addicted members.

Medical research expanded our understanding of the neurobiological underpinnings of addiction, giving us a more precise understanding of how the disease of addiction alters the brain.

In 2004, the U.S. government recognized that family-focused therapy was the exception rather than the rule, and that lack of coordination of treatment was a serious concern. The Substance Abuse and Mental Health Services Administration (SAMHSA) also noted that new models of family systems therapy were being adapted that showed promise in treating families with addicted members, including multidimensional family therapy (Center for Substance Abuse Treatment, 2004). You will find that elements of the 14 FRT Principles described in the next chapter appear in other treatment models (see Appendix B for a list of the 14 FRT Principles).

Addiction specialists began integrating findings from biological, psychological, social, and spiritual perspectives. **However, the addict-centered treatment most commonly practiced resulted in approximately 50 percent of addicts not remaining sober—a fairly major anomaly in treatment outcomes.** Clearly, there is a problem with the current addiction treatment paradigm, as addressed by Thomas Kuhn in his theories of scientific revolutions and paradigm shifts (1962). Kuhn recognized that progress in science often resulted from "anomalies" or facts that were difficult to explain within existing models and theories. As his model suggests, anomalies reveal weaknesses in the original paradigm resulting in the need for a break with the old ways of thinking and necessitating a new paradigm.

In the evolution of addiction treatment, cracks in the old paradigm began in 2008 when insurance began to cover addiction treatment, and much of addiction treatment morphed into a money-making business. The addiction treatment "industry" was born, and profit became a driving force. The Mental Health Parity and Addiction Equity Act of 2008 ruled that insurance reimbursement of addiction treatment be on a par with reimbursement for treatment of other mental and medical disorders (Centers for Medicare & Medicaid Services, n.d.). When insurance companies were suddenly mandated to pay for addiction treatment at levels similar to other medical conditions, new residential treatment centers, intensive outpatient programs, and sober houses sprang up across the country. My colleagues and I observed corporations buying up long established, stand-alone residential programs, resulting in slick marketing to lure vulnerable families to their facilities. We also observed unscrupulous companies going to great lengths to fill beds in order to profit from insurance money. Meanwhile, reputable treatment providers continued their work, and tried to stay afloat, despite severe competition. For a graphic illustration of the sad state of addiction treatment today, see the eye-opening 19-minute YouTube video by comedian John Oliver entitled *Rehab* (Oliver, 2018).

It is estimated that the addiction treatment industry was worth $42 billion in 2020, and with passage of the Affordable Care Act in 2010, "3 to 5 million new patients entered the system in need of substance abuse treatment, resulting in the opening of more treatment centers and 'sober homes,' many of which engaged in overbilling, patient brokering, and deceptive marketing" (LaRosa, 2020). And while some addiction treatment centers rake in large amounts of money for company executives and industry investors, approximately 90 percent of addicts in need of treatment still get no treatment at all (LaRosa, 2020), and the type of treatment an addict receives is far more dependent on chance, financial status, and profit-driven advertising campaigns than informed clinical judgment. Predictably, the 50 percent success rate of addiction treatment hasn't budged.

What has been lacking is an overall plan to address the national addiction crisis, a clear set of principles to establish best practices and minimum standards, and a willingness to aggressively take on a largely unregulated, multibillion-dollar addiction treatment industry that is fragmented and highly resistant to change.

Of course, there are thousands of well-trained professionals striving sincerely for better outcomes. I have visited many dozens of treatment centers across the country, and met with countless reputable clinical directors, addiction therapists, and interventionists. For the past 25 years, I have collaborated with scores of these professionals for the benefit of our mutual clients. Although my treatment model was unfamiliar to them, and I sometimes encountered initial resistance, when the FRT goals and priorities were understood, I received almost universal encouragement and support from colleagues.

The vast majority of them, however, did not invite me to teach my model to other clinicians, nor did they emulate it, despite greatly improved results for our clients. The addict in isolation, rather than the addictive/codependent system, almost always remains the focus of treatment; auxiliary codependency "workshops" and "family weekends" at addiction centers notwithstanding. I do not believe this is conscious resistance on the part of colleagues, but an inability to see beyond the current paradigm, to step outside their comfort zone and take in the larger picture. They are attached to the approach they and the addiction treatment industry have relied on in the past.

In Kuhn's Phase Four, a "scientific revolution" occurs. The old paradigm no longer works, and a paradigm shift ensues. As underlying assumptions are reexamined, and former anomalies are resolved, a new paradigm emerges.

I believe that addiction treatment is at this very threshold. It is time to integrate modern mental and medical health treatment with the long-established residential rehab movement. This book's bold premise is to establish a new paradigm, a new treatment model based on science, research, evidence, and best practices. The information is available, the facts are on the table. The current paradigm has failed *half* the addicts who enter treatment, and has largely ignored the beleaguered family members.

The new treatment model that I propose is based on the 14 FRT Principles presented in Chapter 2. I fully understand that in time, further evolution of science and additional research and outcome studies will suggest a new model to replace FRT, but my experience using this model over the last 25 years points to one clear fact: it is better, by a long shot, at treating addiction than is the addict-focused approach. Instead of only 50 percent of addicts remaining sober, close to 100 percent of the addicts I have worked with from a family systems perspective, using the model described in this book, have maintained sobriety, and are well on their way to developing healthy lives.

This outcome applies, of course, to those who follow the simple, step-by-step treatment plan outlined in these pages. As Gabor Maté poignantly recounts, some addicts' attachment to their drug of choice runs so deep, and their traumatic wounding is so debilitating that they truly cannot imagine life without it (2008). (And, sadly, there are government institutions and legal systems in place that enable addicts to prolong their addiction—for instance, government agencies that give money to addicts who then use that money to purchase drugs.) However, when addicts and those who enable them follow this model, remission and sustained recovery can be achieved.

Here is what the Clinical Director of the Betty Ford Treatment Center replied when I asked him in 2010 about the treatment center's recovery rates: "Those who follow our discharge recommendations have a success rate of staying sober through the critical first year that approaches 100%, and those who do not follow our discharge recommendations have a success rate that approaches zero." I asked him, "What are those discharge recommendations that result in a 'nearly 100% success rate'?" He replied:

> We advise them, upon discharge, to transfer to a family-based intensive outpatient program, go to daily AA meetings—90 meetings in 90 days—and then keep going—and get a sponsor and work the Steps. And that the family members, the codependents, do the same in Al-Anon. And, depending on the circumstances, for the addict to move into a Sober Living Environment.

I further propose we put the addict and the addictive/codependent family system under the care of one mental health professional—instead of shunting the addict from an interventionist to a detox facility to a counselor at a rehab program, then to an IOP (Intensive Outpatient Program) with yet another counselor, and to an SLE (Sober Living Environment) managed by still another individual, while the family's issues are largely ignored (see Figure 1.8). I propose that this one professional case manage the addict and the addict's family in a wrap-around treatment program that extends from the first contact with the FRT therapist through at least the first year of the addict's sobriety. The FRT therapist is uniquely qualified to lead this nascent field into the next treatment paradigm. The clinician who is trained to think systemically and to understand the unconscious dynamics at play in both enabling and perpetuating the disease of addiction is the right person for this job (see Figure 1.9).

We need all of the adjunctive services—doctors, detox facilities, rehab programs, step-down programs, sober living facilities, support groups, etc. But, more

Chapter 1. Addiction Treatment: Introducing a New Paradigm

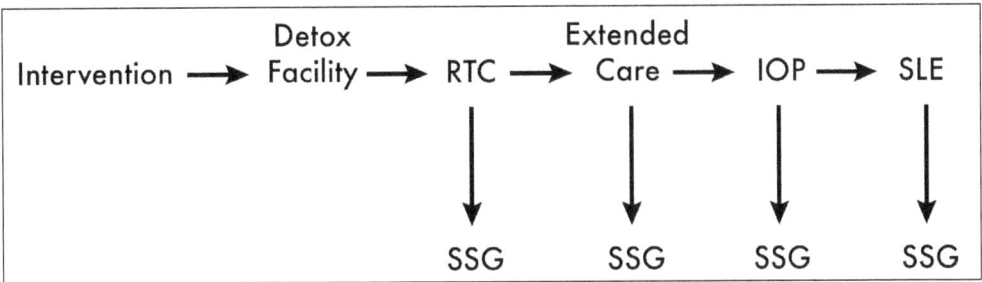

Figure 1.8 *Current Paradigm of Addiction Treatment.* Addiction treatment focuses only on the addict. The addict is shunted from one provider to the next: Interventionist (2 hours to 2 days), Detox physician (3 to 7 days), Residential Treatment Program (RTC) counselor (30 days), Extended Care counselor (30 to 60 days), Intensive Outpatient Program (IOP) counselor (3 to 6 months), and Sober Living Environment (SLE) manager (3 to 6 months). In this model, the addict may attend Social Support Groups (SSG) in multiple locations, some of them far away from home.

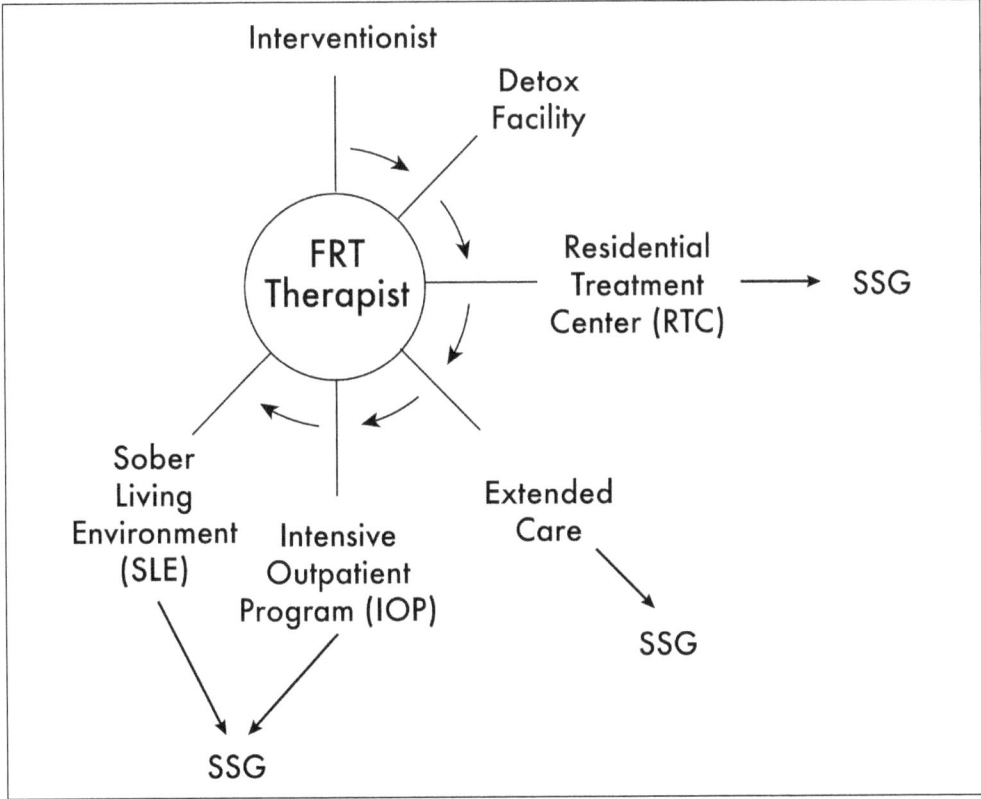

Figure 1.9 *The FRT Treatment Model.* The FRT therapist is the licensed mental health professional who intervenes, beginning with the first phone call, and treats the family system, the addict, and the enabling codependents. The FRT therapist works hand in hand with all therapeutic resources and adjunctive services, coordinating treatment through the initial year of continuous sobriety. In this model, the addict and the codependents (not pictured) will attend social support groups near their home while they are in outpatient treatment. The addict may be living in a sober living environment during outpatient treatment.

than anything, we need an addiction-trained, family-based mental health professional to treat the addict *and* the family, and to guide all aspects of the addiction treatment process, from the first phone call through at least the first year of continuous sobriety.

I have used this FRT model successfully with hundreds of family members over the last twenty-five years, and I describe the specifics of this model in detail in this book. It is my goal to train and enlist other therapists to step into this new, far more effective paradigm, with me. It is my hope that person may be you.

Given the ubiquity and profitability of residential rehab facilities, it is not surprising that I have encountered plenty of pushback when I have maintained that residential treatment is contraindicated in most circumstances. This is my reasoning:

- The real work for the addicted family system will happen at home, where the family members—the system—will recover together. (A common refrain often heard in treatment settings is: "You have to stand up where you fell down.") The recovery work occurs when the addict and the codependents regularly attend social support groups and attend therapy with an FRT therapist. The FRT therapist will guide them in addressing their issues, and coordinate their involvement in social support groups, as they mend the damage done, return to a trajectory of normal development, and begin creating a new future, one day at a time.
- Residential treatment programs are often seen as the "easier, softer way" for addicts. Most families are resistant to looking at the painful issues they have lived with and contributed to, and they want to avoid hard lifestyle changes themselves. "Hey, the problem is the addict, let's just send them away to be fixed." This is commonly known as "IP-ing"—labeling the addict as the "identified patient." This stance allows the codependents to stay in denial and avoid acknowledging their own issues, rather than seeking help for their role in supporting and enabling the unconscious homeostasis of their addictive/codependent family system.
- Many addicts come to see a residential treatment center as a "time-out" in a spa or retreat center, as merely an interlude between periods of addictive behavior.
- Many recovering addicts don't find residential treatment programs cost effective. Overheard at a social support group: "Shit, I could have saved 90K by just going to AA meetings."
- And, if the codependents refuse to "step up," a residential program may fail to keep the addict sober in the months after he or she leaves treatment and returns to the unchanged, enabling, codependent family and peer culture. We see addicts over and over again depleting their families' resources by attending a succession of costly rehabs.

I began my own recovery from alcoholism in 1979, entered graduate school in 1990, began my clinical work in a family-based adolescent outpatient program in

1992, and became a licensed therapist in 1996. Along the way, I have been guided by a number of mentors—all authors and experts in the addiction field—including the family systems-oriented addiction psychologist, Stephanie Brown, Ph.D.; the family systems addiction psychiatrist and addictionologist, Timmen Cermak, M.D.; Brad Reedy, Ph.D., director of a family-based wilderness treatment program; and addictionologist, Kevin McCauley, M.D. These individuals have guided my work during, and since, the time when I founded and directed two family-based outpatient addiction treatment programs—one for teens and one for adults. I've made many mistakes on the road to learning about effective addiction treatment, and figured out along the way what works and what doesn't.

Based on what I have learned during the last two and a half decades, I have developed a program that has produced a nearly 100 percent success rate for those who have followed the guidelines that I established—the same guidelines that I'm proposing in this book. And, like anyone working in this field, I have met many families who, for various reasons, were resistant to take on the serious work needed to change.

As I mentioned, when I have described my treatment model to other addiction treatment providers, they have been interested and receptive, but have expressed little desire to consider adopting it. It was as if they had the elephant's tail in their hands and were happily calling it a rope and were unaware of, or uninterested in, a larger perspective. They were unaware that their paradigm, "normal science" to them, was in crisis. And, if they were aware of the crisis, they did not have any suggestions for what to do to achieve more successful outcomes, so they chose to deny the anomalies they couldn't resolve.

I've come to understand that these treatment providers, doctors, interventionists, and others were, just like addicted families, caught in a systemic homeostasis. Like the treatment field in general, they adhere to an addict-centered approach which has long been the model in addiction treatment. They were simply doing things "the way they have always been done," thinking that tweaks here and there were enough to improve their programs. Meanwhile, half of their patients relapse, return to their addiction, and far too often, die.

Their treatment and interventions were successful—but only in half the cases! All of us feel good when just *one* addict under our guidance does the work to achieve and maintain remission—to return to normal development and create a happy and fulfilling life. We know that there are no guarantees when it comes to recovery for the addict or the codependent. And as a result of the tireless work of all of us in the addiction treatment field, there are many millions of addicts who have put their disease into remission and who have returned to healthy lives.

What about the others? What about the families and children who are still suffering, who are still in the throes of addiction and codependency, the addicts who perhaps have been to multiple treatment programs, but who are still in their disease? Maybe they do not even know they have this brain disorder, and maybe they don't know their families are part of the problem, because we providers have failed to ask the right questions, have failed to include the enablers, have failed to educate medical doctors, and have failed to follow a comprehensive, long-term approach.

In the next chapter, I will outline the 14 Principles of Family Recovery Therapy. I believe that clinicians who apply these principles and use the treatment guidelines described in this book will achieve much higher rates of success—families that become healthier and happier, codependents who heal and grow, and addicts who sustain remission and live fulfilling lives.

In order to do this work, you will need to modify your approach to treating addiction. Or, if you are new to the field, you will need to adopt an approach that is different from the current addict-focused, multiple-provider model you were doubtless trained in. You will need to collaborate closely with the members of your team—the other professionals working with a particular family. You will need to join the team, take the helm, and coordinate with your oarsmen to row together.

More than anything, we need addiction-trained, family systems-based mental health professionals who will treat the family system, the addict *and* the enabling codependents, and who will guide the treatment, from day one. The right person for this job is a therapist/clinician who is trained to think systemically and to understand the unconscious dynamics at play both in the enabling system's support and in its perpetuation of the container in which the addict lives. Just as an air traffic controller saves lives by directing pilots to follow flight paths, and the primary care physician interacts with specialists, addicts and their families are best served when treatment is carefully coordinated.

As the FRT therapist guiding treatment, once you have stepped into the role of team leader, you will oversee the continuum of care for the family members, beginning with the first call from the family through at least the first year of continuous sobriety. I invite you, as someone interested in improving outcomes in your treatment of addiction, to read on, and consider what we tell the newcomer, the addict in early recovery: "Trust the process."

Three key points:

First, throughout this book, I primarily write about substance addiction, but this model can be applied to addiction of any kind—to any condition that meets the criteria for addiction: craving, loss of control, adverse consequences, and chronicity. Compulsive behaviors related to food, gambling, sex, spending, and other repetitive, self-harming behaviors that can be categorized as addictions also benefit from the kind of treatment that I describe in this book. This model can also be applied to new kinds of addiction that have developed with the increased use—and misuse—of technology. The 2013 *Diagnostic and Statistical Manual of Mental Disorders (DSM-5)* (American Psychiatric Association), described Internet Gaming Disorder as a "condition for further study." And on June 18, 2018, the World Health Organization announced that the forthcoming *International Statistical Classification of Diseases and Related Health Problems* (ICD) would include "Gaming Disorder" as a new category. Gamers that meet the criteria for addiction, and other addictive or compulsive users of technology, respond well to treatment with this model.

Second, I talk throughout this book about the "family system." The reality is that each of us lives in a complex web of interpersonal relationships, which also comprise systems. An FRT therapist needs to consider the various important influences on an individual when assessing a family and developing a treatment plan. The "system" surrounding an addict can include work, legal, peer, and other social networks with which they are involved. Comprehensive treatment must include coordination with a variety of entities or communities that may play a role in enabling the addiction.

And third, as therapists, we are not immune to becoming enabling codependents who let our own "stuff" blind us to the reality of the unconscious dynamics at play in working with an addicted family. Murray Bowen is reputed to have said, "After four sessions, we are inducted into a family's system." We addiction therapists need to continue to get consultation, lest we fall prey to the seductive influences of the family members who are caught in a dilemma—they "want to recover," but they are also powerfully affected by their unconscious drive to maintain the previously existing systemic homeostasis, and will predictably tend to resist aspects of recovery. FRT therapists, grounded in the dynamics of addiction and codependency and alert to the potential for induction into addictive family systems, must rely on outside consultation to preserve as much objectivity as possible.

Chapter 2

The Fourteen Principles of Family Recovery Therapy

Most of us feel safer when we know the protocol in each situation: what is likely to happen and what we need to do. We all function best when we are grounded in a stable reality. We rarely think about many of the systems that we take for granted. But our world would be thrown into chaos if, for example, the rules of the road were suddenly abandoned and cars were allowed to drive in either direction on both sides of the road, not heeding red lights or stop signs, and going as fast on city streets as on the highway. In the United States, our federal, state, and local laws, along with generally accepted customs, help provide a relatively safe and reliable environment. And we have placed people in supervisory roles to enforce the laws and statutes.

Treatment of addiction, in my mind, similarly benefits from a structure that is organized and consistent. The Family Recovery Therapy treatment model provides a solid framework, as well as guidelines for a family in crisis, and extends treatment from the initial phone call through the first year of continuous sobriety. The basic principles of this model foster a coherent recovery path for the family suffering from addiction and codependency. These principles are not new, and I am grateful to all those who, over many decades, have contributed to the addiction treatment and family therapy fields. What is unique to the Family Recovery Therapy model is the consolidation of these principles into a comprehensive whole, designed to provide a solid recovery foundation for the entire family—almost doubling the odds of success.

Following is the complete list of the 14 Principles of Family Recovery Therapy, with descriptions and explanations that clarify the thinking that informs each principle, its origin and purpose, and why it is crucial to a successful treatment outcome. Each principle contributes an essential element to the treatment process, and I believe that omission of any one of them undermines the family's potential for solid and lasting recovery, just as leaving out a critical part in manufacturing an automobile, such as the brakes, will fail to produce a functional car.

A note before we start. In 2016, the U.S. government made a comprehensive effort to address the public health crisis caused by the prevalence of alcohol, illicit drugs, and prescription drug misuse. Their findings are elucidated in the 2016 U.S. Department of Health and Human Services compendium, *Facing Addiction in*

America: The Surgeon General's Report on Alcohol, Drugs, and Health (Office of the Surgeon General). This landmark report is based on hundreds of peer-reviewed studies. It presents addiction research and recommendations that cover addiction neurobiology, prevention, treatment, and recovery, and it addresses how to integrate health systems to facilitate treatment. The Surgeon General's extensive study refers, in different language, to the efficacy of each of the first 13 of the 14 Family Recovery Therapy Principles described in this chapter. The report validates decades of our successful work in this field. In Chapter 4, I will compare these 14 Principles with the *Principles of Drug Addiction Treatment (Third Edition)* (2018) published by the National Institute on Drug Abuse (NIDA), the lead federal agency that supports scientific research on drug use and its consequences.

The 14 Principles of Family Recovery Therapy

FRT Principle 1
Addiction is a chronic, relapsing, treatable medical disease with profound mental and physical consequences. Addicts will need long-term, possibly lifelong, recovery support, which can take many forms.

Addictive disorders are chronic, relapsing, medical conditions, just as are diabetes, asthma, and hypertension. Once a chronic disorder develops, it becomes a lifelong fixture—chronic conditions do not go away (Office of the Surgeon General, 2016). Those who suffer from a chronic condition can best be helped with early detection and treatment that includes vigilant medical and psychological management. The treatment protocol and attention required for chronic conditions intensifies during periods of exacerbation or relapse.

Drug and alcohol addiction are often considered "pediatric" disorders, since the majority of chemically dependent individuals began use as minors (Substance Abuse and Mental Health Services, 2012). This means that these disorders can become entrenched at a young age and can be more difficult to treat in older individuals who have a long history of substance use.

As a society, we are still only beginning to be aware that addiction is a pervasive, life-harming, and potentially fatal, brain disease. Most medical doctors in this country receive inadequate education about addiction, and, as a consequence, do not understand that addiction requires comprehensive treatment. I have had to educate my personal physician about the fact that I am an alcoholic, and I'm not sure that he fully gets it. When I began to work with him, almost 15 years ago, I said:

> Hey Doc, you need to know that I'm an alcoholic. My father died of this disease, it killed my son, and it may take out other members of my family. You are my doctor, and you need to know this. I have been sober for a number of years, but I could relapse any day. As long as I'm in active recovery, I think I will be okay. My disease, alcoholism, is a brain disease that tells me that I don't have a disease. The only treatment that works for me, the only

medicine, is for me to be endlessly reminded that my brain can't be trusted on this. I get these reminders by going to meetings with other recovering addicts and hearing, over and over, that today, just today, I need to not drink. Your job, as my doctor, is to remind me to "take my medicine," to go to meetings and to stay in contact with my mentor who is my personal guide on staying sober.

And every time I see my doctor, he asks me, "Are you still going to your support meetings? Still talking to your mentor?" I appreciate this additional support. I have regularly gone to meetings throughout my recovery, and, hopefully, I will continue to for the rest of my life.

As treatment providers, it is our job to get educated, and then to educate our clients and patients. When parents of teens consult me about their drug-using kids, I often tell them:

> At this point, I have no idea whether or not your child's substance use has progressed to addiction. But, just like when a growth pops up on top of your child's head, we need to get it checked out. The odds are that this is not addiction, just like the lump on his head probably is not a tumor. But either could be serious, and both can benefit from early detection and treatment.

Like physicians, mental health practitioners also receive minimal addiction training, which has serious implications for the health of individuals, marriages, and families. Very often, a mental health practitioner doesn't recognize the signs of addiction or codependency in clients, or, if it becomes clear that addiction is an issue, does not understand how to treat it or how to refer to an appropriate provider. This can result not only in ineffective treatment, but in allowing damage from addiction to persist and get worse, both for the addict and the family. Or, if addiction is identified, a therapist unschooled in addiction may focus on getting the addict into treatment, and not recognize or address the complex family dynamics involved, a scenario that can be detrimental to the addict and to the family.

We mental health professionals are trained to help people get more control over their lives. We help them recognize and work with their ego. We help them recover from mental illnesses. We help them improve their relationships—or see that there are irreconcilable differences between partners, in which case, we help them dissolve their relationships. But the disease of addiction runs counter to this approach. The addicted brain is already asserting "control" by responding to the trigger to use and ingesting the substance (Lyvers, 2000). The addict cannot learn to *control* his substance use, and no amount of therapy is going to change this fact. So, applying therapy to help someone "get control" is like adding fuel to a fire, and it can actually strengthen an addict's denial and defenses.

FRT Principle 1 lays the foundation for what comes next. The addict has a disease. A serious, life-threatening disorder that can be treated and put into remission—if the treatment is effective and comprehensive. Understanding addiction is crucial to grasping Family Recovery Therapy.

FRT Principle 2
Effective treatment of addiction usually involves treatment of codependents, because codependents enable addiction. Codependency is a chronic relationship pattern that has profound mental and physical consequences and is characterized by an obsessive focus on other people. Codependents may need lifelong recovery support, which can take many forms.

An addict is often easily identified—a sloppy drunk, someone slurring their words, a person at a party who vomits. An addict's behavior often stands out. Codependency is subtle, not easily noticed, and hard to pinpoint. To an addiction counselor, however, the signs of codependency are readily apparent—the addict and the codependent fit together, hand in glove. Here is how Stephanie Brown described it to me:

> Unhealthy codependency is developing an addictive emotional attachment to another person. The addict has an addictive emotional attachment to alcohol or substances or to being out of control in some way. The codependent develops exactly the same out-of-control emotional investment and attachment to a person. The center of the self of the codependent becomes invested in being able to control somebody else, which is never successful from a recovery frame. The codependent then deepens that intense attachment, abandoning the self to become invested in that attachment or bond to another [personal communication, 2021].

Recovery for the addict means replacing their addictive behavior and thinking with healthy alternatives. Recovery for the codependent means discovering and turning their attention to their self and focusing on their own personal growth and development (Brown & Lewis, 1999).

The *Serenity Prayer* is said by thousands of people in recovery daily: "God, grant me the serenity to accept the things I cannot change, the courage to change the things I can, and the wisdom to know the difference" (Alcoholics Anonymous®, n.d.-c). For the codependent, this prayer can be more complex than for the addict, who is simply not picking up a substance.

God, grant me the serenity to accept the things I cannot change
  (…like other people),
The courage to change the things I can
  (…I can only change myself),
And the wisdom to know the difference
  (…which is very difficult in an enmeshed, emotionally fused, poorly differentiated, family system).

The untreated codependent, like the addict, has yet to come out of denial and understand their role in perpetuating the dysfunctional family dynamics. Think about how you have developed certain views, perhaps about politics or religion. We could certainly have a discussion, you and I, a conversation, in which I *try* to make you think differently, but could I, in an evening or a day or a week, convince you to make a fundamental shift and join another political party? Or reverse your view on religion from being a believer to a non-believer, or vice versa? No, of course not. And the more I pushed, the more defensive you would become, digging in your heels and becoming even more attached to your position.

This pushing-to-make-someone-change is the crux of codependency. Codependents can spend *their whole lives* pursuing the illusion that they can change another person. Their. Whole. Lives. Of course, the codependent isn't trying to change another person simply as an exercise. The codependent typically loves the addict and is terrified of the consequences of the addict's behavior. They see that the addict is harming herself, making a mess of her life, leaving in her wake destroyed relationships, thwarted development, impaired health, and adverse financial consequences. The codependent tries fiercely to prevent the addict from creating more havoc in her life, and more negative repercussions in the lives of those around her. The codependent engages in a single-minded quest for safety and sanity: she believes that if she could *control* the addict, everything would be so much better.

Recovery for the codependent is about slowly redirecting their focus away from the addict and towards themselves. The recovering codependent must first acknowledge that they, themselves, not only have a problem, but that they play a pivotal role—one that might surprise them—in the life and behavior of the addict (Brown, 1995; Beattie, 1986). Without the codependent's interference, the addict quite possibly would get sober on her own. The addict who is no longer supplied with free rent, free food, free transportation, free drugs, free alcohol, endless bailouts, might just have a crisis, might "hit bottom," and might finally reach out for help on her own. Some codependents may continue "to put cushions under the addict"—to prevent them from hitting a bottom—in a vain attempt to prevent their addict from suffering. A codependent's misguided love can do terrible, even deadly things to those they "love."

I often tell the story of a mother who called me, seeking help for her son who had "vomited on her sofa" the previous night. I did not get a chance to treat this family because she, the mother, "didn't need to talk to anyone." She just wanted me to "call her son." Her son, it turned out, was 64 years old! He had lived with his mother his whole life, and his mother had enabled her son with a lifetime of free rent, food, and alcohol—all the while futilely trying to change her son.

The codependent abandons him or herself—their goals, needs, and desires—and invests in the other person, which both prevents the other person from growing up and facing life on life's terms, and robs the codependent of a fulfilling, healthy life of their own. It is cruel, selfish—and blind. Codependents do not understand how their behavior is part of their addict's problem. They have been relentlessly trying to help, to love their addict into sobriety. They monitor the alcohol level in bottles and hide bottles when they can, they lie and cover up for their addict when he is in a pinch, they give him meals and a roof over his head, hoping fervently that their devoted attention will someday cause their addict to wake up and choose recovery. Unfortunately, it does not work this way.

The codependent merges emotionally with another person and can take over directing the other person's life. Murray Bowen, M.D., one of the pioneers in family systems theory, describes this behavior as failing to differentiate a separate self out of an enmeshed, undifferentiated family ego-mass (see Chapter 3, Figure 3.5).

Self-differentiation is a developmental process. Symbiosis and a tendency towards enmeshment are present in all of us, to some degree. When children are young, a healthy parent-child relationship is symbiotic by nature. A parent feels sad at the thought of their child growing up and leaving home, but knows that growing up is a necessary part of life, and understands that this is the best thing for the child—to develop a life of their own.

But in addictive family systems, unhealthy enmeshment and symbiosis impede the growth and development of all family members (Staton et al., 1982; Bowen, 1974). The helpful child may take over responsibilities the addicted parent cannot fulfill, giving up his or her own development to become a "Parentified Child." Or the codependent parent may develop an inappropriately close emotional relationship with their child, who has inadvertently abandoned him or herself in service of becoming the "Spousified Child." In addictive families, there are likely to be several codependents, each playing a role which is in some way dictated by the presence of addiction and codependency—so much so that a husband may hand his wife a drink just after she returns from an addiction treatment center, "forgetting" that his wife is actually an addict. The husband is unconsciously motivated to return to the old family dynamic, which could lead to his supporting his wife's resuming drinking—all to get the family back to "normal." It is critical that codependent, enmeshed family members discontinue sabotaging behaviors and disengage from emotional involvement that actually result in both prolonging addiction and undermining their own lives (Rotunda et al., 2004). It can require extensive, often lifelong, work on the part of codependents to change their attitudes, beliefs, and behavior.

Treatment programs that do not involve and treat the enabling codependents as comprehensively as they treat the addict have high failure rates. The codependent/addictive family system is typically locked in place—treating only the addict fails to address this enmeshed system, which is highly resistant to change.

FRT Principle 2 is the second pillar of FRT's foundation. It is vital for the FRT therapist to understand the dynamics of codependency as well as to recognize the limits of what he or she can do. Clearly, a therapist cannot change another person. As a wise therapist once told me, "our helplessness is our best weapon." We need to accept that the only person we can help is the individual who is willing to acknowledge their problem, ask for help, and choose to follow our guidance.

FRT Principle 3
In Family Recovery Therapy (FRT), the client in treatment is the family system that suffers from both addiction and codependency.

This is a fundamental tenet of Family Recovery Therapy: we treat the system comprised of the addict and those enabling and impacted by his addiction—the codependents and other close family members. To facilitate the change needed for an addicted family to recover, and for each family member to grow and address the developmental tasks appropriate for his or her age, we need to evaluate not only each individual, but also the interplay between individuals—the relationships. The FRT therapist needs solid training in family systems theory and methodology.

Addiction is often multigenerational. Addicts and codependents often come from families already affected by addiction and codependency. Unhealthy family dynamics, norms, and patterns can get entrenched over decades. A family systems therapist understands that estrangements, disruptions, divorces, emotional cutoffs, and family secrets from generations ago can impact present-day family dynamics.

It is interesting to note that an addictive/codependent family can ensnare the unsuspecting FRT therapist into their system. It is important to re-emphasize that Murray Bowen is reputed to have said that it takes only four sessions for a therapist to get inducted into a family's system—which is why it is essential that FRT therapists seek consultation and support when doing this work.

The family system is strong: roles, rules, and rituals are deeply entrenched. Family members may urge the FRT therapist to make exceptions to the treatment guidelines in order to preserve established and traditional family patterns. This may not even be a conscious ploy by the family member who is new to recovery; the individual may be struggling to adapt the treatment specifications to her own situation and be caught between the old and the new, and may simply need compassionate, but clear and informed, direction. The FRT therapist needs to be attuned to the dynamics of an addictive family system.

Relationship patterns in addictive family systems develop in response to the behavior of the addict. A crisis occurs—the addict is too hungover to go to work, or too drunk to pick up the kids at school—and another family member steps in to rescue the addict; nobody in the family wants anyone outside of the family to know what's really going on. The wife calls her husband's boss to say he has come down with the flu and can't come to work; an older child stays home from school so they can pick up the younger kids when the school day is over.

When addiction occurs in a family, codependent family members learn to focus on the person in crisis. Out of love for the addict and fear of bad consequences, they become hypervigilant and wary, on the lookout for the next situation that needs to be fixed. Keeping secrets and "covering up" become endemic, and family members learn to hide what they feel and think, because what they say and do must be in service of keeping up the outward appearance that everything is normal.

Over time, addiction provokes specific, recurring relationship patterns in the family (Brown & Lewis, 1999; Bowen 1974). Often, children or spouses of addicts will never experience a relationship with the parent, or partner, as anything other than a relationship with an addict—disconnected, remote, and unloving—even though that reality may never be voiced out loud.

All relationships, in families as well as in other settings, tend to develop predictable patterns. Knowing how the other person will behave, and how we will act in response, is the homeostatic glue that keeps relationships stable. But "stable" does not necessarily mean healthy. And this is why Family Recovery Therapy sees the family *system* as the client—the relationship patterns, as well as the individual development of the separate family members, can be distorted and derailed by addiction. Not only is it necessary for the addict to change, it is necessary for the family members to change, or the system will maintain its unhealthy homeostasis—the drive to stay the same—which has been maintained with longstanding, often unconscious, beliefs and behaviors (Bowen, 1961).

Recovery takes time, and change will not happen without a person both deciding to change and following through, consciously and repeatedly, and adopting new behaviors that cement the change. This is true for both the addict and the codependent family members. (This is where the current treatment paradigm drops the ball: it fails to consider the complex, often unconscious, influence of family members on an individual's recovery.) Family members of an addict consciously want to help their loved one to recover, and may even believe they know exactly how to do that. However, unconsciously, due to forces they may not even know exist, there is a pull on the family members to create what is familiar and predictable, to revert to well-established behavior patterns from the past. Consider the following two scenarios:

> An alcoholic goes to residential treatment for 60 days, comes home to the same, untreated family and peer group. Everyone welcomes him home, and someone hands him a beer, thinking that treatment must have worked because he was there for 60 days and, in that time, must have learned how to drink occasionally without it being a problem. (True story; this has happened more than once in my practice.)
>
> In another version, the same alcoholic goes to the same treatment program and comes home to a family that has been in treatment while he has been in residential treatment. The family has met consistently with an FRT therapist, gone to regular social support groups like Al-Anon, and learned about addiction, codependency and the "family disease" of addiction. Upon discharge, the alcoholic goes directly to meet with the FRT therapist and his family. In this meeting, he agrees to continue outpatient treatment at home, including family therapy, to do drug testing, perhaps to move into a sober living environment (SLE), and to attend social support meetings.

In which situation will the recovering addict stand the best chance of staying sober? In the families I see, I only work with those who follow the protocol outlined in the second scenario. I know that when the codependents do their work at home at the same time that the addict is doing his in a comprehensive treatment program, the addict stands a very good chance both of staying sober after residential treatment and of developing a healthy, fulfilling life. Fifty percent of the addicts in the first scenario will typically relapse.

What happens if some of the family members do not want to participate in addiction/codependency treatment? The reality is that initially, practically every new family member is resistant—everyone is in pain from the crisis that typically led the family to call our office. If we offer hope, and are confident in our approach, we can point toward a path that most people will follow, particularly as they see positive change occur, over time. Nearly every family member is at least somewhat resistant. Sometimes a family member is highly resistant. We need to work with whoever is willing to do the work. We encourage every family member to participate in treatment, but we understand that we cannot *make* someone choose recovery. If family members are not willing to actively participate in the treatment process and follow the recommendations of the FRT therapist, they will not be part of the process. We will work with those individuals who want to change and are willing to follow our guidance.

Sometimes this means that families and marriages will split apart, temporarily or permanently, as one member seeks recovery and another does not. And sometimes, a family member who initially refuses to participate in treatment, decides at a later point—perhaps when they have hit a bottom of their own or seen a loved one recover—to seek treatment, which may lead to the family reuniting and working together to restore healthy development.

FRT Principle 3 acknowledges an entity larger than the addict or a codependent family member—the family system. Despite the crazy things that may have happened, together they are still a family, a unique, bound-by-relationship group that has been wounded and fragmented. But the family can be fully restored to a functional whole, if the recovery work is embraced. As each individual engages in their personal recovery process, the FRT therapist works to help heal the disrupted bonds between family members, and to build a healthy family.

FRT Principle 4
During the first year of treatment, the FRT therapist monitors, assesses, and guides the family in an integrated treatment process, which addresses biological, psychological, social, and spiritual recovery.

How long do you think it would take for you, as an adult, to learn to read, write, and speak a foreign language well enough that you could live and work in a country where that was the predominant language spoken? Certainly a few months would not do the job. Probably it would take at least a year, more likely even longer.

How long do you think it would take for you, as an adult, to master playing the violin well enough to perform in public? If you were motivated you could do it, but you would have to practice a lot, and for a long time.

So, what about families? Can they change? Evolve, yes, but fundamentally change? Not without a compelling reason, motivation, and hard work! Homeostasis is a powerful force, and preserving the status quo is of paramount importance. Homeostasis preserves stability and provides predictability, and, for better or for worse, provides a semblance of safety in an all too chaotic world (Levin et al., 2001). But homeostasis is the enemy of recovery.

An addictive/codependent family system, surviving from crisis to crisis, may experience a crisis momentous enough to provoke fundamental change. When a family member cries out for help, he or she is motivated to do something different. The individual is aware that continuing to do the same thing isn't working, that the insanity is only getting worse, and that something significant has to shift if things are going to get better.

But the codependent who reaches out may be pretty clueless about what to do, what needs to change, and how those changes can happen. When a codependent calls an FRT therapist, their cry is, "Help! What should I do?" And the job of the FRT therapist, from that first phone call, is to guide the person who is calling, and the other family members, on a path towards recovery. An FRT therapist understands the broad picture, infers the likely history of calamities that has preceded the call, imagines the toll wrought by addiction and codependency and the anguish and distress of family members—some in favor of getting help, and some who are not certain help is needed. The FRT therapist needs to engage the family and coach them forward, step by step, in a process that will be life-changing for everyone involved.

Initially, the FRT therapist is a first responder, called upon to manage the crisis that precipitated the phone call. The FRT therapist is also the counselor who instructs the family members to take the next steps, to stop trying to change the addict, to attend social support groups, to adhere to the treatment plan, to allow the process of recovery to unfold—one day at a time. The FRT therapist is active and directive, spelling out the goals of each phase of treatment and helping family members stay on track through the shifts and changes that occur. In time, as the family members ensconce themselves in recovery (much as a person who wants to learn Italian fluently may live for a time in Italy), the FRT therapist can uncover the intricate interpersonal dynamics that have been in place for years, even decades. The FRT therapist can coach family members to develop healthy, un-enmeshed relationships, helping each family member to individuate and set personal goals in all areas of their lives, and facilitate repair of the wounds and hurts caused by years of dysfunction. The FRT therapist stands by each family member and encourages each one of them to do his or her own work, which will allow the process of recovery to unfold; he or she assists family members as they transition from one phase to the next, ensuring a consistent and stable process.

When we scan the addiction treatment field, it is clear that many parts of it are firmly in place and providing solid services: interventionists, transport services, detox facilities, residential and outpatient programs, sober living houses, drug testing resources, sober coaches, addiction medical and psychiatric doctors, and social support groups. However, what is missing is an entity that can ensure the cohesion of the treatment and recovery process through the span of any one family's journey toward recovery (McLellan et al., 2005). Without a framework that holds the pieces together, treatment can become fragmented: addicts may relapse when bridges that aid transition are absent, family members get left out, the family as a whole—the family system that is the actual client—receives inadequate attention and may descend further into chaos and devastation.

The FRT therapy model pulls together the pieces of the recovery process and holds them in place over an extended time frame—at least for the first year of continuous sobriety. In this way, the addict and the codependents—the family system—can be better served. With fewer cracks to fall through, relapse rates decrease. And when support and guidance for the codependents and the addict are integral components of the process, recovery is more likely to be sustained.

What does the first year of recovery actually look like? Who will be doing what? The answer is specific to each family's situation. An FRT therapist directs the family throughout that first year of continuous sobriety, brings in necessary resources, coordinates other professionals and facilities, and provides comprehensive guidance, counseling, and psychotherapy for each family member and for the whole family. The FRT therapist also makes recommendations to help the family continue to grow and make progress beyond the first year, so that the family can develop a solid foundation for healthy growth and long-lasting recovery.

Recovery is a process that takes time. In social support groups, it is not uncommon to hear statements like:

> When I got to a year of sobriety, I thought I had it all figured out. And then, on my five-year anniversary, I realized that I was just getting started. Now, with two decades of recovery, I realize that the future is going to be full of more growth, more love, more loving relationships—and that is why I keep coming back to my support groups.

Recovering lost development and healing the past needs to be a way of life; therefore, it is a process. Yes, it starts with a decision to follow specific guidelines, but it is the work that follows—one day at a time—that matters. Addiction, of course, is also a way of life. It consists of thoughts and behaviors practiced every day, over and over, that reinforce the addictive lifestyle. Any addict or codependent can make the decision to get into recovery, but only those who follow up that decision with action over the long term, one day at a time, will have a chance of success—just like learning a foreign language or playing a musical instrument (Tiebout, 1944).

FRT Principle 4 outlines the FRT therapist's role. In this recovery process, the FRT therapist is the guide who sees the bigger picture and steers each individual along a prescribed path, working with all aspects of recovery: biological, psychological, social, and spiritual. This process is designed to put addiction into remission and lead each individual, and the family system, towards restored development.

FRT Principle 5

As the treatment team leader, the FRT therapist guides the family throughout the continuum of care and collaborates with all supportive therapeutic services, which may include other treatment providers, interventionists, treatment programs, physicians, and any other adjunctive services.

As already noted, the treatment model customarily practiced today is fragmented. It does not provide a continuum of care for an individual and family recovering from addiction and codependency, because it lacks a lead person to oversee the process (Satz et al., 2008; McLellan et al., 2005). The treatment process often breaks down as the addict transitions into or out of a residential program and through various phases of ongoing care. Generally, there is no licensed, addiction-trained, family systems-trained, mental health professional who has eyes and ears on the family throughout treatment, and certainly not from the initial phone call through the first year of continuous sobriety.

Guiding the family members to disrupt the existing family homeostasis, "the way things have always been done," and to create new family norms is central to this principle. Stephanie Brown and Virginia Lewis describe this process in their book, *The Alcoholic Family in Recovery: A Developmental Model* : "In fact, it is the collapse of the system from inside that is crucial to recovery. Reaching outside the family and relying on external sources of support (treatment programs, 12-steps groups, therapists, religious affiliation) ironically offers the necessary stabilization" (1999, p. 19). We all tend to settle into our lives and, to a great extent, to operate unconsciously. The first year of recovery, if successful, will result in the family changing previously accepted norms. Individuals in treatment will be asked to do things that are uncomfortable, that go against their nature, and are different from their former way of behaving. For the addict—and the family—to "hit bottom" and be willing to move, step by step, towards recovery requires family members to trust a professional who can see and help coordinate the big picture.

The big picture may include other therapists, medical doctors, managers of sober living homes, and employers. It is the job of the FRT therapist to make referrals for auxiliary care and coordinate care with any providers involved in the family's recovery. Chapter 12, "Working with Other Treatment Providers," describes in detail the interactions that an FRT therapist may engage in with various providers. In a private conversation, addiction psychiatrist Timmen Cermak confirmed to me the importance of a coordinated FRT approach, "No one deserves to be a part of this (treatment) continuum unless they do it in a way that's integrated with what came before them and what comes after them. Their services need to be constructed in that way" (personal communication, 2018).

The fact that recovery involves many components is substantiated by the Clinical Director of the Betty Ford Treatment Center, quoted also in Chapter 1, who asserted:

> "Those who follow our discharge recommendations have a success rate of staying sober through the critical first year that approaches 100%, and those who do not follow our discharge recommendations have a success rate that approaches zero."
> And when asked, "What are those discharge recommendations that result in a 'nearly 100% success rate'?" he replied:
> We advise them, upon discharge, to transfer to a family-based intensive outpatient program, go to daily AA meetings—90 meetings in 90 days—and then keep going—and get a sponsor and work the Steps. And that the family members, the codependents, do the same in Al-Anon. And, depending on the circumstances, for the addict to move into a Sober Living Environment.

The job of the FRT therapist is to help the family members in treatment stay on track, from day one through the first year of sobriety—to seek and use available support systems, and to keep turning towards recovery.

In working with addiction, we need to remember that we are treating a distressed, out-of-control, addictive/codependent family system that, over time, has become trapped in dysfunctional thinking and behavior patterns. Every family member needs guidance, encouragement, and loving support to change. The initial hours, the first days, that critical first month, the dangerous first three, "relapse-prone" months, the first year—at all phases—the family needs hands-on care. These individuals are doing what we have prayed they would do—they have finally said, "We need help, tell us what to do!" And, at the very same moment, they are resistant (Levin et al., 2001; Beattie, 1986; Brown & Lewis, 1999). They are frightened, nervous, and confused. The addict knows exactly what will dispel that uncomfortable feeling: resuming their "medicine," their drug, alcohol, porn, gambling, spending, gaming, or overeating. Family members are at risk of falling right into their old, controlling patterns: trying to dissuade the addict from relapsing; taking the focus off themselves. Everyone needs to rely on his or her counselor and sponsor.

When codependent family members ask for help, generally their real hope is that the therapist will "somehow get their addicted family member sober." But from the first meeting, the FRT therapist has challenged their beliefs and urged them to let go of their illusions. The FRT therapist has clearly told them that only the addict can make the decision to "get sober." And the codependent family members need to understand that their new job is to "keep the focus on themselves" and let the FRT therapist and others guide the addict's treatment and recovery.

Here is an example of a fragmented treatment approach in which the lack of therapeutic support for the codependent undermined the recovery process:

> Susan, a 45-year-old alcoholic, agreed, reluctantly, to go to treatment. Her husband, Tom, had said he was tired of her drunken behavior and couldn't tolerate it any longer. They found a solid-sounding, well-known treatment program near their home. Susan entered the 30-day, high-end, expensive program, situated on a scenic meadow surrounded by acres of rolling hills. On Sundays, the program allowed family members to visit, and Tom drove to the treatment center to see Susan. Their relationship, not unlike many addictive/codependent family systems, was highly conflictual, and their time apart hadn't done anything to improve their situation. It was no surprise that the couple started arguing during Tom's visit. Susan stormed off to her room, and Tom drove home, concerned that this treatment wasn't going to work, and that his wife would come home after 30 days and go right back to drinking. Tom was right: Susan came home, and within 24 hours, the two were arguing with each other. In front of Tom, Susan angrily opened a bottle of wine (there was still lots of alcohol in the house) and started drinking.

When I heard the story of Susan's treatment and subsequent relapse, I was not surprised. While Susan was getting major guidance and support, Tom had no contact with the staff at the program, or with any outside therapist or counselor, until he arrived for a "family weekend" three weeks into Susan's stay. During the weekend, he heard lectures on alcoholism and recovery, and a little about codependency, but he did not recognize his behavior as codependent, or as having any relationship to Susan's alcoholism. He and Susan met briefly with her addiction counselor, who told Tom about Susan's wonderful progress, but at no point was there any reference to the care Tom would need going forward.

The current common model of addiction treatment goes something like this:

1. Addict and family meet interventionist; addict is intervened on, typically spending somewhere between four and ten hours in the presence of the interventionist. The interventionist may or may not be certified or licensed as a mental health professional. The interventionist gives the codependent family members a few suggestions—go to Al-Anon meetings and stop rescuing your addict—but rarely are the codependents referred for professional treatment themselves.

2. Addict goes to residential treatment, meets his or her residential drug counselor, who hopefully is a certified addictions counselor but seldom is a licensed mental health professional. Addict spends 30–90 days in the treatment facility with the residential counselor in charge of his treatment. Treatment for the codependents is largely ignored. Rarely will the residential counselor work with the codependent and recommend that she attend social support groups or seek out mentors in recovery. Nor will the residential counselor recommend that the codependent see a therapist who can actively address her part of the family's recovery.

3. Addict is then discharged and referred to a typically 90-day outpatient treatment—again, new strangers to work with. There is often no strategy in place to coordinate the addict's transition from residential to outpatient treatment, and an appropriate living situation for the addict frequently has not been planned—the addict often returns to the same unchanged family dynamics and peer culture, and typically resists moving from there into a "step-down" (Intensive Outpatient Program) or sober living environment.

In this process, at each phase of treatment, the addict is supposed to rely for support on someone they do not know, someone they are aware will serve only as a temporary guide. Treatment becomes fragmented as different individuals take charge of different treatment phases. The transitions are often bumpy, at best.

Let's take a closer look at the transition out of a residential treatment program in the most commonly used model. The residential program has monitored the addict and formed a good picture of what should comprise the next phase of treatment. The discharge staff may recommend that the addict move into a sober living environment, enroll in an intensive outpatient program, and attend daily social support meetings (and perhaps they will suggest that the codependents go to their own social support and mutual aid groups). Sounds good, so far.

Without ongoing support, what often happens is that the addict and codependents resist and "modify" these recommendations. Their recommendations are typically at odds with the previous homeostasis of the family. The addict, instead of moving into a sober living environment, decides to move back home, where the codependent (who found the social support group "uncomfortable" and does not go back) resumes her controlling behavior. The addict, meanwhile, may go to a few AA meetings each week, but sits in the back and does not participate, and eventually stops going altogether.

These dynamics are not unusual and contribute to the high relapse rate in the first year. Let's contrast this to the transition process when an FRT therapist is guiding treatment.

I have found that directors of residential programs, transitional housing managers, and medical doctors are very receptive to having a knowledgeable and skillful professional oversee the long-term treatment process. They understand that consistency is vital to providing effective care, but they are rarely in a position to ensure that it exists when treatment follows the current paradigm. A meeting with some therapists from a residential program confirmed my belief that directors of these programs eagerly welcome coordination of care.

One afternoon, I was sitting in an Italian restaurant across from two field therapists employed by a well-reputed wilderness program that specializes in working with young adults. They were on a marketing tour and had invited me to lunch to pitch their program. In response to their question of how we might work together on a case, I replied, "In my FRT model I would need to be assured of close collaboration. I need your clinical director to understand this up front." I continued, expressing my frustration at what it is often like when a program has "taken over" my case; they have not understood that they are *only one component* of my year-long Family Recovery Therapy treatment model.

I explained that fragmented treatment is an all-too-common experience when referring a client to a residential treatment program. When I refer a client to a residential program, the success of my year-long, family-based approach depends on tight collaboration between the addict's field therapist, the codependent family members, and myself. This wilderness program they were representing could fit into our year-long treatment program, but only if I participated both in weekly phone meetings with the family members and with the wilderness therapist, and I also coordinated—in close consultation with their staff—the transition process after the wilderness program.

When the two field therapists understood my integrated model, they laughed and said, "Our program director would love to have a clinician insist on collaboration, because that close coordination with the referring professional is exactly what he wants!"

With this kind of treatment structure in place, the job of the client's residential program counselor becomes much easier: in the weekly calls, the counselor can dialogue with the FRT therapist and the family members about potential future

Chapter 2. The Fourteen Principles of Family Recovery Therapy

placement for the client. Program directors are well aware that their 30-60-90-day program is only as effective as what comes after discharge—and that many of their clients will return to the same enabling family dynamics and the same drug-using peer culture that existed before treatment, a scenario which will likely undermine the client's recovery chances. But when a coordinated, comprehensive treatment plan is in place, the chance of sustained recovery is significantly greater (Compton et al., 2015).

I have also discovered that medical doctors appreciate the opportunity to collaborate with a family therapist. Generally, therapists defer to medical doctors in coordinating treatment, yet doctors often welcome guidance and collaboration. Doctors want to provide optimal care, but they typically can spend only a brief time with each patient; they gratefully accept a more in-depth perspective on the patient from an involved, well-informed, case-managing therapist.

FRT Principle 5 further delineates the specifics of the FRT therapist's role. In short, a more positive recovery outcome can be achieved when an FRT therapist directs the treatment process, collaborates with physicians and other treatment providers, holds in mind the overall framework and structure of treatment, and makes sure that all components of the treatment process contribute to a healthy recovery for the family system and its members.

FRT Principle 6
The FRT therapist must be well-versed in the 12 Steps and have a thorough understanding and appreciation for the fundamental role that mutual aid programs play in recovery from codependency and addiction.

Addiction is a chronic, relapsing brain disease. The addict, by definition, is powerless over his desire to use drugs and, on his own, cannot control his cravings, impulses, and behaviors related to drug use. The goal is to help the addict first stop drug use, and then refrain from resuming drug use for just one day, while helping the family system find and create a healthy lifestyle. The FRT therapist guides the addict and the family members to take steps forward on a recovery path, providing suggestions and a treatment protocol.

One component of recovery for the addict, which is vital both in the initial phase of treatment and going forward, is social support and mutual aid groups (Erikson. M., 2020). These groups offer the addict a community of recovering peers—others who have been where he has been and who can both model recovery and also support and encourage him to stay on a path of sobriety.

In early recovery, an addict needs peer support to reinforce that recovery is possible. Living a life without drugs is daunting to anyone who has been using for any length of time, and guidance from those who have made it past the early days and weeks of sobriety is invaluable to the newly sober addict. For the addict to walk into a room filled with other recovering people, people who are typically happy and welcoming and who also suffer from the disease of addiction, and who therefore can understand and relate to him, is a huge relief. The opportunity for connection with like-minded individuals is a powerful gift for the recovering addict who has probably been largely surrounded by family, colleagues, even doctors or therapists, who don't understand his disease, may have criticized and shamed him for not being able to control it, and have no clue about the hellish existence of an addict or the challenges of recovery from addiction.

Social support groups consist of recovering peers who can provide empathy, caring, acceptance, and love to the struggling addict at any stage of recovery. They provide connection with other people who have been at the lowest point in their lives and know the desperation, despair, isolation, and hopelessness of being caught in the downward spiral of addiction, and who have moved beyond that demoralizing and seemingly impassable point. It is invaluable for the addict to witness the strength and hope of those who have been where he is.

Social support groups, groups of peers in recovery, provide many other benefits to the addict who is dealing with the challenges of adapting to a new lifestyle and learning new behaviors and new thinking. In groups of her peers, the addict will hear stories of people whose histories, or aspects of them, are familiar and resonate with her own experiences. This provides the sense of belonging—of being with others whose experience she can relate to. She is not alone, her situation is not unique, and she does not have to face sobriety as a solo individual among aliens who do not comprehend the enormity of the task ahead of her.

In addition, the addict will witness recovery—how people have managed, despite their past, to find a way of coping that is different from relying on drugs. She will hear what individuals chose to do instead of turning to drugs when they were besieged with memories of using. She will hear what her peers do to manage cravings. She will hear new ways to think about alcohol or drugs that remind her how important it is to not drink or pick up her drug of choice. She will hear how others in recovery face emotional challenges, and that they can feel feelings and survive the discomfort of feelings without having to drink or use.

Group members remind the newcomer he cannot control his desire to use drugs, but show him that some rudimentary, but essential, behavior changes will help him modify his old patterns and stay sober. The addict's peers tell him not to use, this hour, or this day, to keep going to meetings, and to spend time with others in recovery.

The treatment for addiction, beyond detoxification and stabilization, is to do whatever is necessary to keep the addict from acting on their midbrain's craving. This is something that the addict's prefrontal cortex—by definition—will never, ever, be able to do. The addict's prefrontal cortex—their thinking brain, their wisdom, their knowledge—cannot prevent the addict from relapsing or from resuming their addictive behavior, no matter how smart, how determined, or calculating they may be. In time, nearly every single addict, without support, is at high risk of relapsing. There are those who stop going to social support and mutual aid groups and do not relapse, but for every one of these individuals, there are many, many more who relapse.

As previously mentioned, the most available social support group for addicts is Alcoholics Anonymous, the international mutual aid group that assists people to stop drinking and become sober. It is estimated that more than two million people worldwide are AA members (Alcoholics Anonymous®, n.d.-b). In addition, many people participate in various 12-Step programs that are patterned after AA, including Al-Anon, Narcotics Anonymous, Nicotine Anonymous, Marijuana Anonymous, Cocaine Anonymous, Gamblers Anonymous, Overeaters Anonymous, Sex and Love Addicts Anonymous, and Debtors Anonymous. There are several dozen different kinds of 12-Step programs modeled after AA.

Twelve-Step programs are ubiquitous, but there are other mutual aid groups that can also help addicts get and stay sober. Among the non–AA groups are Life-Ring Secular Recovery, SMART Recovery®, Women for Sobriety, and Secular Organizations for Recovery. In all of these groups, addicts learn new ways of thinking and behaving, just as they do in AA. What secular groups do not have is the concept of a "Higher Power." AA's 12 Steps, as described in *Twelve Steps and Twelve Traditions*, state in Step 1 that the addict is "powerless over alcohol" and in Step 2 that there is a "Power greater than ourselves" which can "restore us to sanity" (Alcoholics Anonymous World Services, 1981, p. 5). Throughout this book as I refer to the 12 Steps they can be found in this same reference, commonly known as the "12 by 12."

This, however, does not mean that AA is a religious group. It is not. But the concept of a "power beyond oneself" is not acceptable to everyone. Some addicts want to avoid anything that even reminds them of unpleasant, religion-related situations from the past.

Probably, AA is the group that most directly speaks to the addict's inability to control their addiction ("powerless over alcohol") and their need to surrender control to something beyond themselves ("Power greater than ourselves"). This is consistent with what we know about the midbrain co-opting the prefrontal cortex. The AA Steps clearly acknowledge that the addict needs something more than the belief system that supported and justified their drinking—the thinking mind of the addict in the throes of craving will rationalize continuing to drink. The "Power greater than ourselves" jargon was based on AA's origins in the Oxford Group, a religious organization in New York that, in the 1930s, helped alcoholics get sober, including AA's co-founder, Bill Wilson.

Clinically speaking, "God" or "Higher Power" could be seen as a placeholder for "something other than my mind," which might be the collective wisdom of the support group itself, or a belief in the basic goodness of the universe, or any entity or concept the addict chooses to value. This concept squarely demonstrates that the alcoholic needs a belief in *something* beyond their ego to counter their addictive and disordered thinking, something outside of themselves that can support them through the ongoing challenges of recovery.

Many individuals recoil from this approach because of the frequent references in AA to "God." This is unfortunate. Those who recoil typically have failed to understand the critical last four words in the Third Step, "as we understand Him." The word "God" and "Him," with a capital H, may certainly be off-putting to some, but what they refer to is simply a power beyond the addict himself. In reality, we all "turn our will and our lives over to" powers other than ourselves. When we are sick or injured, we turn our will and lives over to the doctor. When our house is on fire, we turn our will and our lives over to the firefighters. In FRT, we have found the structure and tenets of 12-Step social support groups to be extremely effective.

At first, caught up in the throes of denial, the addicted/codependent family member fails to understand that their family "is on fire." Without seeking and following treatment recommendations, the dysfunction and pain will continue, and, ultimately, lives could be lost—and certainly, precious lives and relationships will fail to flourish.

From a bird's-eye view, AA's first three Steps are simple to understand. Those addicts and codependents who recover have simply acknowledged that there was a problem (Step One), realized there was a solution (Step Two), and turned for guidance to something greater and other than themselves (Step Three).

AA's first three Steps, as amended by author:

STEP ONE: We admitted we were powerless over (insert specific addiction or codependency)—that our lives had become unmanageable.
STEP TWO: Came to believe that a power greater than ourselves (greater than our ego/thinking mind) could restore us to sanity.
STEP THREE: Made a decision to turn our will and our lives over to the power that we have chosen.

Here is a partial list of those we naturally, at some point in our lives, "turn our will and life over to": doctor, police, boss or supervisor, dentist, hairdresser, 12-Step sponsor, fireman, therapist or psychologist, teacher, religion, self-help groups, parent or spouse, and, for some, God.

There are those who understand the addict's loss of control and those who do not. This is why the vast majority of addiction treatment providers are themselves in recovery from addiction or codependency, because they fully grasp this concept and its implications. It is essential that an FRT therapist both grasps the concept of loss of control and comprehends the role that social support groups play in helping an addict deal with that reality.

Does someone who wants to be an FRT therapist need to be a regular member of a social support or mutual aid group? No, certainly not. But they need to be intimately familiar with them, to understand how they function, and to appreciate their significance to the recovering addict (see Appendix C about AA working with professionals). And, in monitoring the overall progress of the recovering addict, the FRT therapist needs to check in with the addict regarding her participation and progress in the social support groups she attends. The FRT therapist acts in some ways as a cheerleader and needs to encourage the recovering addict to use the groups, and to embrace the concepts and tools and connections she gains by attending them (Timko & DeBenedetti, 2007).

For codependent family members, their own social support groups are an essential aid to their healing, recovery, and wellbeing. Codependency can leave family members overwhelmed, exhausted, and desperate. In Family Recovery Therapy, the initial goal is to help codependents shift their focus away from attempting to change the addict, and instead, to make their own lives and needs their main concern. Social support groups encourage and help the codependent regain a healthy, functional, and loving acceptance of themselves.

The FRT therapist needs to understand the nature of social support and mutual aid groups for codependents, just as they do for addicts, and to comprehend and convey the immense benefit to family members of regular participation in these groups. An FRT therapist can benefit from attending a few different social support meetings in order to better grasp the value, dynamics, and function of these groups.

There are two types of codependents who can benefit from social support groups. The first type consists of fundamentally healthy people whose loved one has become an addict. To have a loved one slide into addiction is traumatic—seeing her personality change, putting her life at risk, and even abusing the very family members who are concerned about her. Unfortunately, when codependents shift their focus away from themselves and their goals, and make the addict the central organizing point of their lives, they can suffer profound mental and physical consequences (Beattie, 1986; Lancer, 2017; Cermak, 1986). Their own self-care and priorities take a backseat to their addict's needs.

The second type of codependent who can benefit from support groups includes those who have had a childhood impacted by addiction and have a very skewed perspective of what healthy relationships look like. They often end up in dysfunctional relationships and frequently choose others from addicted or codependent families as partners. Currently, there may not be active addiction in their relationship or family, but they have absorbed thinking and behavior patterns characteristic of codependency and can suffer from low self-esteem, difficulty prioritizing themselves, strong proclivity to focus on others, and difficulty establishing healthy relationships.

For codependents of either type (and there are those who fit both categories) the benefit of these free social support groups cannot be overstated. It can be a relief for a codependent, just as it is for an addict, to walk into a room of peers and be greeted warmly by others whose experiences have been similar to theirs, and who can understand and empathize with their pain.

Codependents generally feel isolated, distraught, and desperate. They have spent months, probably years, or even decades, worrying about and trying to change their addicted loved one. This impossible task has been met with defeat after defeat, and they often feel like they are failures because they haven't been able to accomplish this unrealizable goal. Codependents can feel guilty and ashamed about having addiction in their lives, and about not being able to "fix" it. They can also feel distraught and despairing, because the addict they haven't been able to fix is still sick and harming himself, creating havoc for those around him, and on a trajectory towards premature death.

When codependents are welcomed by people from families such as their own, and hear stories that are similar to theirs, they feel relieved to learn they are not alone; they are not the only people dealing with the tragedy of addiction. They are among peers who have been where they've been and who can provide comfort, companionship, and connection—they can experience true empathy from others who are or who have been in their shoes. And, they learn that there is a way out. The families in these rooms are recovering peers, people who have made progress freeing themselves from the bondage of a life focused on addiction. Codependents hear how family members have changed themselves and created lives that have meaning, connection, and fun. They feel understood and cared about in ways even their well-meaning friends, who themselves have never struggled in the midst of addiction, could not (Al-Anon Family Groups, 2018).

By listening in meetings, codependents can learn very specific strategies others in situations like theirs have used. This can help guide them out of the morass of codependency. They learn, first and foremost, that they cannot control another person, they cannot change an addict, and it is not their fault—no one can change another person, and no one can fix an addict, no matter how much love, support, and money they pour into the process. Codependents learn that it is okay—actually, necessary—for them to take care of themselves and set boundaries to define what they will and won't tolerate from their addicted loved one. They learn that setting limits may actually help the addict, but that their goal is to protect and heal themselves, and to recover from the devastating consequences of addiction on their lives.

The most available social support group for codependents is Al-Anon, which was established in the 1950s by Lois Wilson, the wife of AA's co-founder, Bill Wilson. Al-Anon, as described by the Al-Anon Family Group Headquarters' *Detachment* brochure, is a "worldwide fellowship that offers a program of recovery for the families and friends of alcoholics, whether or not the alcoholic recognizes the existence of a drinking problem or seeks help" (Al-Anon Family Groups, n.d.-a).

The Al-Anon program was modeled after the AA program, and shares much of the same structure and many of the foundational principles of AA. Some of those who attend Al-Anon object to the concepts of "powerlessness" and a "Power greater than ourselves," but, just as for those attending AA, the core intention of these concepts is to acknowledge that codependents, by themselves, using the same thinking and behaviors they have been relying on unsuccessfully for years, cannot fundamentally change themselves. Codependents, just like addicts and alcoholics, need guidance, support, and a new way of thinking in order to recover. And, just as for recovering addicts, the "higher power" concept is not a religious tenet, but simply confirmation that they are seeking help beyond what they can do on their own.

There are few groups outside of Al-Anon that specifically provide support for the family members of alcoholics. While there are minimal statistics on the number of people who attend Al-Anon worldwide, surveys by the Al-Anon Family Group Headquarters show that members who have attended Al-Anon meetings report improved physical and mental health, better daily functioning, and fewer areas of trouble in their own lives (Al-Anon Family Groups, n.d.-b). Another option is Co-dependents Anonymous, which is a rapidly-growing 12 step program for those wanting to develop healthy relationships.

Through participation in social support groups, codependents learn a new perspective on themselves and their lives and receive guidance in creating more satisfactory and fulfilling lives. A community of peers is an invaluable milieu in which to witness, experiment, and experience new ways of acting and interacting (Ablon, 2018).

FRT Principle 6 states unequivocally that social support groups are vital to recovery. The 12-Step social support and mutual aid groups provide a crucial function in fostering recovery for both addicts and family members. It is essential that the FRT therapist understand the comprehensive role these groups play as a partner in the recovery process.

FRT Principle 7

The FRT therapist, who is a state-licensed medical or mental health professional, must be knowledgeable and experienced in many paths to growth and recovery. Ideally, the therapist is engaged in a personal recovery practice, whether 12-Step or other, in which capacity, the therapist stands shoulder-to-shoulder with the family members.

It is not necessary that FRT therapists themselves be in recovery from addiction or codependency, although many therapists drawn to working with addiction do have some personal experience in recovery. Therapists who are in recovery from addiction like working with addicts. They see themselves in addicts, they know how it feels to be an addict, and they remember the tremendous challenges they faced and overcame on their journey toward healing. They understand addiction from the inside out and know the pitfalls of denial, self-will, and control that addicts wrestle with. They are also aware that treating addicts is challenging: addicts lie, resist treatment, and don't show up for sessions. But therapists, whether or not in recovery from addiction, understand that some potential clients, when initially presented with our model, may simply go away. FRT therapists typically only work with those who seek help and willingly choose this comprehensive recovery path. Therapists understand that working with potential clients' resistance is part of the process.

Addiction includes a number of self-harming, chronic, out-of-control behaviors. A family therapist who is actively pursuing recovery from behavioral addictions, including addiction to food, sex, gambling, debting, gaming, Internet, or other, less well-known addictive activities, qualifies as "in recovery." "In recovery" does not necessarily mean "in 12-Step recovery," although experience in 12-Step programs can be a benefit, given the likelihood that clients will attend these programs because they are the most available social support groups. A therapist—or any person—who has never experienced the angst of a consuming, out-of-control, life-ravaging substance use or a compelling self-harming behavior may have difficulty understanding—and little inclination—to work in the realm of recovery. On the other hand, after reading the concepts outlined in this book, therapists with an interest in addiction but without such firsthand knowledge may be drawn to this work.

Codependency can itself be seen as an addiction. Therapists in recovery from codependency know intimately its subtle complexities. Codependency, unlike substance addiction, is not black and white. The addict has a powerful emotional attachment to alcohol, or substances, or to particular out-of-control behaviors. Recovering codependents have a compulsive emotional drive to focus on others and to try to fix the addict or other afflicted persons. Codependents in recovery know the lengths they have gone to—and continue to go to—to avoid becoming embroiled in obsessive thinking and compulsive behaviors, to avoid the minefields of dysfunctional family dynamics, and to keep their compass pointing towards "self-healing" and "self-recovery," rather than towards "other-fixing" and "other-changing."

There are many paths to personal recovery. While the 12-Step route is probably most well-known, many practices incorporate tenets similar to those of the 12 Steps. Therapists who have followed a personal growth practice generally live many 12-Step principles without having pursued 12-Step recovery. Such practices embrace concepts like differentiating what one can control from what one can't, and accepting reality. Often common to these practices is a belief that something greater than the self—be it one's therapist, the Al-Anon group, universal good, collective wisdom, or simply nature—guides the individual toward taking positive action. The majority of personal recovery practices embrace the values of honesty, integrity, self-responsibility, and compassion. However, because 12-Step programs are so prevalent in the recovery world, it is vital that non–12-Step-oriented individuals who wish to become FRT therapists attend a variety of AA and Al-Anon meetings in order to grasp the 12-Step culture.

FRT Principle 7 brings the concept of professional congruity into the FRT model; it requires the FRT therapist to have a commitment to their own growth and recovery. In standing shoulder-to-shoulder with recovering family members, the FRT therapist keeps a strong foothold in his or her own healing path while accompanying each family member on their personal recovery journey. As an individual dedicated to personal growth, the FRT therapist shares and embodies the philosophy and perspective of other recovering individuals. In this way, the FRT therapist is both an example and a partner to family members in recovery. This helps instill confidence in the family members that their therapist has integrity and solid knowledge of addiction and codependency and can have compassion for the plight of addicts and codependents, as well as reliable knowledge and actual experience of an effective path towards wellness. It is meaningful and reassuring to family members that their FRT therapist not only "talks the talk" but "walks the walk" of recovery.

FRT Principle 8
Since addiction and the codependency that enables it are chronic conditions, it is recommended that the addict and codependents develop ongoing support beyond the first year of continuous sobriety.

Recovery is an ongoing process. It requires significant change to shift from an addictive way of life to a healthy, individuated way of life. It happens "one day at a time," for an extended period, and it's progressive. Just as continuing practice is required to learn and maintain fluency in a foreign language or mastery in playing a musical instrument, the language of recovery requires repetition and reinforcement. Addiction, as we know, is a chronic, relapsing, medical disorder that requires lifelong maintenance. There is no "fix," no silver bullet that reverses the problem and makes it go away, just like there is no "fix" that allows someone to stay skilled in playing a violin without the work to sustain what they've learned. The good news is that, with continual practice, sustained recovery, similar to the violinist's ability, naturally unfolds.

Once again, I applaud many different ways to get and stay sober. I do not claim that the model presented in this book is "the only way." However, I have used this approach with many families, and found it highly successful.

Recovery from codependency is also a process. It takes time, and has its own language that requires repetition and reinforcement. When you've maintained a focus on others for a long time, it's easy to slip back into minimizing your own needs, putting someone else first, helping out in a situation where your help has not been requested, or taking on tasks that aren't in your purview but that you can see clearly need to be handled. Furthermore, codependency is almost always embedded in unconscious thinking and behavior that may go back several generations (Noriega, 2004). This means that, even for the rigorously vigilant, old patterns may creep into their repertoire. Love and fear have fused patterns of behavior in place. Excavating old beliefs, and dismantling the complex behavior patterns built on their foundation, demands courage, patience, and support.

I believe, in the majority of cases, there is never a time that addicts or codependents "finish recovery," or are "fully recovered." Sustained replacement of innate tendencies, chronic behaviors, and long-standing beliefs demands ongoing practice of new ways of thinking and acting. Genetic proclivity toward addiction is well-established; in codependency, generations of family patterns and low levels of differentiation tug codependents to return to previous ways. And dynamics among all family members, addict included, are susceptible to regressing to long-standing, multi-generational, deeply embedded, homeostatic patterns.

The first year of recovery provides a solid beginning, but it is not the end of the road (Dennis & Scott, 2007). The years that follow strengthen that foundation. Recommendations for an addict beyond the first year of recovery may include attending and being active in social support groups, living with sober people, drug-testing, psychotherapy, and engaging in spiritual practices. For codependents, attending and actively participating in their own social support groups is always advocated, and continued therapy for individuals or the family may be beneficial. In social support groups, for both addicts and codependents, there are "old-timers" who have attended meetings for 20 or 30 or more years. Participants in these groups categorically state that they attribute their fulfilling lives, satisfying relationships, and good health to regularly attending groups. If addicts and codependents seek support and practice new behaviors, their foundation grows stronger. But, despite their best efforts, someone in recovery may be just one calamity away from falling back into their past ways of handling crises. Sticking to a practice of attending meetings and helping others can avert just such a slip (McCrady et al., 2004), or "codependent relapse." In these groups, too, are heard the voices of those who say they thought things were going fine, so they stopped attending group meetings, and then they relapsed, slipped back into old patterns and found themselves in their old misery. They add that when they started participating in groups again, their lives got better.

Family members have often spent years—if not decades, even generations—adapting to addiction, and the resulting dysfunctional behaviors and relationship patterns may be deeply entrenched. It is vital that family members understand that, to optimize their recovery path, they need to continue the work of healing and growth beyond the critical first year of treatment.

FRT Principle 8 names the fact that living in recovery requires active attention in order to maintain and enjoy a healthy life. FRT creates a structure that supports the addict and the family in pursuing ongoing recovery.

FRT Principle 9
Treatment includes monitoring for co-occurring mental and physical health problems and providing appropriate referrals as needed.

Addiction goes by many names—alcoholism, drug addiction, substance abuse, chemical dependency, substance dependency, and substance use disorders. These terms are all subsumed under the heading, "Substance-Related and Addictive Disorders," in the American Psychiatric Association's *Diagnostic and Statistical Manual of Mental Disorders Fifth Edition* (*DSM-5*) (2013), or *DSM-5*, which is the reference book mental health practitioners use when diagnosing psychological disorders. The *DSM-5* lists many substances in its description of Substance-Related Disorders, among them alcohol, cocaine, tobacco, hallucinogens, and stimulants, and also includes gambling in the same chapter in a section entitled, "Non-Substance-Related

Disorders" (*DSM-5*, pp. 585–589). It should be noted, however, that the *DSM-5* excludes from its description of Substance-Related Disorders constellations of repetitive behaviors, sometimes referred to as behavioral addictions, such as Internet gaming, exercise addiction or shopping addiction (*DSM-5*, p. 481). Addiction, or a substance use disorder, is a mental (as well as a medical) disorder, but it is common for an addict to suffer from other, co-occurring mental health problems that will also need to be a focus of treatment (Substance Abuse and Mental Health Services Administration, 2020).

Addicts and codependents often suffer from complex issues. Many addicts and codependents experienced long periods of neglect and abuse during childhood, and these damaging dynamics likely impeded their development and continue to affect them in their adult years (Dube et al., 2003). Some issues are long-standing but have not been treated, or still require additional treatment. FRT therapists assess for co-occurring issues, then treat or make referrals to specialists who can provide appropriate care. However, it is not unusual for the newly recovering person to present various mood, anxiety, eating, sleeping, and sexual symptoms, all substance-induced, that will resolve themselves once the individual is substance-free and stable. Nonetheless, when there is a possibility of underlying or coexisting mental disorders, it is important that these be addressed, and the person get treated or referred for appropriate treatment.

It is not uncommon for an addict who enters treatment to be taking psychotropic medicine that had been prescribed to treat the symptoms of addiction. Once the individual is on a solid recovery path, it becomes apparent that the medicine is no longer needed, because the symptoms it treated were caused by active addiction and are no longer present. Stopping medication should be done in consultation with the FRT therapist and the prescribing physician.

When there are questions about the source of symptoms, or it's unclear whether a co-occurring medical or psychiatric condition exists, it is appropriate to refer the individual to an addiction doctor or addiction psychiatrist for assessment (McCauley, 2007) (see Appendix D). An addictions-trained psychiatrist can help sort out which symptoms may resolve on their own in the process of recovery, and which may require ongoing attention, although it may take time for addiction-related symptoms to clear up sufficiently for the psychiatrist to make a thorough diagnosis. Certainly, someone whose addiction had pediatric onset, or who grew up in an unstable home, was traumatized, or had a long course of active addiction, may well benefit from ongoing psychiatric help. Whenever possible, the FRT therapist is well served by developing collegial relationships with addiction-trained psychiatrists and physicians to whom he can make referrals when there are psychiatric or medical problems that need to be addressed.

The FRT Principle 9 speaks to the fact that co-occurring issues often present with addiction. The FRT model recognizes this; the FRT therapist makes referrals as needed, so there is a comprehensive continuum of care.

FRT Principle 10
Medically Assisted Treatment may be necessary, if medication is used in the service of recovery and not as a substitute for recovery.

The Medically Assisted Treatment (M.A.T.) approach is proving to be invaluable in addressing many aspects of addiction treatment, and plays a key role in the treatment both of addiction itself and of the many co-occurring physical and mental health problems caused by addiction. But the M.A.T. approach, by itself, has not had much success in putting the majority of addicts into long-term remission, and certainly does not address the often multi-year, multi-faceted rehabilitation that is required for sustained recovery (Galanter, 2018). It is not uncommon for an addict to be severely impaired emotionally, psychologically, and physically. An addict taking a pill—without robust social support—will not get "a fix" for the multiple issues at play in addiction. M.A.T. doctors must fully understand addicts' complex needs in order to coordinate their services with those of other professionals and entities that contribute to sustained recovery.

According to the Substance Abuse and Mental Health Services Administration (2021), "as with all medications used in M.A.T, buprenorphine should be prescribed as part of a comprehensive treatment plan that includes counseling and other behavioral therapies to provide patients with a whole-person approach." Within these guidelines, using buprenorphine in combination with the integrated treatment approach of Family Recovery Therapy could be valuable, but its use needs to be incorporated into the context of the overall treatment plan, with clear communication and collaboration between the FRT therapist and the prescribing physician. Certain medications may be helpful in the early stages of addiction treatment, but it is vital for the prescribing physician to understand and support the FRT treatment plan and process.

FRT Principle 10 states that M.A.T. is helpful and even necessary, in some instances. Just as each family is unique, so too is the FRT treatment plan, which is specifically tailored for each family system. It is this individualized and highly integrated approach that allows the FRT therapist to comprehensively and effectively guide the recovery of an addict and their family.

FRT Principle 11
Regular drug testing is a powerful tool and will be used in addiction treatment.

A sober addict is a miracle. Biologically, addicts' midbrains are just one fix away from instant pleasure or relief of pain—addicts are wired to use substances, despite pleas from their "rational" prefrontal cortex (their executive function brain) to heed their best intentions, fervent hope, and promises to the contrary. In 1979, when I was in my first year of recovery, my recovery guide told me the following: "Larry, there is an 800-pound gorilla inside your head, doing push-ups every day, whose only job is to get alcohol into your mouth!" More recent brain science has backed this up. Craving is real; it never completely disappears. Our brain never forgets the euphoric experiences of getting high or the instant removal of pain.

An addict is vulnerable to relapse, particularly in the initial year of sobriety. Drug testing effectively discourages an addict from using, and can quickly detect a relapse, if one occurs (Kilmer et al., 2013).

I am aware of many instances where illicit drug use has gone undetected in residential treatment programs or sober living homes because of lax drug-testing procedures. Nothing upsets a sober living house or residential treatment program more than the drama of substance use by some residents. It is foolish not to regularly drug test this population. Addicts need help and support to recover, and drug testing supports sobriety. During the first days and weeks of sobriety, I recommend performing urine tests every two to four days (addicts know how to fake urine tests), random saliva tests, and, when alcohol has been an issue, a regular Breathalyzer™ test. The frequency of testing may be decreased over time as a client demonstrates investment in recovery. A wily addict knows the retention rate for every drug he uses, and may employ that information to plan his drug use, if he thinks the substance will be out of his system before the next test.

FRT Principle 11 makes no bones about the fact that drug testing is required if real recovery is the goal of treatment for the addict. Addicts will go to amazing lengths to get high and avoid detection of drug use. They have been known to catheterize themselves or inject urine into their bladder. Such drastic measures are propelled by a biological imperative, driven by a hijacked brain, not simply willful actions by a resistant client. An addict who lacks strong, consistent support not to use can easily revert to drug-using behavior. Regular drug testing is one of our best tools to help the addict, day to day, as they detox and stabilize (Jarvis et al., 2017).

FRT Principle 12
All members of the family seeking treatment must be fully informed of, and understand, the therapeutic goals, as well as understand and agree to the treatment plan, which includes specific recommendations for different stages of treatment.

The FRT therapist is intimately familiar with the treatment protocol and the trajectory of recovery. The therapist needs to hold in mind the whole picture and the larger narrative, while simultaneously gently guiding the family to take the next right action. As therapists, we need to impart to the family members every step of the way that we are very clear about what needs to happen, and in what order, both in the next moments and in the overall scheme of treatment—we need to instill confidence in them that we've "got this." We need to reassure them that we know how this will work—that we see the path and its many forks, and that at each juncture we will confidently choose the best direction for them as well as clarify the reasons for our suggestions (Dekkers et al., 2020). Denial and resistance on the part of the addict and the codependents can pull them to choose what AA members call "an easier, softer way." Denial is a strong force, and an authoritative and directive FRT therapist needs to be sure and steady in steering the family forward, as well as clear and confident in explaining the rationale for treatment recommendations (Brown & Lewis, 1999).

For example, codependents may balk at the idea of attending social support groups and assert that "the addict has the problem." The skillful FRT therapist not only reminds them that the family system is the client, and that attending social support groups is a condition of treatment, but that the groups offer family members support and relief at a time when they are experiencing significant stress—a social support group is a place where there are other individuals who have weathered similar stressors and are available to share their experiences. The FRT therapist assures the codependents that they will hear stories they can relate to, and they will come to realize that they are not the only ones who've had to deal with the craziness of addiction. At each stage of treatment, the FRT therapist needs to convey, plainly and confidently, the value and purpose of every treatment recommendation so that family members understand the importance of following the guidance provided. By laying out the path clearly to the whole family, the FRT therapist creates a "new normal" where transparency, respect, and clarity are the norms. In this way, the therapist establishes a foundation of trust with the family members.

Those who do this work know that great breakthroughs can occur in recovery. They have witnessed many examples of these in the various social support groups. It is important that we embody and hold the hope of recovery, and that we transmit this to our clients. FRT Principle 12 ensures that they are clear about and make an informed choice to participate in this process.

FRT Principle 13
Optimal recovery is achieved when family members commit to all aspects of the treatment program.

Treatment is challenging for those recovering from addiction and codependency. The addict is asked to stop enacting addictive behavior, to cease trying to "control" (i.e., "reduce" or "limit") substance use or self-harming behavior, to surrender and give up a known lifestyle, and to adopt ways of thinking and acting that are totally foreign to them. Codependents are asked to shift their perspective 180 degrees, from "the other" to "the self," to embrace the concept of hitting bottom, and to surrender their life view and conviction that they must fix, rescue, and control the person in crisis: the addict. Again, as Stephanie Brown explained, "It is the collapse of the family structures and defense mechanisms that protected and maintained the drinking that clears the ground for the transformative process of recovery" (Brown & Lewis, 1999, p. 19).

These are big changes for every family member to embrace. And it is no wonder that some family members balk at embarking on change of this magnitude, and resist the FRT therapist's treatment recommendations.

The job of the FRT therapist does not include changing other people. It does not entail trying to convince someone who is opposed to these principles to buy into the plan. A basic premise of recovery is that you cannot change another person—only the addict can change himself or herself, and the only person the codependent can alter is him or herself.

If a family member refuses to go along with treatment recommendations, but still wants to be a part of the treatment process, the FRT therapist turns the focus to the resistant individual to explore his or her resistance, answer his questions, and clarify anything he might not understand about the treatment process. However, within a reasonable time, the individual must either agree to the treatment protocol, or not be a part of it. Otherwise, treatment will encounter one obstacle after another. The not-committed-to-treatment family member will attempt to derail the recovery process, and the consulting room is likely to feel more like a lawyer's office than a therapist's office. This dynamic undermines the work of the family members who are committed to following through with treatment—any ambivalence or reservations they have may be reinforced by the uncommitted individual.

Instead, if a family member is unwilling to commit to the treatment plan, she needs to not be a part of the treatment process. Then the other family members can stay on track with the work they need to do. The family members who are committed to treatment will become stronger and clearer in their boundaries and more able to stay on their own recovery path, in and out of the therapist's office, without a dissenting voice in the mix.

The dissenting individual is not a bad person because he refuses to go along with the plan. He simply is not ready to adopt the treatment path outlined by the FRT therapist, and therefore is disqualified from participating in treatment at the present time. The person who initially refuses to commit to treatment may change his mind at a later point, but he will still be invited to participate in treatment only if he is willing to commit to all aspects of the treatment plan.

The FRT Principle 13 makes clear that sustainable recovery can be optimized when everyone involved is on board with the treatment plan outlined by the FRT therapist—the team leader. I have seen this work, and work well, in family systems treatment.

FRT Principle 14
Typically, a member of the enabling subsystem contacts the treatment provider. It is vital that the provider begin to engage the caller in the Family Recovery Therapy treatment model during this first contact.

It is noteworthy that there are no references available to support FRT Principle 14. The Family Recovery Therapy model differs from other addiction treatment modalities in prescribing a new and different paradigm, one that to my knowledge has not yet been the subject of scientific research. I propose this model based on my experience and work in the field, and this is the first clinical publication that describes it in detail. Crucial to this model is the thesis that the client in treatment is the *family system*, and, furthermore, that addiction treatment typically *starts* with someone other than the addict, as stated in FRT Principle 14. The approach of beginning treatment with the enablers does not appear in the Surgeon General's report cited above precisely because it is a radical departure from the treatment paradigm that is currently in use.

A codependent is often the first person in the family to seek help and is the person most likely to call a treatment provider. Optimally, that first call is to an FRT therapist who begins to join with the caller, who is probably an integral player in the system, and to introduce the concept of a systemic treatment model.

If we fail to engage the codependent enablers in treatment, we cannot apply the FRT model. The codependent is typically unaware of the role they play in sustaining the homeostasis of the addicted family system. The codependent enablers often view the addict as the only family member with a problem and generally cannot see the extent of their contribution to the addict's addictive behavior.

I have been using this approach successfully for many years. When I meet with the codependent enablers, and educate them about Family Recovery Therapy, I have found that they are very open to the idea of "helping" me treat the addict. They are willing to come to individual and family therapy, and to attend social support and mutual aid groups, all in service of treating the addict. Over time, they come to understand that addiction has impacted them as well as the addict, and they learn they can benefit from getting help, not only for the addict's sake, but also for themselves and their family.

This FRT approach is in stark contrast to the current addiction treatment paradigm which focuses on the addict and gives scant attention to the long-term, entrenched, and pervasive enabling system that surrounds the addict. The "addict-centered" approach colludes with the codependent caller's view that the addict is the Identified Patient (IP). Treatment of the addict using the currently common approach further solidifies the codependents' perspective that "the addict is the problem," and does not alert the addict's family members to their role in sustaining the problem or to the reality that the "addictive/codependent system" is at issue.

This is why it is critical to engage the codependent from day one. If the codependents observe that interventionists, doctors, and treatment programs focus only on the addict's treatment, they may continue to be unaware of their role in the addictive system and not understand that they, too, may require help.

Social support and mutual aid groups are an integral component of long-standing, highly regarded Residential Treatment Centers (RTCs) for addicts. It is not unusual for an addict in residential treatment to attend a group meeting in the local community each evening. And, it is virtually always the case that RTCs invite the codependents to some sort of one- to four-day "Family Program," at which family members may be introduced to the idea of getting support for themselves. However, in my 25 years of working with dozens of RTCs, I have never heard of *any* program that includes in its curriculum the recommendation that codependents go to a social support or mutual aid group *while attending* the family program.

The difference between the dominant paradigm and the FRT treatment model is obvious. One approach treats the individual; the other treats the family system.

In the FRT model, if the addict attends a 30-, 60-, or 90-day residential program, the codependents, during the same period, attend 30, 60, or 90 days of social support or mutual aid groups at home, and also participate in 30, 60, or 90 days of weekly therapy with the FRT therapist. In addition, during this time, the family takes part in weekly phone therapy sessions that include both the addict's counselor and the FRT therapist, and in some instances may also include the addict. The codependents, just like the addict, will get help to fundamentally change their lives and make up for their own years of lost development.

Let's again compare the "coming home" experience of an addict who is receiving treatment within the current addiction treatment paradigm (A.) to that of an addict who is receiving treatment that is based on the FRT model (B.).

A. Addict coming home when treatment follows the current addiction treatment paradigm:

- The enabling codependents are not in recovery, are not doing any daily work to change the unconscious dynamics that support the prior homeostasis; the homeostasis that existed in the home during active addiction persists.
- The family focus will be on the addict changing, while at the same time, the addict will be returning to the family dynamics, conscious and unconscious, that supported his substance-using lifestyle in the past and that promote the household's continuation of "the way things used to be."
- Whatever aftercare recommendations the residential center has suggested for the addict may not be supported by the family and may even be discouraged as disruptive to the prior homeostasis.

B. Addict coming home when treatment follows the Family Recovery Therapy model:

- Addict has been informed about, and in some cases, participated in weekly family therapy on the phone with the FRT therapist and the treatment center counselor. Addict knows that each family member is in a process of change and is taking responsibility for themselves and their own recovery.
- Addict and the family are aware of and supportive of the addict's ongoing treatment plan and recovery protocol at home.
- Addict knows that his family members have been attending their own social support and mutual aid groups while he has been in treatment, and both the addict and family members will continue attending these groups.

- Addict understands that the enabling codependents will no longer enable him.
- Addict knows that the former homeostasis of the home is changing and will be replaced with the dynamics of a "family in recovery."

When treatment follows the dominant paradigm, the odds are much lower that the addict will maintain sobriety, or create a recovery-focused life, than when the family is engaged in the FRT model. It is the FRT model that supports changing the system, the very substrate which nurtured the addiction. And it is the FRT model that fosters growth of a true recovery environment in which both the addict and the codependent family members can grow and flourish. This is why I have seen a nearly 100 percent success rate, when all family members adhere to the FRT treatment recommendations.

Periodically, it is the addict who makes the initial call to my office. I have come to see that this call could be a trap, and may undermine the possibility of engaging the whole family in my model. The addict may have been pressured by the codependent "to call someone." Typically, when I have met with this caller, I have seen them only once. I suspect they have gone back to the codependent and reported, "I saw the addiction therapist, and he said I'm fine."

In these situations, over the years, I have learned to ask the caller the following questions: "Who else is concerned?" And, "Are they available to talk with me?" The concerned family member will almost always agree to talk to me by phone, and then to come in for an individual session as well. I then ask to see the two of them together. It is in this session that we have an opportunity to see the whole picture and also I have the chance to make some recommendations which could lead to beginning FRT treatment.

FRT Principle 14 shifts the paradigm to a new, systems-based way of treating addiction. Engaging the codependent is key to the success of the FRT model.

Chapter 3

What Is Addiction?

It is helpful to view addiction through a few lenses. This chapter contains several different perspectives. Section One contains a detailed discussion of scientific advances in our understanding of addiction (and substance abuse, generally), an overview of the bio-psycho-social-spiritual damage an addict suffers, and a description of the extensive impact of addiction on the family.

Section Two contains four foundational definitions of addiction. The first of these definitions is based on the chapter, "Substance-Related and Addictive Disorders," in the American Psychiatric Association's *Diagnostic and Statistical Manual of Mental Disorders Fifth Edition* (*DSM-5*) (2013). The *DSM-5* is considered the principal authoritative source for psychiatric diagnoses and is the culmination of many years' work by a number of psychiatrists and other mental health professionals. The description included here is a very brief summary of the *DSM-5* text.

The last three definitions of addiction in Section Two were written by addiction-trained medical doctors and published by the American Society of Addiction Medicine (ASAM). The first of these is the most recent ASAM definition (2019). It is concise, and replaced ASAM's previous two definitions (one short, one long) published in 2011. ASAM determined that a revised definition was warranted in 2019, based on changes since 2011 both in the public's acceptance of addiction as a brain disease and in what addiction specialists had learned about addiction prevention, treatment, remission, and recovery. The 2019 definition is followed by ASAM's former, 2011 descriptions: the Short and Long Definitions of Addiction. These latter two are included here, in part for historical reasons, but also because they provide substantial detail about the nuances and complexities of addiction.

Part One: What Is Addiction? A Clinical Overview

Addiction is a serious and potentially life-threatening disease. It is a disease of faulty brain chemistry and structure. Understanding the science of addiction is helpful in grasping its complex nature.

Addiction has been sorely misunderstood for millennia. But since the 1990s, thanks to modern neuroimaging tools and the work of skilled research scientists, we know the following: for the addict, ingesting certain substances and/or engaging in particular behaviors trigger the reward center in the midbrain to release a surge of the neurotransmitter dopamine, which overrides the biochemical pathways governing the rational, thinking part of the brain—the prefrontal cortex and its executive function. The reward center sends out signals, telling the addict to ingest more of the substance or repeat behaviors to acquire the substance and "get high." Any rational decisions the addict may make related to his substance use or behaviors are quickly overpowered by his midbrain's messages; the addict is no longer "in control," because the rational, decision-making part of his brain is no longer governing his choices.

This concept is difficult for a non-addict or an addict in denial to comprehend. The following example may help. As teenagers, my friend and I would see if we could hold our breath for three minutes. Our rational, thinking minds decided to stop breathing, but at some point, an instinctive, survival-driven part of our brains took charge, basically saying, "I'm not interested in what you want, I am going to start breathing again." It is like that for addicts. We can decide not to drink, and our midbrain says, "Whatever, I'm going to have a drink." This is devastating to the ego and to our rational, thinking self, and the addict's only recourse is to use the most primitive defense mechanisms: denial and rationalization. Addicts deny reality and slip from the bonds of sanity, much to the chagrin of those who care about them.

While we typically think of addiction as applying to drugs and alcohol, its scope is much larger. Many non-drug-related behaviors can also trigger the brain's reward system to create an unquenchable craving for more—more food, more spending, more gambling, more video gaming, more social media, more work. The prefrontal cortex, which normally sets reasonable limits on how much of something is enough, gets hijacked by the dopamine-based, "I've got to get more" part of the brain.

It is not clear why some people are susceptible to addiction and others are not; or why some people are susceptible to some *kinds* of addiction but not to other kinds. Physician and author Dr. Gabor Maté, in his book *In the Realm of Hungry Ghosts: Close Encounters with Addiction* (2010), offers a compelling argument that the cause of addiction for many people is rooted in an emotionally barren early childhood. Maté reminds us that humans need to be loved, nurtured, and protected in the first months and years of life. But when this intimate, calm, and consistent attention from early caregivers is lacking, the nervous system fails to develop normally. Individuals who have not received sufficient early nurturing or who have experienced abuse are unusually vulnerable to stress. When these individuals mature, they lack sufficient internal resources and security to "self soothe" when stressed. They have difficulty regulating their emotions when upset, irritable, or restless. Many of these individuals may actually have a deficit of dopamine, the brain neurotransmitter that is largely responsible for feelings of calmness and pleasure, and will seek ways to artificially increase their dopamine levels. They turn to substances (like alcohol, nicotine, heroin) and behaviors (like computer gaming, overeating, compulsive spending, compulsive sex, watching endless TV) to numb themselves and feel less pain.

While an emotionally impoverished, or worse, abusive, childhood may play a part in the genesis of addiction, it's not the whole story. The idea that addiction (or at least alcoholism, the addiction which was first subjected to scrutiny) has a biological basis was conjectured in the 1930s by Dr. William Silkworth, director of a large hospital in New York City. In his career as a physician, Dr. Silkworth had treated numerous alcoholics, many of whom had suffered repeated relapses, and he developed a theory about the nature of alcoholism. In the book *Alcoholics Anonymous*, which was first published in 1939, Dr. Silkworth described alcoholism as the manifestation of an allergy. He understood that alcohol was a substance that alcoholics could not metabolize normally. According to Silkworth, alcoholics who repeatedly relapsed were subject to the phenomenon of craving, and could not drink without experiencing the unstoppable desire for more. Silkworth's description—without benefit of neuroimaging and modern scientific research—was a prescient explanation of how the addiction cycle works. These are the words of Dr. Silkworth:

> Men and women drink essentially because they like the effect produced by alcohol. The sensation is so elusive that, while they admit it is injurious, they cannot after a time differentiate the true from the false. To them, their alcoholic life seems the only normal one. They are restless, irritable, and discontented, unless they can again experience the sense of ease and comfort which comes at once by taking a few drinks—drinks which they see others taking with impunity. After they have succumbed to the desire again, as so many do, and the phenomenon of craving develops, they pass through the well-known stages of a spree, emerging remorseful, with a firm resolution not to drink again. This is repeated over and over, and unless the person can experience an entire psychic change there is very little hope of his recovery.
>
> On the other hand—and strange as this may seem to those who do not understand—once a psychic change has occurred, the very same person who seemed doomed, who had so many problems he despaired of ever solving them, suddenly finds himself easily able to control his desire for alcohol, the only effort necessary being that required to follow a few simple rules [Alcoholics Anonymous 2001, "The Doctor's Opinion" pp. xxviii–xxix].

I think Dr. Silkworth would agree that the most important recovery rule for the alcoholic is to get together with other sober alcoholics and to get the support to not drink that day—and the next day, and the next, one day at a time.

Research on alcoholism over the past 70 years has furthered our understanding of the biological factors contributing to alcoholism. The first twin studies, conducted in Sweden in the 1950s, found significantly higher rates of alcoholism among twins, and higher rates among identical twins than fraternal twins, suggesting there is a genetic basis to alcoholism (Kaij & Rosenthal, 1961). More recent studies in the U.S. found that adopted boys whose biological families had alcohol problems were more likely to become alcoholics than boys adopted from families without alcohol abuse in their families of origin (Cadoret et al., 1980; Cadoret et al., 1987; Cadoret, 1994).

During the 1990s, psychiatrist and addiction specialist Marc Schuckit and his colleagues published studies showing that male offspring of an alcoholic male are four times more likely to develop the disease than are male offspring of non-alcoholic fathers. In an interview with Bill Moyers on addiction, Schuckit also said that it is unlikely that the propensity toward alcoholism depends on a single gene, but that it involves several genes—some that mediate impulsivity and risk-taking behavior, and others that relate directly to metabolism of the drug (Moyers, 1998). Clearly, there are biological differences between the addict and the non-addict.

As mentioned earlier, brain scans have provided scientists with visual evidence of the parts of the brain that are affected in alcoholism, as well as in other addictions that have been studied (including cocaine and methamphetamine). From studying the location and function of neurotransmitters in the brain, neurophysiologists have been able to map how addiction works in the nervous system. These studies clearly show that the brain of an individual in the throes of addiction operates differently than the brain of a non-addict. Unfortunately, we don't know how an addict brain looks *before* developing addiction, but we do know that as addiction progresses, it changes the brain (figures 3.1–3.3 on next page).

Whether the culprit is genetics, other biological abnormalities, childhood experiences, and/or an individual's particular psychological makeup (which is impacted by biological and social factors), we have a clearer scientific understanding today than we did fifty years ago about what addiction is and how addiction works. The most recent definition of addiction formulated by the American Society of Addiction Medicine (2019) is a useful reference:

> Addiction is a treatable, chronic medical disease involving complex interactions among brain circuits, genetics, the environment, and an individual's life experiences. People with addiction use substances or engage in behaviors that become compulsive and often continue despite harmful consequences.
>
> Prevention efforts and treatment approaches for addiction are generally as successful as those for other chronic diseases.

Addiction treatment professionals use a shorthand version of the ASAM's definition and describe the criteria for addiction in terms of "the four Cs":

> *Craving.* The addict has an urgent, unquenchable desire to self-medicate with a substance or behavior.
>
> *Control (Loss of).* The addict continues to use the substance or engage in the behavior, even after fervently deciding not to.
>
> *Continuing* despite adverse consequences. The addict continues the behaviors, even though bad things happen as a consequence.
>
> *Chronicity.* The behaviors persist, and, even if stopped for a while, they recur.

Or, as renowned spiritual teacher and author Eckhart Tolle says in characterizing addiction, "...you no longer feel that you have the power to stop. It seems stronger than you. It also gives you a false sense of pleasure, pleasure that invariably turns into pain" (Tolle, 1999, p.18).

Tolle's words are apt. They speak to a central characteristic of addiction: lack of control. An addict, though he thinks he is in control, is not. When someone is

Chapter 3. What Is Addiction?

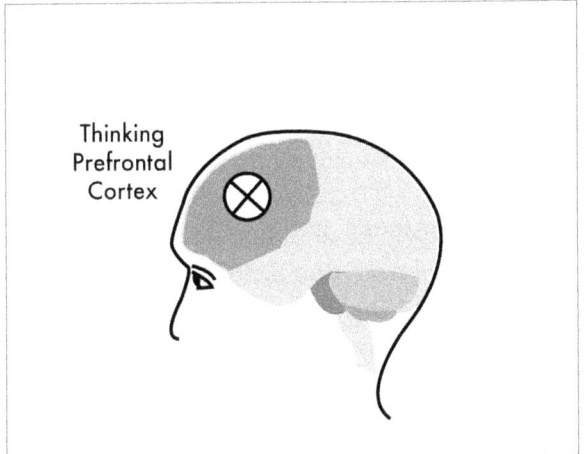

◀ Figure 3.1 *The Normal Human Brain.* The thinking prefrontal cortex is intact and the executive part of the brain reasons well and makes sound decisions.

▶ Figure 3.2 *The Addicted Human Brain.* Craving originates in the midbrain, which overrides the rational prefrontal cortex, leading to impulsive decisions and loss of control over substance use.

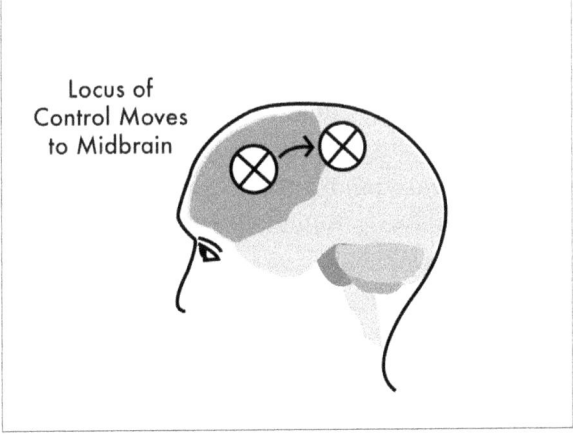

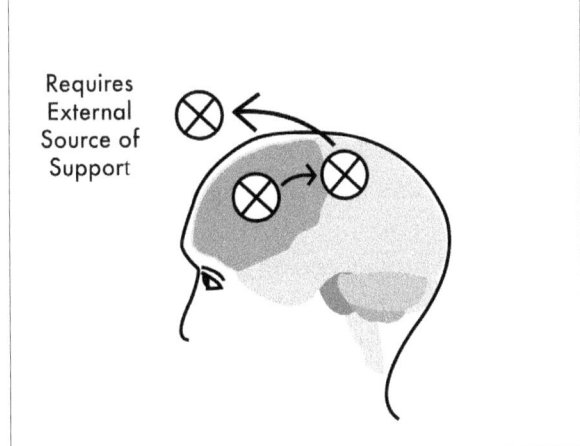

◀ Figure 3.3 *The Addict's Prefrontal Cortex and External Support.* The addict's prefrontal cortex—the rational, thinking brain—has been hijacked by the midbrain, and the addict requires external support to refrain from substance use.

exercising "control," it means the part of the brain that thinks and makes decisions is in charge. For an addict, that decision-making part is at the mercy of the brain's reward center. The thinking, rational part of the addict's brain is not in control. The addict, in fact, is in denial—denying that he is out of control, denying that he can't stop, even denying that there is a problem, despite what may be massive evidence to the contrary.

Tolle's words also acknowledge another problem in addiction—that the "pleasure" derived from the substance or behavior is elusive. The addict's pleasure system is defective. An addict often is not so much seeking pleasure as pursuing *relief from pain*. However, using the drug leads to more pain. While the drug temporarily assuages pain, it provokes craving for more of the drug to relieve more pain, and a vicious cycle ensues.

Addictionologists understand that addiction is a chronic medical disorder, not unlike diabetes, hypertension, and asthma—it is a disease of an organ, the brain. And because addiction is chronic, it requires life-long management. There are certainly many substance users and substance abusers who do not meet the criteria for addiction, and there are many substance abusers who *appear* to meet the criteria for severe abuse or addiction, but who at a later point in their lives are able to return to social drinking without reverting to patterns of substance abuse. These scenarios raise a question for the treatment professional: what treatment best serves the substance-abusing individual and his or her family?

Degrees of abuse can be murky to define, and the subject of what constitutes addiction, and hence what constitutes effective treatment, is controversial. Where is the line between substance abuse and substance addiction, or the delineation between mild, moderate, and severe abuse? The *Diagnostic and Statistical Manual of Mental Disorders, Fourth Edition* (*DSM-4*) (American Psychiatric Association), published in 1994, considered two general categories of problematic substance use, abuse, and dependence, with dependence being equivalent to addiction and requiring addiction treatment. The *DSM-5* (American Psychiatric Association, 2013) determines severity of addiction with more specificity according to the number of criteria met, and describes substance use disorder on a continuum from mild to severe. The eleven *DSM-5* criteria for substance use disorder are grouped into four categories: impaired control, social impairment, risky use, and pharmacological indicators (withdrawal and tolerance).

In viewing substance abuse, some treatment providers refer to the "Desistance Theory" of recovery. This term is borrowed from criminal justice terminology and refers to the capacity of a criminal to stop engaging in criminal behavior. When applied to substance abuse, desistance theory holds that there are addicts who, at some point, can desist from addictive behavior. In contrast to the belief, "once an addict, always an addict," this theory holds that some alcoholics can, in fact, recover and become social drinkers. This doubtless is true for some substance-abusing individuals, but I think these individuals are probably not true addicts, but rather are serious substance abusers who were not genetically, innately, temperamentally, or in some other way predisposed to developing addiction. In my experience, the vast majority of clients are best served by using the disease model not only to achieve remission, but to stabilize their lives, restore growth, and resume normal development. Serious substance abuse can significantly damage health, relationships, work, finances, and other vital aspects of life. Those in recovery from debilitating substance use, whether or not their substance-related behavior can be clinically classified as addiction, can benefit from a recovery model that supports positive change and growth in all these areas. Perhaps a few non-addicts are "caught in the net of addiction treatment" and later, after sobriety, stabilization, and addressing other problems, are able to use substances without ill effect. This does not disprove the disease model, which is based on the chronicity of addiction, but highlights the complexity of diagnosing and treating addiction.

Problematic substance abusers, who can look like addicts in their initial presentation, may respond favorably to a range of treatment approaches that collectively fall under the heading, "Harm Reduction." Harm reduction models can include psychodynamic, cognitive, motivational, and behavioral therapy, and are effective for some substance users who have not crossed the line to addiction. Stopping all substance use may not even be required for these individuals to refrain from abusing substances.

Dr. Lance Dodes, in his book, *The Heart of Addiction: A New Approach to Understanding and Managing Alcoholism and Other Addictive Behaviors* (2002), writes about treating substance abuse from a psychodynamic perspective, viewing unconscious drives as the source of maladaptive behaviors and substance use patterns. These drives can be explored and ameliorated through psychodynamic psychotherapy. For some individuals, substance use has been a coping mechanism for dealing with problems that stem from childhood family dynamics or painful life events. When the problems that led to the maladaptive behavior have been examined and resolved in psychotherapy, and the individual has learned healthy, effective ways to manage life stressors, he or she no longer needs to rely on drinking or drugs to cope.

Cognitive behavioral therapy as a harm reduction approach is appropriate for someone who experiences symptoms of substance abuse and responds to treatment. Lance Dodes' approach, using psychodynamic therapy, works well if the substance use and self-harming behavior ceases to be problematic. I support these and other approaches to treatment when they work within a reasonable period of time.

Different treatment approaches are helpful for different non-addict users. Some substance abusers can stop with cognitive behavioral help, some will need addiction treatment, and some who receive addiction treatment are unable to stop, and die premature deaths. And certainly, there are some substance abusers who are able to stop substance abuse on their own, without assistance from any type of treatment.

The issue in treating substance abuse or addiction is determining what approach achieves resolution of problematic substance use as well as restoration and maintenance of health. Obviously, if treatment has not succeeded in assuring cessation of problematic substance use within six to twelve months, then the level of treatment needs to be escalated until remission can be achieved and sustained.

Many of the clients I work with have engaged in a long and frustrating struggle to resolve their addiction. I believe that these clients are best served by viewing addiction as doctors do, as a chronic brain disorder which requires comprehensive, long-term treatment and recovery work. Family Recovery Therapy is particularly useful for those addicts whose families are willing to engage in a comprehensive, family-based, approach to recovery. Treatment of the entire family system is effective and long-lasting, whether it is determined that the addict has severe addiction issues or not.

Addiction in Families

The above descriptions of addiction and substance abuse address what goes on for the addict/user. But there is a core aspect of addiction that these descriptions do not address: the social network of the addict. An addict does not live in a vacuum. An addict is almost always part of a social system that allows or enables him or her to continue addictive behaviors, despite their negative consequences. Partners, family members, friends, employers, medical doctors, social service agencies, and even drug treatment programs may play a role in shoring up, covering up, or in some way obfuscating the damage the addict leaves in his wake; they can protect the addict from experiencing and having to face the consequences of his behavior.

An addict's social network is usually comprised of her partner, her children, and possibly other family members such as the addict's parents or siblings. That is why we say addiction is a *family disease*; it affects the family and is often perpetuated by family members, although unintentionally and with the hope of making things better. Spouses or family members are scared by the addict's behavior, afraid of what might happen to the addict, as well as frightened by the aftermath of the addict's behavior. Their compulsion to control the addict is often as intense as the addict's compulsion to get her drug (or "fix" of overspending, or gambling, or eating excess food, or other addictive, self-harming behaviors). Because the family members are as dependent on their need to control the addict as the addict is on her addiction, they are described as "codependent." Just as addicts are in denial of their addiction, people in relationship with addicts are also typically in denial—of how they actually enable the addiction, allow it to continue and to progress, and of their own unhealthy attachment to "control/helping." Many codependents develop mental and medical disorders themselves, largely because they have taken on an impossible task, that of controlling another person, and have turned away from their own lives. It has been conjectured that the mortality rate for codependents, due to the consequences of their disease, may be even higher than it is for addicts. The codependent's angst can manifest in numerous stress-related conditions. Stress is implicated in a wide range of medical conditions such as anxiety, depression, obesity, heart disease, and diabetes, many of which can become severe and even lead to premature death (Griffin, 2014).

Members of a family (or larger system) may say that they want the addict to stop his addictive behavior, but often there is an unconscious force at work in the family system that leads family members to undermine the addict's attempts at recovery. This force is the pull to maintain homeostasis—"the way it's always been." In some families, the addict fulfills the role of "the problem person." In a family in which the alcoholic father is the apparent problem, a child getting ready for school in the morning is not surprised to see her father sprawled out, asleep and disheveled, on the sofa. She thinks to herself, "Uh oh. I guess it was one of those nights that Dad came home so drunk he crashed on the living room couch. Mom's going to be really upset today." She sees the distress in her mother's face, and knows her mom is going to make some excuse to her dad's boss for why he can't come to work today. The family constellates around the father not being available or responsible.

In most cases, if the addict starts to get well, the family is thrown out of balance. To maintain homeostasis, the other family members sometimes need to keep the addict sick and restore the old, familiar family roles. The family members resume their focus on the addict, instead of looking at their own part in supporting the dysfunctional system, or at their own lives. These codependent family members are the enablers who prop up the addictive system in which both addict, and family are emotionally enmeshed.

A note about families with teens or young adults who suffer from addiction: while it may be apparent how codependency operates when the addict is an adult, it is less obvious, but very much a problem, when a young person—a teen or a young adult—becomes an addict. In the case of a minor, codependents in his network may include: a teacher, a doctor, a school official who is willing to overlook signs of a problem, and well-meaning or uninformed parents who rationalize that, "Every teen gets high. I did when I was a kid." It is not until the codependents get help to see their part in potentially enabling addiction that recovery can begin. Please see my book, written with Avis Rumney, *My Addicted Child: Codependency, Enabling, and the Road to Recovery* (2015), for a more detailed description of treating teens and young adults using Family Recovery Therapy.

It is important to point out that adults who develop addiction may have started abusing substances in their teen or young adult years. Rarely does addiction leap out of the woodwork.

Codependency, too, may have a long, if not obvious, history in a family. Often, codependent dynamics in an addictive family system, especially with a multi-generational lineage of addiction, seem so natural and commonplace within the family setting that they become the unconscious map for family interactions.

Below, I describe briefly some of the damage that results from addiction.

Damage to the Addict

Addiction is a bio-psycho-social-spiritual disorder, and an addict can experience severe impairment in each of these aspects of his life.

Biological damage results when addicts ingest substances and engage in behaviors that alter brain chemistry and brain wiring, and that harm body organs and body functioning. The amount and extent of damage due to addiction depends on the individual's drug or addictive behavior history: which drug, which behavior, how much, how often, and for how long. In some cases, there can be irreversible damage to the brain or other organs. Decades of nicotine addiction leading to lung cancer is a well-known example.

Psychological damage in addiction results in part from the addict's single-minded focus on the next "fix," which has deprived him of interacting with reality on real world terms. The parts of the brain that manage self-development and growth of interpersonal relationships have had little activity. How much damage occurs, of course, depends upon the individual and the nature and extent of his addiction.

The addict experiences social impairment because healthy social interactions have been supplanted by drug-seeking and drug-using behavior. The addict's most meaningful social relationships are often related to drug use (or to gaming, food, etc.)—to getting and using drugs, and getting and using more. "Drug buddies" do not interact with each other in the same way as do people who are not using and who are developing normally.

The spiritual aspect of addiction is probably best understood in terms of what the addict deems most important in her life. Love, transcendence, and joy, for the addict, reside in the bottle, or in the drug of choice. There is little room in her world for a healthy spirituality, or a deeper sense of purpose and fulfillment.

Damage to the Family

The family members of an addict suffer from their own addictive behaviors. Codependency is a form of addiction—the codependent family members are often as "addicted" to the addict as the addict is to his drug. Here is Stephanie Brown's description of codependency, also included in Chapter 2:

> Unhealthy codependency is developing an addictive emotional attachment to another person. The addict has an addictive emotional attachment to alcohol or substances or to being out of control in some way. The codependent develops exactly the same out-of-control emotional investment and attachment to a person. The center of the self of the codependent becomes invested in being able to control somebody else, which is never successful from a recovery frame. The codependent then deepens that intense attachment, abandoning the self to become invested in that attachment or bond to another [personal communication, 1997].

Codependency is also devastating in its biological, psychological, social, and spiritual repercussions. Rarely is it a single family member who develops codependency, but several—a spouse, a child, a parent. Both the extended family, as a whole, and the individual family members are drawn into the drama of addiction.

Codependents stress and worry about their loved one's wellbeing, behavior, and the consequences, feared or real, of the behavior. Physiologically, prolonged stress can result in insomnia, headaches, and digestive problems, depending on the individual. And chronic stress—which occurs for many codependents because their loved one suffers from a chronic disease—can wear on various organs and organ systems. Some codependents develop self-harming coping mechanisms, such as overeating or compulsive spending, which may themselves have negative physical consequences. And, as mentioned earlier, children of an addict are more susceptible than those who grew up in non-addictive family systems to developing a substance use problem themselves.

Codependents are, of course, affected psychologically by their relationship with their addicted loved one. Frequent bouts of frustration, anger, and fear are inevitable, and a codependent's mood is often dependent on their perception of how their addict is doing. Anxiety and depression, from mild to severe, can develop. The life of a codependent is challenging, because hoping or trying to change an addict is not only difficult and unsatisfying, it is impossible. Only the addict can change his or her behavior (see Figure 3.4 *Emotional Acre*, which demonstrates that each separate person is responsible for their own wellbeing, and will not find serenity until they take responsibility only for themselves).

Social damage for the codependent manifests both in the family and in outside relationships. The codependent family system gets mired in reacting to the addict, and many rituals and family events can be disrupted by an addict's behavior. Family members often cease focusing on their own needs and goals, and their quality of life suffers. It is not unusual for an addict's children or partner to isolate from social contact and withdraw from interacting with friends "whose families are different" and "who just don't understand." Children internalize these thoughts and feel ashamed of their addicted parent and of their family. They can feel helpless to fix the situation, and discouraged, resentful, or ashamed that they can't. The life of the individual codependent, as well

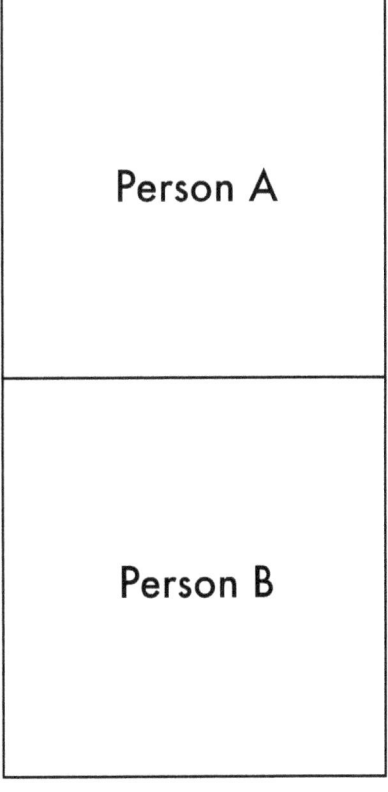

Figure 3.4 *Emotional Acre*. We are each responsible for only our own emotional wellbeing (and not another person's).

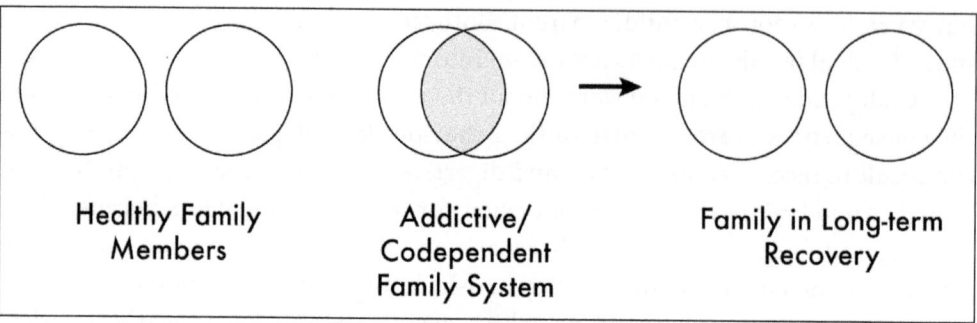

Figure 3.5 *Perspective on Addiction, Codependency, and Recovery.*

as of the codependent family, can shrink into an isolated, unhappy, and unhealthy existence.

Spiritually, the codependent unwittingly makes the addict a higher power, someone more important than themselves. For a child particularly, the addicted parent becomes a central focus. Children of any age expect their parents to be the strong ones, the ones who are there for them; they have been there since the day the child was born. And children can believe, unconsciously, "If I can fix mom, then she will love me and take care of me," when the child, of course, needs the environment of a healthy family to grow and develop. Not being able to "fix" the poorly functioning parent can result in the child feeling inadequate and incompetent.

When one person centers his life around another person and gets mired in trying to control or protect the other, as so often happens in the families of addicts, things do not unfold the way the children, spouse, or other family members hope they will. There is little room within the family to open into more expansive, loving, playful, and spiritual experiences. Each individual in the family is affected, and there is a void, an emptiness, in the family as a whole. Codependents usually seem constricted energetically, and tend to be unhappy and anxious, rather than living a life that is fun and replete with joy, loving relationships, and meaning.

Unless and until the codependents get help to unwind their part in propping up and enabling the addictive system, the addict will not experience the natural consequences of his behavior and will lack motivation to change. Recovery from addiction means recovery not just for the addict, but for the entire family system (see Fig. 3.5).

Part Two: Definitions of Addiction

Following are four clinical definitions of addiction, presented in two sections.

Section One is a brief summary of some key points described in the chapter, "Substance-Related and Addictive Disorders," in the American Psychiatric Association's *Diagnostic and Statistical Manual of Mental Disorders Fifth Edition* (*DSM-5*) (2013). As noted earlier, the *DSM-5* is the primary diagnostic resource used by psychotherapists and therefore is an important guide for assessing psychiatric and behavioral symptoms. Section Two contains the American Society of Addiction Medicine's (ASAM's) three definitions of addiction.

Section One

—*DSM-5* Diagnostic Criteria for Substance Use Disorders

In the chapter, "Substance-Related and Addictive Disorders," the *DSM-5* distinguishes between substance-induced disorders, which can include intoxication, withdrawal, and other physical and mental problems caused by substance use, and substance use disorders, which include the physical, behavioral, and psychological issues generally associated with repeated use of substances. Substance use disorders include ten classes of drugs any one of which, if taken in excess, can activate the brain's reward system and thereby reinforce behavior and memories. In addition, drugs of abuse can directly affect reward pathways, often causing pleasure or at least reducing pain. The *DSM-5* also includes gambling disorder in this section, under the heading of "Non-Substance-Related Disorders," because gambling behaviors activate reward systems similar to those activated by substance abuse, and gambling also produces some behavioral symptoms similar to those resulting from substance use disorders. However, the *DSM-5* specifically excludes Internet gaming, because the evidence of behavioral patterns is less clear.

The *DSM-5* also excludes other "groups of repetitive behaviors, which some term *behavioral addictions*, with such subcategories as 'sex addiction,' 'exercise addiction,' or 'shopping addiction'" because there is "insufficient peer-reviewed evidence to establish the diagnostic criteria and course descriptions needed to identify these behaviors as mental disorders" (*DSM-5*, p. 481).

According to the *DSM-5*, a salient feature of substance use disorders is that the individual continues to use despite having significant substance-related problems. This is one of the classic "4 Cs" that has long been considered a criterion for substance abuse or addiction, continued use despite adverse consequences. Brain changes that can occur with continued use can lead to craving and relapse. The *DSM-5* notes that "These persistent drug effects may benefit from long-term approaches to treatment" (*DSM-5*, p. 483).

The diagnosis of substance use disorder "is based on a pathological pattern of behaviors related to use of the substance" (*DSM-5*, p. 483). Among the ten classes of drugs that the *DSM-5* includes in its description of substance use disorders are alcohol, cannabis, hallucinogens, opioids, tobacco, and cocaine (*DSM-5*, pp. 481–585). For each class of drugs, the *DSM-5* uses the same set of eleven criteria for the purpose of differential diagnosis to aid in assessing the level of severity of the problem. Among the different classes of drugs, these eleven criteria may not all be equally significant, and their manifestation is likely to vary from one class of drugs to another.

The eleven criteria fall into four different categories: Impaired Control, Social Impairment, Risky Use, and Pharmacological Indicators (tolerance and withdrawal).

Impaired Control may manifest as:

1. Using for longer periods of time than intended, or using larger amounts than intended.
2. Persistent desire or unsuccessful attempts to reduce use.
3. Spending a lot of time obtaining the substance.
4. Craving.

Social Impairment may include:

1. Use impeding ability to fulfill obligations at work, home, or school.
2. Continued use despite social or interpersonal problems caused or exacerbated by use.
3. Important social, occupational, or recreational activities are given up or reduced.

Risky Use includes:

1. Use in situations where it is physically hazardous.
2. Continued use even knowing use is causing or exacerbating persistent physical or psychological problems.

Pharmacological Indicators (the body makes physical adjustments to adapt to the continued use of a substance):

1. Tolerance, as evidenced by the need for markedly increased amounts to achieve desired effect, or by markedly diminished effect with continued use of the same amount.
2. Withdrawal, with symptoms specific to a particular drug. This is the body's response to sudden cessation of a drug once the individual has used it repeatedly and developed some level of tolerance to it.

Severity of substance use disorder is assessed based on the number of symptom criteria that are met. Generally, the presence of two or three symptoms suggests a mild substance use disorder, the presence of four or five symptoms suggests a moderate substance use disorder, and the presence of six or seven symptoms suggests a severe substance use disorder. The *DSM-5* does not use the term addiction, but rather uses the term substance use disorder to describe the broad range in which a substance use disorder may manifest, from mild to severe or chronic.

Let's consider a hypothetical case of a married man in his 40s who has begun to increase his alcohol intake over a period of several months. The eleven criteria of the *DSM-5* can be used to assess whether his alcohol use warrants diagnosis as a substance use disorder. First, consider whether he has any signs of impaired ability to control his use. He finds that it takes more alcohol to achieve the desired effect than it used to, and he tends to use more alcohol than he generally plans to. He wants to reduce his use, and has successfully stopped drinking altogether for several weeks at a time, but each time returns to drinking, and to drinking as much as or more than before he stopped. He is exhibiting signs of impaired control—greater use than intended and unsuccessful attempts to stop.

His social impairment largely revolves around exacerbation of marital discord—when he drinks, he becomes argumentative with his wife. However, his drinking has not affected his ability to carry out work, family, or recreational activities.

As for whether his use entails risk, he does not drink and drive or drink in situations that put him or others in physical danger. However, he is aware that drinking aggravates his emotional ups and downs, and that he often feels depressed and remorseful on a day when he has had a lot to drink the night before.

As for tolerance and withdrawal, the fact that he needs to drink more in order to achieve the effect he wants is an indication of at least a mild level of tolerance. He has been able to stop drinking for periods of several weeks at a time without difficulty, so seems not to exhibit notable withdrawal symptoms. In summary, he shows two of signs of impaired control, one sign of impairment socially, some impact on his physical and mental well-being, and signs of tolerance, exhibiting in total five symptom criteria of substance use disorder. While this is only a superficial look at his situation with respect to alcohol, and needs to be considered in the context of other aspects of his life, his behavior, and his physical and psychological concerns, it appears that he may suffer from a moderate substance use disorder.

Section Two—American Society of Addiction Medicine (ASAM)

As noted earlier, in 2011, the American Society of Addiction Medicine (ASAM) published two definitions of addiction, a short version and a long version. Several years later, ASAM determined that a revised definition of addiction was warranted, both because the public's view of addiction had changed, and because new findings had emerged in the prevention and treatment of addiction. In 2019, ASAM updated its earlier definitions and created a briefer, more accessible definition of addiction.

Below is ASAM's 2019 definition. This is followed by ASAM's short and long definitions from 2011. The earlier versions are presented here because their breadth provides a comprehensive view of the nature and complexity of addiction.

ASAM's 2019 Definition of Addiction[1]

Addiction is a treatable, chronic medical disease involving complex interactions among brain circuits, genetics, the environment, and an individual's life experiences. People with addiction use substances or engage in behaviors that become compulsive and often continue despite harmful consequences.

Prevention efforts and treatment approaches for addiction are generally as successful as those for other chronic diseases [Adopted by the ASAM Board of Directors, September 15, 2019].

---

1. "Definition of Addiction," 2019. (https://www.asam.org/Quality-Science/definition-of-addiction). Copyright 2019 by The American Society of Addiction Medicine. Reprinted with permission.

ASAM'S 2011 Definition of Addiction, Short Version[2]

Addiction is a primary, chronic disease of brain reward, motivation, memory and related circuitry. Dysfunction in these circuits leads to characteristic biological, psychological, social and spiritual manifestations. This is reflected in an individual pathologically pursuing reward and/or relief by substance use and other behaviors.

Addiction is characterized by inability to consistently abstain, impairment in behavioral control, craving, diminished recognition of significant problems with one's behaviors and interpersonal relationships, and a dysfunctional emotional response. Like other chronic diseases, addiction often involves cycles of relapse and remission. Without treatment or engagement in recovery activities, addiction is progressive and can result in disability or premature death. [Adopted by the ASAM Board of Directors April 12, 2011].

ASAM's 2011 Definition of Addiction, Long Version (see Footnote 2)

Addiction is a primary, chronic disease of brain reward, motivation, memory and related circuitry. Addiction affects neurotransmission and interactions within reward structures of the brain, including the nucleus accumbens, anterior cingulate cortex, basal forebrain and amygdala, such that motivational hierarchies are altered and addictive behaviors, which may or may not include alcohol and other drug use, supplant healthy, self-care related behaviors. Addiction also affects neurotransmission and interactions between cortical and hippocampal circuits and brain reward structures, such that the memory of previous exposures to rewards (such as food, sex, alcohol and other drugs) leads to a biological and behavioral response to external cues, in turn triggering craving and/or engagement in addictive behaviors.

The neurobiology of addiction encompasses more than the neurochemistry of reward. (1) The frontal cortex of the brain and underlying white matter connections between the frontal cortex and circuits of reward, motivation and memory are fundamental in the manifestations of altered impulse control, altered judgment, and the dysfunctional pursuit of rewards (which is often experienced by the affected person as a desire to "be normal") seen in addiction—despite cumulative adverse consequences experienced from engagement in substance use and other addictive behaviors. The frontal lobes are important in inhibiting impulsivity and in assisting individuals to appropriately delay gratification. When persons with addiction manifest problems in deferring gratification, there is a neurological locus of these problems in the frontal cortex. Frontal lobe morphology, connectivity and functioning are still in the process of maturation during adolescence and young adulthood, and early exposure to substance use is another significant factor in the development of addiction. Many neuroscientists believe that developmental morphology is the basis that makes early-life exposure to substances such an important factor.

Genetic factors account for about half of the likelihood that an individual will develop addiction. Environmental factors interact with the person's biology and affect the extent to which genetic factors exert their influence. Resiliencies the individual acquires (through parenting or later life experiences) can affect the extent to which genetic predispositions lead to the behavioral and other manifestations of addiction. Culture also plays a role in how addiction becomes actualized in persons with biological vulnerabilities to the development of addiction.

Other factors that can contribute to the appearance of addiction, leading to its characteristic bio-psycho-socio-spiritual manifestations, include:

---

2. "Public Policy Statement: Definition of Addiction," 2011. (*https://www.asam.org/docs/default-source/public-policy-statements/1definition_of_addiction_long_4-11.pdf?sfvrsn=a8f64512_4*). Copyright by the American Society of Addiction Medicine 2011. Reprinted with permission.

- *The presence of an underlying biological deficit in the function of reward circuits, such that drugs and behaviors which enhance reward function are preferred and sought as reinforcers;*
- The repeated engagement in drug use or other addictive behaviors, causing neuroadaptation in motivational circuitry leading to impaired control over further drug use or engagement in addictive behaviors;
- Cognitive and affective distortions, which impair perceptions and compromise the ability to deal with feelings, resulting in significant self-deception;
- Disruption of healthy social supports and problems in interpersonal relationships which impact the development or impact of resiliencies;
- Exposure to trauma or stressors that overwhelm an individual's coping abilities;
- Distortion in meaning, purpose and values that guide attitudes, thinking and behavior;
- Distortions in a person's connection with self, with others and with the transcendent (referred to as God by many, the Higher Power by 12-steps groups, or higher consciousness by others); and
- The presence of co-occurring psychiatric disorders in persons who engage in substance use or other addictive behaviors.

Addiction is characterized by (2):

- **Inability to Consistently Abstain**
- **Impairment in Behavioral Control**;
- **Craving**; or increased "hunger" for drugs or rewarding experiences;
- **Diminished Recognition of Significant Problems** with one's behaviors and interpersonal relationships; and
- **A Dysfunctional Emotional Response**.

The **power of external cues** to trigger craving and drug use, as well as to increase the frequency of engagement in other potentially addictive behaviors, is also a characteristic of addiction, with the hippocampus being important in memory of previous euphoric or dysphoric experiences, and with the amygdala being important in having motivation concentrate on selecting behaviors associated with these past experiences.

Although some believe that the difference between those who have addiction, and those who do not, is the quantity or frequency of alcohol/drug use, engagement in addictive behaviors (such as gambling or spending) (3), or exposure to other external rewards (such as food or sex), a characteristic aspect of addiction is the qualitative way in which the individual responds to such exposures, stressors and environmental cues. A particularly pathological aspect of the way that persons with addiction pursue substance use or external rewards is that preoccupation with, obsession with and/or pursuit of rewards (e.g., alcohol and other drug use) persist despite the accumulation of adverse consequences. These manifestations can occur compulsively or impulsively, as a reflection of impaired control.

Persistent risk and/or recurrence of relapse, after periods of abstinence, is another fundamental feature of addiction. This can be triggered by exposure to rewarding substances and behaviors, by exposure to environmental cues to use, and by exposure to emotional stressors that trigger heightened activity in brain stress circuits. (4)

In addiction there is a significant impairment in executive functioning, which manifests in problems with perception, learning, impulse control, compulsivity, and judgment. People with addiction often manifest a lower readiness to change their dysfunctional behaviors despite mounting concerns expressed by significant others in their lives; and display an apparent lack of appreciation of the magnitude of cumulative problems and complications. The still developing frontal lobes of adolescents may both compound these deficits in executive functioning and predispose youngsters to engage in "high risk" behaviors, including engaging in alcohol or other drug use. The profound drive or craving to use substances or engage in apparently rewarding behaviors, which is seen in many patients with addiction, underscores the compulsive or avolitional aspect of this disease. This is the connection with "powerlessness" over addiction and "unmanageability" of life, as is described in Step 1 of 12 Steps programs.

Addiction is more than a behavioral disorder. Features of addiction include aspects of a person's behaviors, cognitions, emotions, and interactions with others, including a person's ability to relate to members of their family, to members of their community, to their own psychological state, and to things that transcend their daily experience.

Behavioral manifestations and complications of addiction, primarily due to impaired control, can include:

- Excessive use and/or engagement in addictive behaviors, at higher frequencies and/or quantities than the person intended, often associated with a persistent desire for and unsuccessful attempts at behavioral control
- Excessive time lost in substance use or recovering from the effects of substance use and/or engagement in addictive behaviors, with significant adverse impact on social and occupational functioning (e.g., the development of interpersonal relationship problems or the neglect of responsibilities at home, school or work);
- Continued use and/or engagement in addictive behaviors, despite the presence of persistent or recurrent physical or psychological problems which may have been caused or exacerbated by substance use and/or related addictive behaviors;
- A narrowing of the behavioral repertoire focusing on rewards that are part of addiction; and
- An apparent lack of ability and/or readiness to take consistent, ameliorative action despite recognition of problems.

Cognitive changes in addiction can include:

- Preoccupation with substance use;
- Altered evaluations of the relative benefits and detriments associated with drugs or rewarding behaviors; and
- The inaccurate belief that problems experienced in one's life are attributable to other causes rather than being a predictable consequence of addiction.

Emotional changes in addiction can include:

- Increased anxiety, dysphoria and emotional pain;
- Increased sensitivity to stressors associated with the recruitment of brain stress systems, such that "things seem more stressful" as a result; and
- Difficulty in identifying feelings, distinguishing between feelings and the bodily sensations of emotional arousal, and describing feelings to other people (sometimes referred to as alexithymia).

The emotional aspects of addiction are quite complex. Some persons use alcohol or other drugs or pathologically pursue other rewards because they are seeking "positive reinforcement" or the creation of a positive emotional state ("euphoria"). Others pursue substance use or other rewards because they have experienced relief from negative emotional states ("dysphoria"), which constitutes "negative reinforcement." Beyond the initial experiences of reward and relief, there is a *dysfunctional emotional state* present in most cases of addiction that is associated with the persistence of engagement with addictive behaviors. The state of addiction is not the same as the state of intoxication. When anyone experiences mild intoxication through the use of alcohol or other drugs, or when one engages non-pathologically in potentially addictive behaviors such as gambling or eating, one may experience a "high," felt as a "positive" emotional state associated with increased dopamine and opioid peptide activity in reward circuits. After such an experience, there is a neurochemical rebound, in which the reward function does not simply revert to baseline, but often drops below the original levels. This is usually not consciously perceptible by the individual and is not necessarily associated with functional impairments.

Over time, repeated experiences with substance use or addictive behaviors are not associated with ever increasing reward circuit activity and are not as subjectively rewarding. Once a person experiences withdrawal from drug use or comparable behaviors, there is an anxious, agitated, dysphoric and labile emotional experience, related to suboptimal reward and the recruitment of brain and hormonal stress systems, which is associated with withdrawal from virtually all pharmacological classes of addictive drugs. While tolerance develops to the "high," tolerance does not develop to the emotional "low" associated with the cycle of intoxication and withdrawal. Thus, in addiction, persons repeatedly attempt to create a "high"—but what they mostly experience is a deeper and deeper "low." While anyone may "want" to get "high," those with addiction feel a "need" to use the addictive substance or engage in the addictive behavior in order to try to resolve their dysphoric emotional state or their physiological symptoms of withdrawal. Persons with addiction compulsively use even though it may not make them feel good, in some cases long after the pursuit of "rewards" is not actually pleasurable. (5) Although people from any culture may choose to "get high" from one or another activity, it is important to appreciate that addiction is not solely a function of choice. Simply put, addiction is not a desired condition.

As addiction is a chronic disease, periods of relapse, which may interrupt spans of remission, are a common feature of addiction. It is also important to recognize that return to drug use or pathological pursuit of rewards is not inevitable.

Clinical interventions can be quite effective in altering the course of addiction. Close monitoring of the behaviors of the individual and contingency management, sometimes including behavioral consequences for relapse behaviors, can contribute to positive clinical outcomes. Engagement in health promotion activities which promote personal responsibility and accountability, connection with others, and personal growth also contribute to recovery. It is important to recognize that ***addiction can cause disability or premature death, especially when left untreated or treated inadequately.***

The qualitative ways in which the brain and behavior respond to drug exposure and engagement in addictive behaviors are different at later stages of addiction than in earlier stages, indicating progression, which may not be overtly apparent. As is the case with other chronic diseases, the condition must be monitored and managed over time to:

- Decrease the frequency and intensity of relapses;
- Sustain periods of remission; and
- Optimize the person's level of functioning during periods of remission.

In some cases of addiction, medication management can improve treatment outcomes. In most cases of addiction, the integration of psychosocial rehabilitation and ongoing care with evidence-based pharmacological therapy provides the best results. Chronic disease management is important for minimization of episodes of relapse and their impact. Treatment of addiction saves lives [3]

Addiction professionals and persons in recovery know the hope that is found in recovery. Recovery is available even to persons who may not at first be able to perceive this hope, especially when the focus is on linking the health consequences to the disease of addiction. ***As in other health conditions, self-management, with mutual support, is very important***

---

3. *See* ASAM Public Policy Statement on **Treatment for Alcohol and Other Drug Addiction**, Adopted: May 01, 1980, Revised: January 01, 2010.

in recovery from addiction. Peer support such as that found in various "self-help" activities is beneficial in optimizing health status and functional outcomes in recovery.[4]

Recovery from addiction is best achieved through a combination of self-management, mutual support, and professional care provided by trained and certified professionals.

Explanatory footnotes:

1. The neurobiology of reward has been well understood for decades, whereas the neurobiology of addiction is still being explored. Most clinicians have learned of reward pathways including projections from the ventral tegmental area (VTA) of the brain, through the median forebrain bundle (MFB), and terminating in the nucleus accumbens (Nuc Acc), in which dopamine neurons are prominent. Current neuroscience recognizes that the neurocircuitry of reward also involves a rich bi-directional circuitry connecting the nucleus accumbens and the basal forebrain. It is the reward circuitry where reward is registered, and where the most fundamental rewards such as food, hydration, sex, and nurturing exert a strong and life-sustaining influence. Alcohol, nicotine, other drugs and pathological gambling behaviors exert their initial effects by acting on the same reward circuitry that appears in the brain to make food and sex, for example, profoundly reinforcing. Other effects, such as intoxication and emotional euphoria from rewards, derive from activation of the reward circuitry. While intoxication and withdrawal are well understood through the study of reward circuitry, understanding of addiction requires understanding of a broader network of neural connections involving forebrain as well as midbrain structures. Selection of certain rewards, preoccupation with certain rewards, response to triggers to pursue certain rewards, and motivational drives to use alcohol and other drugs and/or pathologically seek other rewards, involve multiple brain regions outside of reward neurocircuitry itself.

2. These five features are not intended to be used as "diagnostic criteria" for determining if addiction is present or not. Although these characteristic features are widely present in most cases of addiction, regardless of the pharmacology of the substance use seen in addiction or the reward that is pathologically pursued, each feature may not be equally prominent in every case. The diagnosis of addiction requires a comprehensive biological, psychological, social and spiritual assessment by a trained and certified professional.

3. In this document, the term "addictive behaviors" refers to behaviors that are commonly rewarding and are a feature in many cases of addiction. Exposure to these behaviors, just as occurs with exposure to rewarding drugs, is facilitative of the addiction process rather than causative of addiction. The state of brain anatomy and physiology is the underlying variable that is more directly causative of addiction. Thus, in this document, the term "addictive behaviors" does not refer to dysfunctional or socially disapproved behaviors, which can appear in many cases of addiction. Behaviors, such as dishonesty, violation of one's values or the values of others, criminal acts etc., can be a component of addiction; these are best viewed as complications that result from rather than contribute to addiction.

4. The anatomy (the brain circuitry involved) and the physiology (the neurotransmitters involved) in these three modes of relapse (drug- or reward-triggered relapse vs. cue-triggered relapse vs. stress-triggered relapse) have been delineated through neuroscience research.

Relapse triggered by exposure to addictive/rewarding drugs, including alcohol, involves

---

4. *See* ASAM Public Policy Statement on **The Relationship Between Treatment and Self Help: A Joint Statement of the American Society of Addiction Medicine, the American Academy of Addiction Psychiatry, and the American Psychiatric Association**, Adopted: December 01, 1997.

the nucleus accumbens and the VTA-MFB-Nuc Acc neural axis (the brain's mesolimbic dopaminergic "incentive salience circuitry"—see footnote 1 above). Reward-triggered relapse also is mediated by glutamatergic circuits projecting to the nucleus accumbens from the frontal cortex.

Relapse triggered by exposure to conditioned cues from the environment involves glutamate circuits, originating in frontal cortex, insula, hippocampus and amygdala projecting to mesolimbic incentive salience circuitry.

Relapse triggered by exposure to stressful experiences involves brain stress circuits beyond the hypothalamic-pituitary-adrenal axis that is well known as the core of the endocrine stress system. There are two of these relapse-triggering brain stress circuits—one originates in noradrenergic nucleus A2 in the lateral tegmental area of the brain stem and projects to the hypothalamus, nucleus accumbens, frontal cortex, and bed nucleus of the stria terminalis, and uses norepinephrine as its neurotransmitter; the other originates in the central nucleus of the amygdala, projects to the bed nucleus of the stria terminalis and uses corticotrophin-releasing factor (CRF) as its neurotransmitter.

5. Pathologically pursuing reward (mentioned in the Short Version of this definition) thus has multiple components. It is not necessarily the amount of exposure to the reward (e.g., the dosage of a drug) or the frequency or duration of the exposure that is pathological. In addiction, pursuit of rewards persists, despite life problems that accumulate due to addictive behaviors, even when engagement in the behaviors ceases to be pleasurable. Similarly, in earlier stages of addiction, or even before the outward manifestations of addiction have become apparent, substance use or engagement in addictive behaviors can be an attempt to pursue relief from dysphoria; while in later stages of the disease, engagement in addictive behaviors can persist even though the behavior no longer provides relief.

Adopted by the ASAM Board of Directors April 12, 2011

CHAPTER 4

Effective Treatment—FRT's Fourteen Principles and the Federal Guidelines for Addiction Treatment

The consequences of drug abuse and addiction currently cost our society over a trillion dollars each year (Altarum, 2018). While this nation spends hundreds of millions of dollars annually on addiction treatment, we know that *effective* treatment reaches perhaps only 10 percent of still-suffering addicts. And we know that half of those who engage in treatment will relapse within one year of "completing" treatment in a residential or outpatient program. *The reality is that the current model of addiction treatment has not made a significant dent in America's addiction crisis.*

Here is a snapshot of several ineffective ways that individuals, treatment providers, and government agencies attempt to address this national tragedy today:

- A frightened family member brings together other family members and friends to "do an intervention," which often increases family stress, alienates members, and rarely works to get sustained help for the addict and the family members.
- Interventionists meet with an addict and their family for only a day or two, refer the addict to a 30-day program, have minimal follow-up with the addict or the family. Even if the addict goes to treatment, at best there is only a fifty percent chance of the addict achieving remission for a full year.
- Treatment programs, in spite of their slick marketing materials, fail to fully inform their clients and their families that half of their clients relapse.
- Doctors prescribe addictive medicines to replace addictive street drugs, but fail to engage the addict and the addict's family members in a robust, long-term, comprehensive, and systemic treatment.
- Governments, often politically motivated, fund "programs" that sound good, but are not grounded in effective, evidence-based treatment practices.
- The government often criminalizes drug use, which fuels the war on drugs, and addicts get sent to prison, not to treatment, and rarely get the addiction treatment they need.

Treatment providers are doing their best. But dedicated and hopeful professionals work in a field that is burdened by fragmented and ineffective approaches, and treatment reaches only a small percentage of addicts. In spite of our best efforts, we continue to watch the death tolls rise from this treatable, but sorely misunderstood, disease.

I believe we need to follow the science. I believe we now know what is necessary to radically improve outcome rates. And I know that the Family Recovery Therapy (FRT) model, the new paradigm of addiction treatment I describe in this book, works.

Clinically, FRT's tenets are fully supported by the Federal Government's National Institute on Drug Abuse (NIDA). NIDA describes their drug treatment guidelines in their publication, *Principles of Drug Addiction Treatment: A Research-Based Guide (Third Edition*, [2018]). NIDA's principles comprise the government's current gold standard for addiction treatment. The Principles of Family Recovery Therapy are aligned with NIDA's principles—which are based on science and best practices.

Nearly all doctors, treatment providers, addiction counselors and others working in this field, agree with NIDA's principles and their decades-long research findings. NIDA's conclusions spell out the principles we must consider if we are to effectively treat addiction. In this chapter, I compare NIDA'S research-based findings with the 14 Principles of Family Recovery Therapy.

NIDA's principles and the Principles of Family Recovery Therapy differ on two critical points. Two factors central to FRT go a step beyond NIDA's prescription for effective drug treatment, while the FRT approach still incorporates all the basic components of NIDA's guidelines.

First, FRT includes *a single case manager*, the FRT therapist, who monitors and oversees the continuum of care throughout the first year of sobriety. In contrast, the NIDA report reflects the current treatment paradigm in which the treatment process for an addict includes many different treatment providers, each of whom attends to one phase of an addict's recovery. This approach resembles the parable of the blind men and the elephant that I alluded to in Chapter 1: there is no one overseeing the recovery process as a whole, each provider deals with one aspect of treatment, and there is little coordination among the various providers. In contrast, FRT implements a comprehensive treatment approach: removing the blinders by assigning one individual, the FRT therapist, to supervise and monitor the recovery process, including facilitating coordination and cooperation among different providers.

Second, NIDA's principles do not focus on the vital role of *the family* in the healing process; FRT involves the, typically enabling, family from the very beginning of treatment. This difference between NIDA's principles and FRT is crucial to FRT's efficacy, because addiction is central to the family system, as well as to the life of the addict. Family participation and family recovery are typically essential for sustained recovery for the addict. The thrust of my treatment model is to engage not only the addict, but also those with whom the addict is in relationship: the family members affected by addiction—some of whom may be codependent enablers—whose love and care can lead to an improved recovery outcome. Including these impacted family members from the beginning of treatment is essential. From a clinical standpoint, I believe that failing to include and treat these relationships is one of the most important reasons that current addiction treatment has such a low success rate.

Although family work is not an essential component of NIDA's principles, they do reference the family at several points. NIDA's guidelines note that family counseling can be a part of drug abuse treatment, as can behavioral therapy that addresses "facilitating better interpersonal relationships" (NIDA Principle 6). The terms "family therapy," and "parenting instruction" also are mentioned in NIDA's recommendations.

While two aspects of Family Recovery Therapy—the role of the FRT therapist and the substantial involvement of family in treatment—set FRT apart from other drug addiction approaches, the foundational approach of FRT is very much in line with NIDA's guidelines. Below, I list each of the thirteen points included in NIDA's *Principles of Drug Addiction Treatment* (2018), and describe the specific FRT Principles that correlate with it.

> *NIDA Principle 1:*
> *Addiction is a complex but treatable disease that affects brain function and behavior. Drugs of abuse alter the brain's structure and function, resulting in changes that persist long after drug use has ceased. This may explain why drug abusers are at risk for relapse even after long periods of abstinence and despite the potentially devastating consequences.*

Two FRT Principles speak to the chronic nature of addiction and the need for long-term support:

FRT Principle 1
Addiction is a chronic, relapsing, treatable medical disease with profound mental and physical consequences. Addicts will need long-term, possibly lifelong, recovery support, which can take many forms.

FRT Principle 8
Since addiction and the codependency that enables it are chronic conditions, it is recommended that the addict and codependents develop ongoing support beyond the first year of continuous sobriety.

Family Recovery Therapy addresses the chronic nature of addiction, the potential for relapse, and the addict's probable need for lifelong support. Furthermore, the value of ongoing support extends to those in relationship with the addict—the chronicity of codependency is also at issue, and the recovery of family members can be key to the recovery of the addict.

> *NIDA Principle 2:*
> *No single treatment is appropriate for everyone. Treatment varies depending on the type of drug and the characteristics of the patients. Matching treatment settings, interventions, and services to an individual's particular problems and needs is critical to his or her ultimate success in returning to productive functioning in the family, workplace, and society.*

In the FRT model, a single, state-licensed mental or medical health professional, the FRT therapist, treats the addict and their family from day one. This individual is trained not only to assess and treat a wide variety of issues, but can also bring in additional providers as needed, and coordinate treatment with them. The FRT therapist is both the primary treating clinician and the case manager for the treatment process. "Case manager," as used in this book, describes the role of the FRT therapist throughout the different phases of treatment and in handling situations the addict and their family may encounter during the course of treatment. Phases of treatment can include: intervention, detox, treatment at a Residential Treatment Center, Intensive Outpatient Treatment, and placement in a Sober Living Environment. Situations may include a medical problem that arises for the addict or a family member that requires a medical evaluation, or someone in the family with job issues or who needs financial, legal, educational, or employment guidance. The FRT therapist recognizes the breadth of treatment options and resources that any addict, or addict's family members, may benefit from in the course of recovery, and coordinates care with any other providers involved. FRT Principle 5 describes the role of the FRT therapist as overseer, guide, and coordinator of the addict and family's recovery process:

FRT Principle 5
As the treatment team leader, the FRT therapist guides the family throughout the continuum of care and collaborates with all supportive therapeutic services, which may include other treatment providers, interventionists, treatment programs, physicians, and any other adjunctive services.

> *NIDA Principle 3:*
> *Treatment needs to be readily available. Because drug-addicted individuals may be uncertain about entering treatment, taking advantage of available services the moment people are ready for treatment is critical. Potential patients can be lost if treatment is not immediately available or readily accessible. As with other chronic diseases, the earlier treatment is offered in the disease process, the greater the likelihood of positive outcomes.*

Availability of treatment is essential to ensure that an addict can get help when he reaches out for assistance. There are a great many county and non-profit mental health agencies throughout the United States that offer some kind of addiction treatment. And, of course, support groups such as AA are widespread in large and small communities. My hope is that there will be more and more FRT therapists—licensed mental health providers, grounded in family therapy and trained in addiction—working at agencies or in private practice, who can provide the family-based addiction treatment that I recommend. Until then, many city, county, and non-profit agencies have the capacity to alter their treatment focus and include the codependent family members in the recovery process. This alone could significantly help treatment outcomes, even if there is no single licensed individual who can oversee all phases of treatment.

Confusion abounds in the public regarding what constitutes addiction treatment. What comes to mind for many people when they hear the term "addiction treatment" is "rehab," a destination "where addicts go." In my experience, it is not unusual for a potential client—the family member of an addict—to have already Googled "rehabs" or "addiction treatment" before calling me. Often, their hope is that I will somehow engineer a way to get their loved one to go to rehab, or tell them which rehab center to contact. Many residential treatment programs (RTCs) may be geographically far away from where the family or addict lives. Part of the challenge is to educate the public that "addiction treatment" is not synonymous with "rehab" or "residential treatment," and that an RTC may or may not be useful as a phase of treatment, but it is not a substitute for the long-term support and guidance required for recovery.

A family therapist can be your local *"immediately available or readily accessible"* mental health professional—if they are trained in both family therapy and addiction treatment. Moreover, implementing FRT Principle 14 makes treatment for the addict and family members a priority. The FRT therapist, well-versed in the efficacy of and access to social support groups, can direct an individual seeking help to this readily available support. The addict or codependent may be able to find such a therapist close to home, and there are usually social support and mutual aid groups nearby. I have been treating addictive/codependent families for 25 years, working out of my private practice office, recommending local social support groups, and sometimes coordinating the addict or a codependent's treatment at a residential center as part of treatment.

> NIDA Principle 4:
> *Effective treatment attends to multiple needs of the individual, not just his or her drug abuse. To be effective, treatment must address the individual's drug abuse and any associated medical, psychological, social, vocational, and legal problems. It is also important that treatment be appropriate to the individual's age, gender, ethnicity, and culture.*

Unlike the typical drug counselor, the FRT therapist is trained, as is every licensed mental health professional, to assess for "medical, psychological, social, vocational, and legal problems." Licensed mental health professionals treat within their scope of practice, making referrals to appropriate ancillary providers, as needed, to address issues beyond their expertise. The FRT therapist, in addition to making referrals, coordinates the referral process, communicates and collaborates with any involved professionals, and, if needed, educates them about the treatment plan, and oversees the recovery process for the addict and the family. With the FRT therapist as case manager, it maximizes the potential for a cohesive treatment process and minimizes the possibility of the addict or family getting conflicting directives or opinions from different sources. It is incumbent upon the FRT therapist, as it is for any licensed mental health professional, to work with clients whom he or she deems appropriate. If age or gender or some aspect of the addict's or family's culture is not a workable match for the therapist (e.g., if the therapist does not speak the client's language), the therapist should make an appropriate referral.

Three FRT Principles speak to the role of the FRT therapist in monitoring and addressing the wide range of issues they may encounter in working with an addict and his family:

FRT Principle 4
During the first year of treatment, the FRT therapist monitors, assesses, and guides the family in an integrated treatment process, which addresses biological, psychological, social, and spiritual recovery.

FRT Principle 5
As the treatment team leader, the FRT therapist guides the family throughout the continuum of care and collaborates with all supportive therapeutic services, which may include other treatment providers, interventionists, treatment programs, physicians, and any other adjunctive services.

FRT Principle 9
Treatment includes monitoring for co-occurring mental and physical health problems and providing appropriate referrals as needed.

> NIDA Principle 5:
> *Remaining in treatment for an adequate period of time is critical. The appropriate duration for an individual depends on the type and degree of the patient's problems and needs. Research indicates that most addicted individuals need at least 3 months in treatment to significantly reduce or stop their drug use and that the best outcomes occur with longer durations of treatment. Recovery from drug addiction is a long-term process and frequently requires multiple episodes of treatment. As with other chronic illnesses, relapses to drug abuse can occur and should signal a need for treatment to be reinstated or adjusted. Because individuals often leave treatment prematurely, programs should include strategies to engage and keep patients in treatment.*

The key sentence here is: "*Research indicates that most addicted individuals need at least 3 months in treatment to significantly reduce or stop their drug use and that the best outcomes occur with longer durations of treatment.*" From my experience, few residential programs offer this "longer duration" of treatment unless the addict is willing to live near the treatment program and attend the step-down program affiliated with the residential program—often far from home, family, and the essential local support groups. And none of the residential treatment centers (RTCs) offers a long-term program that includes family members in weekly treatment through the initial year of continuous sobriety. Yes, RTCs recognize the need for longer treatment and will "recommend" the addict seek additional help when returning home. However, in a large number of cases, the addict is discharged after 30, 60, or 90 days, with only a phone number for local aftercare treatment—which, in far too many cases, they fail to call, leading to risk of relapse. The FRT model provides treatment and continuity of care for an addict and their family, from day one, through at least the first year of continuous sobriety, and in many cases, even longer. I may continue to work with some of my clients for several years as they pursue recovery work to restore healthy, age-appropriate development. Both the addict and the family members benefit significantly from extended treatment. Two FRT Principles address the recovering addict's—as well as the family's—need for continued support through the critical first year of recovery and beyond:

FRT Principle 4

During the first year of treatment, the FRT therapist monitors, assesses, and guides the family in an integrated treatment process, which addresses biological, psychological, social, and spiritual recovery.

FRT Principle 8

Since addiction and the codependency that enables it are chronic conditions, it is recommended that the addict and codependents develop ongoing support beyond the first year of continuous sobriety.

> NIDA Principle 6:
> *Behavioral therapies—including individual, family, or group counseling—are the most commonly used forms of drug abuse treatment. Behavioral therapies vary in their focus and may involve addressing a patient's motivation to change, providing incentives for abstinence, building skills to resist drug use, replacing drug-using activities with constructive and rewarding activities, improving problem-solving skills, and facilitating better interpersonal relationships. Also, participation in group therapy and other peer support programs during and following treatment can help maintain abstinence.*

The FRT therapist is well-versed in behavioral therapy, and behavioral change is an integral part of the recovery process for all family members. The advantage of a therapy which extends for more than 30, 60, or 90 days is that the addict can receive substantial ongoing support and reinforcement for solidifying new behavior patterns that replace old habits that may have existed for years, or even decades. In the process of recovery, it generally becomes apparent that there is a broad range of life areas in which adopting new behaviors will benefit the addict. Over time, there is room for more nuanced and extensive change, as well as the opportunity to build additional life skills.

Conducting family therapy is essential to the work of the FRT therapist, who is skilled at working with a wide range of interpersonal relationships. The first sentence in the above principle includes the phrase, "family, or group counseling." Long-term family counseling, which is central to the FRT model, is necessary to address and change the enabling homeostasis of the addict's family. In the course of a one-to three-day family program at a residential treatment center, behavioral change on the part of family members may well be discussed. But change happens over time, and the process of shifting old, entrenched patterns and adopting new ones needs much longer than a few days to establish. Just as the addict's addictive behavior patterns may have existed for decades, the family's codependency may have become established over years of attempting to deal with addiction, and indeed, may have been present for generations.

Group therapy is also integral to the FRT model. The FRT therapist is very familiar with the local "peer support programs," and attendance at group meetings is required as part of the treatment process. Support programs encourage and model behavior change, which is fundamental to the recovery process. The therapist can facilitate entry of the addict or family member into a local support group and can often introduce the newcomer to other recovering individuals who attend a particular meeting.

The following FRT Principles speak to the therapist's need to understand the breadth of different therapy approaches and the variety of paths to recovery, including group support programs:

FRT Principle 4
During the first year of treatment, the FRT therapist monitors, assesses, and guides the family in an integrated treatment process, which addresses biological, psychological, social, and spiritual recovery.

FRT Principle 6
The FRT therapist must be well-versed in the 12 Steps and have a thorough understanding and appreciation for the fundamental role that mutual aid programs play in recovery from codependency and addiction.

FRT Principle 7
The FRT therapist, who is a state-licensed medical or mental health professional, must be knowledgeable and experienced in many paths to growth and recovery. Ideally, the therapist is engaged in a personal recovery practice,

whether 12-Step or other, in which capacity, the therapist stands shoulder-to-shoulder with the family members.

> NIDA Principle 7:
> Medications are an important element of treatment for many patients, especially when combined with counseling and other behavioral therapies. For example, methadone, buprenorphine, and naltrexone (including a new long-acting formulation) are effective in helping individuals addicted to heroin or other opioids stabilize their lives and reduce their illicit drug use. Acamprosate, disulfiram, and naltrexone are medications approved for treating alcohol dependence. For persons addicted to nicotine, a nicotine replacement product (available as patches, gum, lozenges, or nasal spray) or an oral medication (such as bupropion or varenicline) can be an effective component of treatment when part of a comprehensive behavioral treatment program.

In Family Recovery Therapy, medical doctors, including physicians and psychiatrists specializing in addiction, are often part of the treatment team. The significant issue, to both FRT and NIDA, is that medications can be used to *support* recovery, but not to *replace* robust addiction treatment. NIDA suggests medications can be "an important element of treatment ... when combined with counseling and other behavioral therapies" and that medication "can be an effective component of treatment when part of a comprehensive behavioral treatment program." Similarly stated:

FRT Principle 10
Medically Assisted Treatment may be necessary, if medication is used in the service of recovery and not as a substitute for recovery.

It is important to note that, unfortunately, some of the drugs prescribed to aid treatment can themselves become addictive. And, sadly, medical doctors have played a role in over-prescribing drugs, particularly Oxycontin and other narcotics. This is not news. On January 31, 2018, the *Washington Post* reported that doctors prescribed 20.8 million narcotic pills to residents of Williamson, West Virginia, a town with a population of 3,200 (Bever). That worked out to 6,500 pills per resident! And, some years ago, several recovering clients in my practice told me of a local medical doctor who would, for fifty dollars in cash, write a prescription for any narcotic—which could be resold at a hefty profit. This doctor, as well as many, many others, have become virtual "drug dealers," fueling part of our opioid crisis, and leading to untold suffering, immense costs, and numerous deaths.

Today, opiate addicts in treatment are typically prescribed buprenorphine. Buprenorphine, itself, is an addictive drug, not unlike methadone. Yes, it is better to have an addict get reliable drugs from a known source instead of from drug dealers on the streets. And, yes, some addicts will benefit from this medical stabilization as long as it is part of a robust treatment, just as would any individual who has medical or mental health needs.

The FRT therapist collaborates with psychiatrists and medical doctors to guide addicts through the long-term treatment they will need to achieve and sustain sobriety. This issue is complex, but an ethical doctor would agree that the long-term goal of addiction recovery is to help the addict maintain a stable and healthy lifestyle, hopefully without reliance on addictive drugs. There are situations that are exceptions, such as when an individual suffers from chronic pain, in which continued use of a prescribed, but addictive, substance is warranted, and is medically monitored, so as to provide the needed pharmacological assistance without risk of provoking relapse.

> NIDA Principle 8:
> *An individual's treatment and services plan must be assessed continually and modified as necessary to ensure that it meets his or her changing needs. A patient may require varying combinations of services and treatment components during the course of treatment and recovery. In addition to counseling or psychotherapy, a patient may require medication, medical services, family therapy, parenting instruction, vocational rehabilitation, and/or social and legal services. For many patients, a continuing care approach provides the best results, with the treatment intensity varying according to a person's changing needs.*

Of course, reputable Residential Treatment Programs (RTCs) and Intensive Outpatient Programs (IOPs) understand that their 30-, 60-, or 90-day programs are only the beginning of treatment, and program staff will recommend that the addict "seek some form of long-term continuing care." As NIDA states, "*A patient may require varying combinations of services and treatment components during the course of treatment and recovery.*" And although NIDA's eighth principle names the fact that several other therapies, including "family therapy," may be useful, the primary focus is still on the addict. The transfer from short-term detox and stabilization in residential treatment to the next phase, long-term continuing care, is precisely where the current addiction treatment paradigm often drops the ball. Rarely is it clearly established before the addict leaves the residential program what will constitute the next phase of care, and even less frequently is there a seamless transfer from one program to the next. Again, in the words of addiction psychiatrist Timmen Cermak, also quoted in Chapter 2, "No one deserves to be a part of this (treatment) continuum unless they do it in a way that's integrated with what came before them and what comes after them. Their services need to be constructed in that way" (personal communication, 2018).

In the current, addict-focused treatment approach, when the addict—the "problem person"—is "sent away," the codependents and family members typically hope that the "problem" will be "fixed" and that their anxiety and all their difficulties will diminish. This is generally deemed a "success" by the family: the "addict is sober." Commonly, the family system has not been engaged in treatment, nor have family members received the help they need to address their codependency, mistrust, lack of intimacy, and fear. Simply taking alcohol away from an alcoholic will leave the family dynamics unchanged, and the alcoholic and the family members will still be in dire need of help. In addition, in poorly differentiated families, a multi-generational unconscious projection process can take place in which the alcoholic *must* be "the problem." In this situation, the family will resist treatment and balk at change, and will unconsciously undermine the alcoholic's recovery in order to maintain or re-establish the pre-existing homeostasis.

How would the typically impaired, newly sober addict, and their unrecovered family, find the "various combinations of service and treatment" that NIDA recommends? With difficulty, and, in some cases, not at all. The majority of the time, the addict goes through detox and a short course of stabilizing treatment, and is discharged with a piece of paper listing "recommendations." Both the addict and the family are left without sufficient support and resources to effectively point them to the next step or to help them grapple with the complex and extensive damage to their bio-psycho-social-spiritual development which possibly has been derailed by years—even decades, or generations—of addiction and codependency. Neither the addict nor the family is firmly on a path of recovery.

In my case, I was an active addict who, in 1979, simply walked into a social support group and followed the guidance I was given to not drink, one day at a time. It took nearly three years of sobriety, and continuing to go to social support groups, for me to benefit from additional resources—physicians, psychotherapists, outpatient treatment—that I needed to address the developmental deficits resulting from growing up in a loveless, alcoholic home and spending 25 years as an active addict.

When I was 18, my mother went to an Al-Anon meeting. She listened and learned and realized that she did not have to live with an angry drunk. After attending a few meetings, she said to my father, "Either you stop drinking or I will divorce you." Of course, without help, he could not stop. My mother divorced him, he continued to drink and use, and 15 years later, at the age of 56, he died an early death as a result of his substance dependence.

For purposes of illustration, I'd like to compare my own family's experience with what could have happened when I was a child, had the FRT model been in existence and had my family been in treatment with an FRT therapist. I'd like to imagine myself as the FRT therapist who actually treated my family many years ago.

If I were an FRT therapist treating my family of origin, I would have initiated treatment with my mother (FRT Principle 14). I would have educated her about addiction, introduced her to social support and mutual aid groups (Al-Anon, in this case), and described my proposed course of treatment for her and her family. In time, I would have worked with her to bring in my father, and educated him about addiction and treatment. Since my father would have wanted to keep his family intact—his wife and four children—I imagine the odds are good that he would have entered addiction treatment and begun his recovery. (His wife telling him he had to get sober or she would leave him was a great motivator.) I would have referred him to a social support group, conducted therapy with both of my parents, and coordinated with any other professional or support services they needed. Once the parents were stabilized, we would have turned our attention to their teenage son (me), who had already been demonstrating early signs of alcoholism. I would have proposed ways to work with him to stop him from using alcohol and to curb his acting-out behavior, and I would have educated him about addiction. And this intervention on him in his early teen years would possibly have significantly impacted the future trajectory of his life and his decades-long struggle with alcohol.

Sadly, the FRT model did not exist then. My father died a painful, early death, my mother lived out the rest of her life as a resentful and bitter woman, and their son (me) was an active addict for 25 years who nearly died a number of times.

Several FRT Principles refer to aspects of addiction treatment included in NIDA's Principle 8. FRT Principles 1, 2, and 8 address the chronic nature of addiction and codependency, the need for long-term support for both, and the fact that recovery can be multi-faceted:

FRT Principle 1
Addiction is a chronic, relapsing, treatable medical disease with profound mental and physical consequences. Addicts will need long-term, possibly lifelong, recovery support, which can take many forms.

FRT Principle 2
Effective treatment of addiction usually involves treatment of codependents, because codependents enable addiction. Codependency is a chronic relationship pattern that has profound mental and physical consequences and is characterized by an obsessive focus on other people. Codependents may need lifelong recovery support, which can take many forms.

FRT Principle 8
Since addiction and the codependency that enables it are chronic conditions, it is recommended that the addict and codependents develop ongoing support beyond the first year of continuous sobriety.

Additional FRT Principles address the breadth of ancillary resources mentioned in NIDA's Principle 8 that can be helpful in the recovery process for the addict and their family. FRT Principle 4 speaks to the role of the FRT therapist in guiding an integrated treatment process that embraces biological, psychological, social, and spiritual recovery, and FRT Principle 5 describes the breadth of therapeutic resources which an addict or their family may benefit from in the course of recovery. FRT Principle 9 addresses the role of the FRT therapist in monitoring and referring the addict or a family member to other providers for specialized help with medical, mental health, or other problems:

FRT Principle 4
During the first year of treatment, the FRT therapist monitors, assesses, and guides the family in an integrated treatment process, which addresses biological, psychological, social, and spiritual recovery.

FRT Principle 5
As the treatment team leader, the FRT therapist guides the family throughout the continuum of care and collaborates with all supportive therapeutic services, which may include other treatment providers, interventionists, treatment programs, physicians, and any other adjunctive services.

FRT Principle 9
Treatment includes monitoring for co-occurring mental and physical health problems and providing appropriate referrals as needed.

> *NIDA Principle 9:*
> *Many drug-addicted individuals also have other mental disorders. Because drug abuse and addiction—both of which are mental disorders—often co-occur with other mental illnesses, patients presenting with one condition should be assessed for the other(s). And when these problems co-occur, treatment should address both (or all), including the use of medications as appropriate.*

FRT Principles 9 and 10 speak directly to the issues of assessing and treating mental health disorders that may appear in the process of recovery:

FRT Principle 9
Treatment includes monitoring for co-occurring mental and physical health problems and providing appropriate referrals as needed.

FRT Principle 10
Medically Assisted Treatment may be necessary if medication is used in the service of recovery and not as a substitute for recovery.

An addict entering addiction treatment may suffer from multiple substance-induced mental disorders (psychological problems caused by the addictive substances and a substance-using lifestyle) in addition to their presenting substance use disorder. These can include anxiety and/or depression, issues with eating or sleeping, sexual problems, and personality disorders, as well as problems with relationships. How can the substance-induced mental disorders, that will subside in time when remission has been established, be differentiated from ongoing mental disorders? It is probably unlikely that any non-substance use-related mental health problems will be accurately diagnosed during the brief time an addict is in a residential program.

In the FRT model, a licensed mental health professional, the FRT therapist, monitors the addict and family members throughout the first year of continuous

Chapter 4. Effective Treatment—FRT's Principles and Federal Guidelines

sobriety. The FRT therapist can observe and differentiate symptoms that resolve from those that do not, *both* for the addict *and* for the family members, and can make referrals for further assessment and treatment. While NIDA does not address the mental health needs of the codependents, in addiction recovery, these needs require attention and treatment, if the addict and the codependents are to achieve and sustain recovery. And, as noted in FRT Principles 4 and 5, the FRT therapist coordinates treatment with doctors and other adjunctive professionals to address the long-term mental health needs of both the addict and the family members:

FRT Principle 4
During the first year of treatment, the FRT therapist monitors, assesses, and guides the family in an integrated treatment process, which addresses biological, psychological, social, and spiritual recovery.

FRT Principle 5
As the treatment team leader, the FRT therapist guides the family throughout the continuum of care and collaborates with all supportive therapeutic services, which may include other treatment providers, interventionists, treatment programs, physicians, and any other adjunctive services.

> NIDA Principle 10:
> *Medically assisted detoxification is only the first stage of addiction treatment and by itself does little to change long-term drug abuse. Although medically assisted detoxification can safely manage the acute physical symptoms of withdrawal and can, for some, pave the way for effective long-term addiction treatment, detoxification alone is rarely sufficient to help addicted individuals achieve long-term abstinence. Thus, patients should be encouraged to continue drug treatment following detoxification. Motivational enhancement and incentive strategies, begun at initial patient intake, can improve treatment engagement.*

FRT Principle 10 reflects a philosophy similar to that expressed in NIDA's Principle 10:

FRT Principle 10
Medically Assisted Treatment may be necessary if medication is used in the service of recovery and not as a substitute for recovery.

Detoxification is only the first phase of treatment. By itself, it does not change the long-standing behavior patterns and complex developmental, relationship, and other problems that commonly accompany addiction. Medical assistance may be required in order to assure an addict's safety in the detox process. When an FRT therapist is the "case manager" from the beginning of treatment, "medically assisted detoxification" occurs in the context of comprehensive, long-term, family-system treatment.

It is natural for doctors and other staff at a detox facility to "take charge," create treatment plans, and make referrals. This is typical of the current, established, and fragmented system of addiction treatment that has endured for decades. In the standard continuum of care, there is no one individual who is evaluating and coordinating the long-term process. In contrast, when an FRT therapist oversees treatment from the beginning, going forward, it both minimizes diversion of the addict and family to facilities and resources that are not a good fit, and eliminates the risk of fragmentation and confusion, which can happen if the addict or family is pointed in a variety of directions at the same time. This process is addressed in FRT Principles 4 and 5:

FRT Principle 4
During the first year of treatment, the FRT therapist monitors, assesses, and guides the family in an integrated treatment process, which addresses biological, psychological, social, and spiritual recovery.

FRT Principle 5
As the treatment team leader, the FRT therapist guides the family throughout the continuum of care and collaborates with all supportive therapeutic services, which may include other treatment providers, interventionists, treatment programs, physicians, and any other adjunctive services.

It is essential that the FRT therapist, as "case manager," is assertive, and coordinates treatment with the detox facility staff. We need to let the detox facility know that this is "our" case, and that the addict, upon stabilization and discharge, will be relying on our guidance as we determine the next phase of treatment. Once the detox facility staff understands that "someone else is the case manager," they will generally gladly cooperate in coordinating decisions about future treatment. Working with the detox facility staff can be challenging, however, since the facility's medical director, who is generally the person with the power to authorize collaboration, is often difficult to reach. Multiple phone calls, patience, and diligent effort may be required to reach the medical director of a detox center. Without the focused attention of the FRT therapist, the addict and family may find themselves in a state of confusion about next steps, which can hinder or even stop the recovery process in its tracks.

> NIDA Principle 11:
> *Treatment does not need to be voluntary to be effective. Sanctions or enticements from family, employment settings, and/or the criminal justice system can significantly increase treatment entry, retention rates, and the ultimate success of drug treatment interventions.*

While none of the FRT principles directly address the issue of sanctions and enticements, these are inherent in the work of Family Recovery Therapy. An FRT therapist works with the *family system*, and may include the wider community the addict is a part of: colleagues, peers, and recreational groups, for example.

The fact that FRT begins with treating the codependents is significant, because it is their boundaries and conditions that can affect the behavior of the addict. "Sanctions and enticements" can be created and supported by the FRT therapist, who can guide the enablers to stop enabling, thus leaving the addict to face a new and often painful reality of life without cushions—the lights are turned on, the addict's addiction is not only acknowledged, but confronted, and will no longer be enabled. Here are some examples:

- A spouse who says, "Either you enter treatment, or I will divorce you."
- An employee whose boss says, "Either you enter treatment, or I will fire you."
- A parent of an adult child who says, "Either you enter treatment, or I will cut you off."
- A court that says, "Either you enter treatment, or I will put you in jail."

Family Recovery Therapy usually begins with the codependents: they typically make the first call to the therapist. The FRT therapist must help the codependents reach the point where they will no longer tolerate addiction in their lives. As stated earlier, codependent family members typically are in denial of their role in perpetuating the family system's homeostasis, and the first task is to enlist them in the, often slow, unfolding process of education and psychotherapy. Initially, they are looking for help to "fix the addict," and we—acting in a role similar to the social structures named in NIDA Principle 11—need to educate them about the reality of the systemic disorder of addiction and how Family Recovery Therapy works. Several scenarios are possible, depending on the recovery level of the codependents involved:

- Some codependents quickly understand and we can move directly into including the addict in the process.
- Some codependents may need to be in treatment for a long time, perhaps for years, as they utilize psychotherapy and social support groups to strengthen themselves, learn to establish boundaries, and prepare for an intervention process that may facilitate the addict's recovery, or may require them to let go of the relationship with their addict, if he or she resists help.
- Some codependents, for various reasons, never find the self-agency to change. They continue to live in enmeshed, poorly differentiated, addicted families, enabling the addict, and possibly passing this disease on to the next generation.

FRT Principles 2 and 3 speak to the chronic nature of codependency, and the fact that the family *system* suffers from addiction and codependency:

FRT Principle 2
Effective treatment of addiction usually involves treatment of codependents, because codependents enable addiction. Codependency is a chronic relationship pattern that has profound mental and physical consequences and is

characterized by an obsessive focus on other people. Codependents may need lifelong recovery support, which can take many forms.

FRT Principle 3
In Family Recovery Therapy, the client in treatment is the family system that suffers from both addiction and codependency.

> **NIDA Principle 12:**
> **Drug use during treatment must be monitored continuously, as lapses during treatment do occur. Knowing their drug use is being monitored can be a powerful incentive for patients and can help them withstand urges to use drugs. Monitoring also provides an early indication of a return to drug use, signaling a possible need to adjust an individual's treatment plan to better meet his or her needs.**

FRT Principle 11 speaks directly to the significance of drug testing in addiction treatment:

FRT Principle 11
Regular drug testing is a powerful tool and will be used in addiction treatment.

Drug testing serves as a prophylactic, as an intervention to support remission and sobriety, and as a way to quickly discover and intervene when a relapse has occurred. It is not unusual for addicts to relapse in early recovery. Catching a relapse quickly, and applying consequences immediately, is often the turning point in an addict's commitment to treatment. And relapse for an addict who has been substance-free for a while may offer, for the first time, an opportunity for the addict to finally acknowledge that they are powerless over their addiction, and to ultimately commit to treatment. It is important to remember that an addict in early recovery is only a substance-free addict struggling to adjust to a world without drugs. It may take a considerable length of time for an addict's prefrontal cortex to develop the neuronal pathways necessary to understand their disease.

> *NIDA Principle 13:*
> *Treatment programs should test patients for the presence of HIV/AIDS, hepatitis B and C, tuberculosis, and other infectious diseases as well as provide targeted risk-reduction counseling, linking patients to treatment if necessary. Typically, drug abuse treatment addresses some of the drug-related behaviors that put people at risk of infectious diseases. Targeted counseling focused on reducing infectious disease risk can help patients further reduce or avoid substance-related and other high-risk behaviors. Counseling can also help those who are already infected to manage their illness. Moreover, engaging in substance abuse treatment can facilitate adherence to other medical treatments. Substance*

> *abuse treatment facilities should provide onsite, rapid HIV testing rather than referrals to offsite testing—research shows that doing so increases the likelihood that patients will be tested and receive their test results. Treatment providers should also inform patients that highly active antiretroviral therapy (HAART) has proven effective in combating HIV, including among drug-abusing populations, and help link them to HIV treatment if they test positive.*

The FRT therapist understands that addicts engage in high-risk behavior and therefore they need to be evaluated for, and receive appropriate treatment for, a variety of drug use-related or other medical issues. Several FRT Principles (4, 5, 9, and 10) speak to the ongoing need to assess and refer the addict for appropriate medical or psychiatric care in the course of treatment:

FRT Principle 4
During the first year of treatment, the FRT therapist monitors, assesses, and guides the family in an integrated treatment process, which addresses biological, psychological, social, and spiritual recovery.

FRT Principle 5
As the treatment team leader, the FRT therapist guides the family throughout the continuum of care and collaborates with all supportive therapeutic services, which may include other treatment providers, interventionists, treatment programs, physicians, and any other adjunctive services.

FRT Principle 9
Treatment includes monitoring for co-occurring mental and physical health problems and providing appropriate referrals as needed.

FRT Principle 10
Medically Assisted Treatment may be necessary if medication is used in the service of recovery and not as a substitute for recovery.

The FRT therapist recognizes that the family members of addicts are also subject to severe stress and may engage in risky and potentially harmful activities themselves, although, unless drug use is a compensatory behavior for a family member, the actual medical issues are likely to be different from those an addict may exhibit. However, just as for addicts, family members are monitored for co-occurring mental and physical problems, and given appropriate referrals.

I can't imagine that any trained and ethical individual working in the addiction treatment industry would disagree with NIDA's principles. Doubtless, both independent drug counselors and treatment programs are familiar with the principles and use them to guide their work. However, even when counselors and treatment centers are well grounded in NIDA's principles, there remain some significant drawbacks to the current addict-focused treatment approach. I have pointed out the problems: an addict who is intervened on, sent to detox, then on to an IOP or RTC, would typically come into short-term contact with a number of providers, some perhaps only once. And these providers would come into contact only briefly with many short-term clients. Typically, treatment would entail little or no contact between treatment staff and the rest of the family, the codependent enablers, and other impacted family members. The process lacks cohesion, consistency, and efficacy.

The missing piece, of course, is what this book is about—an FRT therapist, a single professional, hand-holding and guiding the impaired, medically and mentally ill individuals in an addicted family system, from day one, through the myriad steps to remission and restored development. Family Recovery Therapy both incorporates the concepts contained in NIDA's *Principles of Drug Treatment* and takes addiction treatment a few steps further toward improving outcomes by ensuring continuity of care, not just for the addict, but for the entire family system.

And, notably, Family Recovery Therapy takes addiction treatment beyond NIDA's principles in stating that treatment will almost always begin with the enablers. NIDA views treatment through the current, dominant, addict-centered paradigm. Proponents of this prevailing treatment approach fail to recognize that addiction is a *systemic* problem—and that it is usually a family member who first reaches out for help. This concept, central to FRT, is spelled out in FRT Principle 14:

FRT Principle 14
   Typically, a member of the enabling subsystem contacts the treatment provider. It is vital that the provider begin to engage the caller in the Family Recovery Therapy treatment model during this first contact.

CHAPTER 5

Bowen's Theory of Family Systems

An FRT therapist is a licensed mental health professional who has been through a process of graduate school education, supervised internships, and state licensing exams, and is trained to understand and treat relationships, particularly couples and families, as well as to work with individuals. There are many theoretical approaches to working with families, but the Bowen Theory (Bowen, 1966) stands out as perhaps the most coherent and applicable to treating families in the throes of addiction. In the course of their studies, interns on a path to becoming therapists are encouraged to choose a theoretical orientation. The state licensing exam process in California requires candidates to base their presentation of a case on their preferred theoretical orientation. Many of my fellow classmates and I chose the Bowen Theory as a perspective for our assessment and treatment planning, both for the licensing exam, and for our future work as therapists. For ease of understanding, I include below a summary of Bowen's work, which serves as a foundation for my work, and informs my thinking in the case studies, which are presented in Part Two of this book.

The first section of this chapter presents the work of Murray Bowen in an unedited 10-page excerpt of Chapter 8, "Transgenerational Models," Section 8, "Interlocking Theoretical Concepts" from *Family Therapy, Ninth Edition* (Goldenberg et al., pp. 194–203 © 2017 South Western, a part of Cengage, Inc. Reproduced by permission. www.cengage.com/permissions). The excerpt from Chapter 8 is included here, both as a resource and as vital foundational material for understanding the FRT model. In the second section, "Bowen's Theory of Family Systems: A Foundation of Family Recovery Therapy," I describe how Bowen's views inform the work of FRT.

Section 1—Excerpt from Family Therapy, ninth edition (Goldenberg et al., 2017)

Chapter 8: Transgenerational Models
LO 2—Eight Interlocking Theoretical Concepts

Bowen's theory of the family as an emotional relationship system consists of eight interlocking concepts. Six address emotional processes taking place in the nuclear and extended families; two concepts—emotional cutoff and societal regression—speak to the emotional processes across generations in a family and in society. All eight constructs are interlocking, so none is fully understandable apart from the others (Kerr, 2003).

The eight concepts are tied together by the underlying premise that *chronic anxiety is omnipresent in life. While it may manifest itself differently, and with different degrees of intensity depending on specific family situations and differing cultural considerations, chronic anxiety is an inevitable part of nature. Bowen viewed chronic anxiety as a biological phenomenon that humans have in common with all forms of life* (Friedman, 1991). *From this natural systems perspective, past generations transmit chronic anxiety, which impacts family members as they balance togetherness and individual self-differentiation.*

Anxiety is the sense of arousal in an organism when it perceives a real or imagined threat. In humans, anxiety stimulates the emotional system, overriding the cognitive system and leading to behavior that is automatic or uncontrolled (Kerr, 2003). *Anxiety is inevitably aroused as families struggle to balance the pressures toward togetherness as well as toward individuation. If greater togetherness prevails, imbalance results and the family moves toward increased emotional functioning and less individual autonomy, leading the person to experience increased chronic anxiety.*

Consider the case of a high school senior who comes from a working-class family in which a sense of togetherness prevails over an appreciation of the individuality of its members. She has just been accepted to a college in another state and has been offered a scholarship. As the family has only limited financial means, the scholarship represents a major opportunity. In a family such as this, the other members might subtly or explicitly pressure the young woman not to take this chance. Let's say that part of her wants to go while a part of her understands (because of the submerged ebb and flow of family dynamics) that she shouldn't go. The chance exists that the family demands for togetherness could keep this young woman feeling anxious, from finding herself as an individual and achieving important life goals. Chronic anxiety, then, represents the underlying basis of all symptomatology; its only antidote is resolution through differentiation (see next section), the process by which an individual learns to chart his or her own direction rather than perpetually following the guidelines of family and others.

LO 3—According to Family Systems Theory, Eight Forces Shape Family Functioning:

1. *Differentiation of self*
2. *Triangles*
3. *Nuclear family emotional system*
4. *Family projection process*
5. *Emotional cutoff*
6. *Multigenerational transmission process*
7. *Sibling position*
8. *Societal regression*

LO 4—Differentiation of Self

The cornerstone of the Bowen family systems theory is the notion of forces within the family that lead to individuality and the opposing forces that make for togetherness. Both intrapsychic and interpersonal issues are involved here. In the former, the person must, in the face of anxiety, develop the ability to separate feelings from thinking and to choose whether to be guided in a particular instant by intellect or emotion. In the latter, he or she must be able to experience intimacy with others but separate as an autonomous individual from being caught up in any emotional upheaval sweeping the family. The well-differentiated person is able to balance thinking and feeling (adhering to personal convictions while expressing individual emotions) and at the same time retain objectivity and flexibility (remaining independent of the family's emotional pressures).

Differentiation of self, says Bowen, reflects the extent to which a person is able to distinguish between the intellectual process and the feeling process of what he or she is experiencing. Differentiation of self is demonstrated by the degree to which a person can think, plan, and follow his or her own values or convictions, particularly around anxiety-provoking issues, without having behavior automatically driven by the emotional cues from others. One way people can demonstrate (especially to therapists) their degree of relative differentiation is through speaking in I-statements (reflective of I-positions), that is, statements that verbalize the degree of separation an individual feels vis-à-vis others.

BOX 5.1 CLINICAL NOTE

A Feminist Challenge

Some feminists such as Hare-Mustin (1978) and Lerner (1986) dispute Bowen's contentions regarding the differentiation of self. They argue that what Bowen seems to value here are qualities—being autonomous, relying on reason above emotion, being goal directed—for which men are socialized, while simultaneously devaluing those qualities—relatedness, caring for others, nurturing—for which women typically are socialized. However, Bowenians McGoldrick and Carter (2001) maintain that by distinguishing between thinking and feeling, Bowen was addressing the need for controlling one's emotional reactivity in order to control behavior and think about how we choose to respond and was not arguing for the suppression of authentic or appropriate emotional expression.

The degree to which one separates emotionally from parents in growing up is key to differentiation. In extreme cases, the attachment becomes a symbiosis in which parents and child cannot survive without one another. Such unresolved emotional attachment is equivalent to a high degree of undifferentiation in a person and in a family (Papero, 1995). (In other cultures, particularly those that focus on family togetherness, individuality and differentiation may be expressed differently.)

The ideal here is not to be emotionally detached or fiercely objective or without *feelings, but rather to strive for balance, achieving self-definition but not at the expense of losing the capacity for spontaneous emotional expression. Individuals should not be driven by feelings they do not understand.* As Hargrove (2009) notes, "The person who balances emotional reactivity and thinking without regard to the family's emotional process is thought to be functioning at a higher level of differentiation of self" (p. 290).

As Papero (1990, p. 48) *summarizes, "To the degree that one can thoughtfully guide personal behavior in accordance with well-defined principles in spite of intense anxiety in the family, he or she displays a level or degree of differentiation." For example, suppose our high school student mentioned previously chooses to go to college. After living away, she goes home at midyear to attend her sister's wedding. Amid the tensions that typically occur around such an event, to what degree is she drawn into family feuds, conflicts, coalitions, or emotional turmoil? Her differentiation can be gauged by the degree to which she is able to remain sufficiently involved to enjoy the pleasures of this family event while sufficiently separated so as not to be drawn into the family emotional system.*

Individuals with the greatest **fusion** between their thoughts and feelings (e.g., schizophrenics dealing with their families) *function most poorly; they are likely to be at the mercy of automatic or involuntary emotional reactions and tend to become dysfunctional even under low levels of anxiety. Unable to differentiate thought from feeling, such persons have trouble differentiating themselves from others and merge easily with whatever emotions dominate or sweep through the family. Highly fused persons, with few firmly held positions of their own, are apt to remain emotionally "stuck" throughout their lives in the position they occupied in their families of origin* (Bowen, 1978).

Bowen (1966) *early on introduced the concept of* **undifferentiated family ego mass**, *a term derived from psychoanalysis. The term conveys the idea of a family emotionally "stuck together," one in which "a conglomerate emotional oneness ... exists in all levels of intensity"* (p. 171). *The classic example of the symbiotic relationship between mother and child may represent the most intense version of this concept (in such families, a father's detachment may be the least intense). The degree to which any one member is involved in the family from moment to moment depends on that person's basic level of involvement in the family ego mass. Sometimes the emotional closeness can be so intense that family members feel they know each other's feelings, thoughts, fantasies, and dreams. This intimacy may lead to uncomfortable "overcloseness" and ultimately to a phase of mutual rejection between members. So emotional tensions in a family system shift over time (sometimes slowly, sometimes rapidly) in a series of alliances and splits.*

Bowen later recast the term undifferentiated family ego mass *into systems language as* fusion-differentiation. *Both terms underscore the transgenerational view that maturity and self-actualization demand that an individual become free of unresolved emotional attachments to his or her family of origin.* To illustrate his point, Bowen (1966) *proposed a theoretical scale (not an actual psychometric instrument) for evaluating an individual's differentiation level. As noted in Figure 5.1, the greater the degree of undifferentiation (no sense of self or a weak or unstable personal identity), the greater the emotional fusion into a common self with others (the undifferentiated family ego mass). A person with a strong sense of self ("These are my opinions.... This is who I am.... This is what I will do, but not this") expresses convictions and clearly defined beliefs. Such a person is said to be expressing a* solid self. *He or she does not compromise that self for the sake of marital bliss, to please parents, or to achieve family harmony.*

People at the low end of the scale are those whose emotions and intellect are so fused that their lives are dominated by the feelings of those around them. As a consequence, they feel anxious and are easily stressed into dysfunction. Fearful and emotionally needy, they sacrifice their individuality in order to ensure acceptance from others. They are expressing an undifferentiated pseudo self, *which they may deceive themselves into thinking is real but which is composed of the opinions and values of others. Those far fewer individuals at the high end are emotionally mature. They can think, feel, and take actions on their own despite external pressures to fall in line. Because their intellectual or rational functioning remains relatively (although not completely) dominant during stressful periods, they are more certain of who they are and what they believe, freer to make judgments independent of any emotional turmoil around them. In the midrange are persons with relative degrees of fusion or differentiation. Note that the scale eliminates the need for the concept of normality. It is possible for people at the low end of the scale to keep their lives in emotional equilibrium and stay free of symptoms, thus appearing "normal." However, they are more vulnerable to stress and, under stress, may develop symptoms from which they recover far more slowly than those at the high end of the scale.*

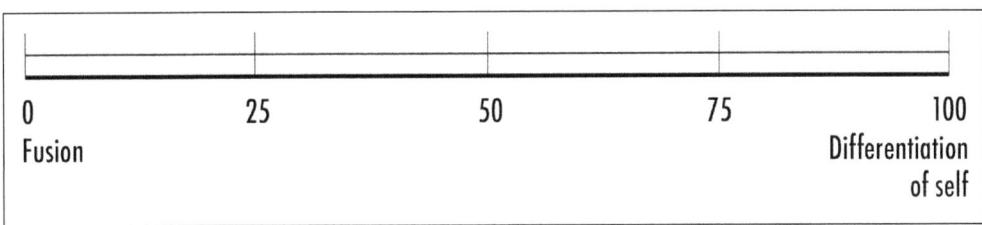

Figure 5.1 Bowen's theoretical differentiation-of-self scale distinguishes people according to the degree of fusion or differentiation between their emotional and intellectual functioning.

- Those at the lower level (0–25) are emotionally fused to the family and others, and lead lives in which their thinking is submerged and their feelings dominate.
- Those in the 25–50 range are still guided by their emotional system and the reactions of others; goal-directed behavior is present but carried out in order to seek the approval of others.
- In the 50–75 range, thinking is sufficiently developed so as not to be dominated by feeling when stress occurs, and there is a reasonably developed sense of self.

- *Those rare people functioning between 75 and 100 routinely separate their thinking from their feelings; they base decisions on the former but are free to lose themselves in the intimacy of a close relationship. Bowen (1978) considers someone at 75 to have a very high level of differentiation.*
- *Those over 60 constitute a small percentage of society.*

To summarize:

- Below 50 (low differentiation): tries to please others; supports others and seeks support; dependent; lacks capacity for autonomy; primary need for security; avoids conflict; little ability to independently reach decisions or solve problems.
- 51–75 (midrange differentiation): definite beliefs and values but tends to be overconcerned with the opinions of others; may make decisions based on emotional reactivity, especially whether significant others will disapprove.
- 76–100 (high differentiation): clear values and beliefs; goal directed; flexible; secure; autonomous; can tolerate conflict and stress; well-defined sense of solid self and less pseudo self (Roberto, 1992).

A person's level of differentiation also relates to the person's relative independence from others outside the family group. A moderate to high level of differentiation permits interaction with others without fear of fusion (losing one's sense of self in the relationship). While all relationships ranging from poorly to well-differentiated ones are in a state of dynamic equilibrium, the flexibility in that balance decreases as differentiation decreases. Figure 5.2 illustrates the varying degrees to which a person's functioning can be influenced by the relationship process.

Bowen family systems theory assumes that an instinctively rooted life force in every human propels the developing child to grow up to be an emotionally separate person, able to think, feel, and act as an individual. At the same time, a corresponding life force propels the child and family to remain emotionally connected. Because of these counterbalancing forces, no one ever achieves complete emotional separation from the family of origin. There are considerable differences in the amount of separation each of us accomplishes, including differences between siblings in the degree to which they emotionally separate from the family. The latter is due to characteristics of the different parental relationships established with each child, which we elaborate on later in this section.

LO 5—Triangles

Bowen family systems theory also emphasizes the emotional tension within an individual or in that person's relationships. For example, the greater the fusion in a couple, the more difficult it is to find a stable balance satisfying to both. One way to defuse such an anxious two-person relationship, according to Bowen (1978), is to triangulate—draw in a significant family member to form a three-person interaction. Triangulation is a common way that two-person systems under stress attempt to achieve stability (Hargrove, 2009).

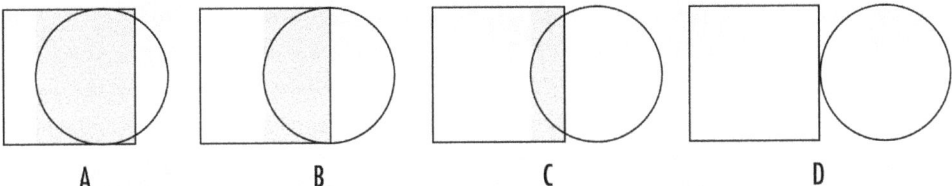

Figure 5.2 *Relationship A is one where the functioning of each person is almost completely determined by the relationship process. The degree to which individual functioning is either enhanced or undermined by the relationship is indicated by the shaded area. The clear area indicates the capacity for self-determined functioning while in a relationship. Relationships B and C are progressively better differentiated. Individual functioning, therefore, is less likely to be enhanced or undermined by the relationship process. Relationship D is theoretical for the human. It represents two people who can be actively involved in a relationship yet remain self-determined. Source:* Kerr and Bowen (1988), p. 71.

Think of a couple in therapy that are considering divorce. After weeks of hostility and mutual blaming, the therapist invited the couple to bring in their 16-year-old son and asks the young man, "What do you think of your parents getting a divorce?" The young man, looking very sad, says, "Finally, someone has asked me for my opinion." Each parent looks at each other and realizes that in their fused state of rage and anxiety, they have both neglected their son. They both take deep breaths and for the first time start talking more honestly about all their thoughts and feelings. As this example suggests, the basic building block in a family's emotional or relational system is the **triangle**. *During periods when anxiety is low and external conditions are calm, the dyad or two-person system may engage in a comfortable back-and-forth exchange of feelings. However, the stability of this situation is threatened if one or both participants get upset or anxious, either because of internal stress or from stress external to the pair. When a certain moderate anxiety level is reached, one or both partners often will involve a vulnerable third person.*

Let's continue the example of the divorcing couple and their son by suggesting that throughout their lives together, the son has often played the role of his parents' referee. A few weeks of family therapy go by, and the son tells his parents and the therapist that he feels that his father's frequent absences from home due to his sales job are the cause of his parents problems. The father becomes defensive and angry, and the mother becomes anxious. She now turns to the therapist and says, "That is one of the most important problems between us. He's never home. Certainly you see how painful this has been for me." Now the mother, perhaps with the son's collusion, wants to create a new triangle, this time with the therapist. The therapeutic goal is for the clients to view themselves as individual, differentiated selves as well as family members. However, if the therapist (as the third person in the triangle) loses emotional contact with the other two, the twosome will proceed to triangulate with someone else.

Bowen (1976) refers to the triangle as the smallest stable relationship system. By definition, a two-person system is unstable and forms a three-person system under stress as each partner creates a triangle in order to reduce the tension in their relationship.

When anxiety is so great that the three-person triangle can no longer contain the tension, the distress may spread to others (as when the family in our example tried to triangulate with the therapist). As more people become involved, the system may become a series of interlocking triangles, in some cases heightening the very problem the triangulations sought to resolve. For example, a distraught mother's request for help from her husband in dealing with their daughter is met with withdrawal by the father. As the mother–daughter conflict escalates, she communicates her distress to a son, who proceeds to get into conflict with his sister for upsetting their mother. What began as a mother–daughter conflict has now erupted into interlocking conflicts—between mother and daughter, brother and sister, and mother and father. Thus, triangles extend and interlock into ever-larger groups as tension increases (Kerr, 2003). Sometimes such triangulation can reach beyond the family, ultimately encompassing social agencies or the courts.

Generally speaking, the higher the degree of family fusion, the more intense and insistent the triangulating efforts will be. The least-well-differentiated person in the Family is particularly vulnerable to being drawn in to reduce tension. Often this person winds up being the identified patient. The higher a family member's degree of differentiation, the better that person will manage anxiety without creating triangles (Papero, 1995). Beyond seeking relief of discomfort, the family relies on triangles to help maintain an optimum level of closeness and distance between members while permitting them the greatest freedom from anxiety. Perhaps in our example, the father and mother might discuss the prospect of divorce with their son.

Kerr and Bowen (1988; Kerr, 2003) point out that triangulation has at least four possible outcomes: (a) a stable twosome can be destabilized by the addition of a third person (e.g., the birth of a child brings conflict to a harmonious marriage); (b) a stable twosome can be destabilized by the removal of a third person (a child leaves home and thus is no longer available to be triangulated into parental conflict); (c) an unstable twosome can be stabilized by the addition of a third person (a conflictual marriage becomes more harmonious after the birth of a child); and (d) an unstable twosome can be stabilized by the removal of a third person (conflict is reduced by getting a third person, say a mother-in-law who has consistently taken sides, out of the picture).

In another familiar example, conflict between siblings quickly attracts a parent's attention. Let us assume that the parent has positive feelings toward both children. If the parent can control his or her emotional responsiveness and manage not to take sides while staying in contact with both children, the emotional intensity between the siblings will diminish. As McGoldrick and Carter (2001) observe, involvement in triangles and interlocking triangles represents a key mechanism whereby patterns of relating to one another are transmitted over generations in a family.

Nuclear Family Emotional System

Bowen (1978) contends that people choose mates with levels of differentiation equivalent to their own. The relatively undifferentiated person will be attracted to a person who is equally fused to his or her family of origin. These poorly differentiated people, now married, likely will become highly fused and produce a family with the same characteristics. Bowen indicates that the resulting **nuclear family emotional system** will be unstable and will seek to reduce tension and maintain stability. *The greater the nuclear family's fusion, the increased likelihood of anxiety and potential instability, and the greater the family's propensity to seek resolution through fighting, distancing, exploiting the compromised functioning of one partner, or banding together over concern for a child* (Kerr, 1981).

Kerr and Bowen (1988) *note three possible symptomatic patterns in a nuclear family when partners are intensely fused. The greater the level of fusion in the marital dyad, the more frequently are these mechanisms likely to occur. Similarly, in a family with a high level of chronic anxiety, these mechanisms are at work continuously, their intensity or frequency changing in response to acute anxiety being experienced at the moment* (Papero, 1990). Each pattern described here is intensified by anxiety and, when the intensity reaches a sufficient level, results in a particular form of symptom development. The person (or relationship) who manifests the symptom is largely determined by the patterns of emotional functioning that predominate in a family system. The three patterns are as follows:

1. Physical or emotional dysfunction in a spouse, *sometimes chronic, an alternative to dealing directly with family conflict; the anxiety generated by the undifferentiated functioning of every family member is absorbed disproportionately by a symptomatic parent.*

2. Overt, chronic, unresolved marital conflict, *in which cycles of emotional distance and over closeness occur; both the negative feelings during conflict and the positive feelings for one another during close periods are likely to be equally intense in roller-coaster fashion; the family anxiety is being absorbed by the husband and wife.*

3. Psychological impairment in a child, *enabling the parents to focus on the child and ignore or deny their own lack of differentiation; as the child becomes the focal point of the family problem, the intensity of the parental relationship is diminished. Thus the family anxiety is absorbed in the child's impaired functioning; the lower a child's level of differentiation, the greater his or her vulnerability to increases in anxiety and dysfunction.* Furthermore, dysfunction in one spouse may take the form of an overadequate-underadequate reciprocity, *in which one partner takes on most or even all family responsibilities (earning a living, caring for the children, cooking, shopping, arranging a social life, and so on) while the other plays the counterpart role of being under-responsible (can't drive without anxiety, can't choose clothes, can't have friends to the house). Fused together, the two pseudo selves develop an arrangement in which one partner increasingly underfunctions while the other takes up the slack by assuming responsibility for them both.* When the tilt gets too great, according to Singleton (1982), the one giving up more pseudo self for the sake of family harmony becomes vulnerable to physical or emotional dysfunction.

In some cases, this pattern intertwines with marital conflict, as when the underadequate one complains of dominance, inconsiderateness, and so forth from the spouse. The overadequate one is more comfortable with the arrangement until the underadequate one complains or becomes so inadequate as to cause difficulties for the overadequate one. This problem is likely to be seen by the unsophisticated eye as belonging to the unhappy underadequate spouse rather than as a relationship problem for which both need help.

Almost any family will have one child who is more vulnerable to fusion than the others and thus likely to be triangulated into parental conflict. Any significant increase in parental anxiety triggers this child's dysfunctional behavior (in school, at home, or both), leading to even greater anxieties in the parent. In turn, the child's behavior becomes increasingly impaired, sometimes turning into a lifelong pattern of poor functioning.

The nuclear family emotional system is a multigenerational concept. Family systems theorists believe individuals tend to repeat in their marital choices and other significant relationships the patterns of relating learned in their families of origin and to pass along similar patterns to their children. The only effective way to resolve current family problems is to change the individual's interactions with his or her family of origin. As that person changes, others in emotional contact with him or her will make compensatory changes (McGoldrick & Carter, 2001). *As differentiation proceeds, all become less overreactive to the emotional forces sweeping through the family.*

Family Projection Process

Parents do not respond in the same way to each child in a family, despite any claims to the contrary. That is, they pass on their level of differentiation to the children in an un-even fashion: some emerge with a higher level than their parents, some with a lower level, and others with a more or less identical level (Papero, 1995). *In particular, those children more exposed to parental immaturity tend to develop greater fusion to the family than their more fortunate siblings and have greater difficulty separating smoothly from their parents. Responding to their mother's anxiety, they remain more vulnerable to emotional stresses within the family and consequently live lives more governed by emotional upheavals than do their brothers or sisters.*

*The fusion-prone, focused-on child is the one most sensitive to incipient signs of instability and other disturbances within the family. Bowen (1976) believed that poorly differentiated parents, themselves immature, select as the object of their attention the most infantile of all their children, regardless of his or her birth order in the family. This child receives the parents' own low levels of differentiation and becomes that way him- or herself. Bowen calls this transmission experience the **family projection process**. In many cases, this child is physically or mentally handicapped or psychologically unprotected in some fashion and pays the price by becoming poorly self-differentiated.*

The intensity of the family projection process is related to two factors: the degree of immaturity or undifferentiation of the parents and the level of stress or anxiety the family experiences. In a triangulating scenario described by Singleton (1982), the child responds anxiously to the mother's anxiety as principal caretaker. The mother becomes alarmed at what she perceives as the child's problem and becomes overprotective. Thus, a cycle is established in which the mother infantilizes the child, who in turn becomes demanding and impaired. The third leg of the triangle is supplied by the father, who is frightened by his wife's anxiety and by needing to calm her but, without dealing with the issues, plays a supportive role in her dealings with the child. As collaborators, the parents have now stabilized their relationship around a "disturbed" child and in the process perpetuated the family triangle. That person will be less able to function autonomously in the future.

LO 6—Emotional Cutoff

Children less involved in the projection process are apt to emerge with a greater ability to withstand fusion, to separate thinking and feeling. Those who are more involved try various strategies to separate upon reaching adulthood, or even before. They may attempt to insulate themselves from the family by geographic separation (moving to another state), through the use of psychological barriers (cease talking to parents), or by the self-deception that they are free of family ties because actual contact has been broken off. This latter experience was charmingly portrayed in the 2002 romantic comedy My Big Fat Greek Wedding, in which a Greek-American woman falls in love with a non–Greek man. The overly close family can't tolerate this relationship and at first fights to stop it. The movie is about the young woman's experience in separating. In time, everyone seems to come together in mutual respect. However, during the last scene, the bride's parents give the newly married couple a new house as a wedding gift, which is, of course, right next door to theirs. While cultural issues certainly play a role here, we witness a situation in which psychological gains of separation might be seen to have been mitigated by lingering family dynamics of overinvolvement.

Bowen (1976) considers such supposed freedom an **emotional cutoff**—*a flight of extreme emotional distancing in order to break emotional ties*—and not true emancipation. In Bowen's formulation, cutting oneself off emotionally from one's family of origin often represents a desperate effort to deal with unresolved fusion with one or both parents—a way of managing the unresolved emotional attachment to them. More likely than not, the person attempting the cutoff tends to deny to himself or herself that many unresolved conflicts remain with family-of-origin members. Kerr (1981) contends that emotional cutoff reflects *a problem* (underlying fusion between generations), solves *a problem* (reducing anxiety associated with making contact), and creates *a problem* (isolating people who might benefit from closer contact). As McGoldrick and Carter (2001) note, cutting off a relationship by physical or emotional distance does not end the emotional process but actually intensifies it. Cut off from siblings or parents, those individuals are apt to form new relationships (with a spouse or children) that are all the more intense and that may lead to further distancing and cutoffs from those new relationships.

Cutoffs occur most often in families in which there is a high level of anxiety and emotional dependence (Bowen, 1978). As both factors increase and greater family cohesiveness is expected, conflicts between family members may be disguised and hidden. Should the fusion-demanding situation reach an unbearable stage, some members may seek greater distance, emotionally, socially, perhaps physically, for self-preservation. When a family member insists on communication, it is apt to be superficial, inauthentic, and brief (short visits or phone calls during which only impersonal topics are discussed).

Bowen insisted that adults must resolve their emotional attachments to their families of origin. In a revealing paper (1972), he openly described his personal struggles to differentiate from his own family of origin. Without differentiation, Bowen argued, family therapists may unknowingly be triangulated into conflicts in their client families (much as they were as children in their own families), perhaps overidentifying with one family member or projecting onto another their own unresolved family conflicts. Family therapists need to ensure that unfinished business from their past does not intrude on current dealings with client families.

Section 2—Bowen's Theory of Family Systems:

A Foundation of Family Recovery Therapy

Many counselors and providers in the field of addiction treatment are recovering individuals who have completed the credentialing process to become Certified Alcohol & Drug Counselors. What differentiates the FRT therapist from other addiction treatment providers who work in the field is the breadth of their education and training—they are licensed mental health providers in addition to being educated in addiction. As a licensed mental health professional, the FRT therapist, at a minimum, has obtained a master's level degree in counseling or psychotherapy, and has received extensive education in diagnosing mental illness, psychological development, family systems theory, marriage and family relationships, cultural competency, ethics and the law, and a variety of approaches to psychotherapy. In addition, in order to become a licensed therapist, in California, for example, it is necessary both to accrue several thousand supervised intern hours working with individuals and families, and to pass rigorous state licensing exams.

Someone who has gained mastery of a subject can educate and pass on to others what they have learned. Drug and alcohol counselors often are addicts in recovery who have worked rigorously to achieve sobriety and establish a sober lifestyle. A drug counselor in a residential treatment program can hold the hand of the newly sober client and guide them through the initial days and weeks of sobriety. These counselors provide essential guidance and education in the early stages of an addict's path to achieve and sustain sobriety, and contribute a significant component to addiction treatment.

The FRT therapist, whether or not personally in recovery from addiction, has received some graduate training in drug and alcohol counseling as well as in psychotherapy. This preparation gives the therapist the capacity to foresee and address "what comes next" in the recovery process after the addict has detoxed and stabilized. When an addict has been using substances for some time, perhaps even for decades, and has built a lifestyle around feeding their addiction, their normal development has almost always been interrupted and delayed. Their addiction has taken their personal development "off-line," and their bio-psycho-social-spiritual growth has been impacted, especially if their addiction began before age 25. For the individual with a long history of addiction, possibly beginning at a young age, simply staying sober will not address the profound gaps in their development. The recovering addict will benefit from doing the work needed to acquire these missing elements in order to approach a level of development they would have achieved had addiction not interrupted their lives (see Appendix A).

In my case, I started drinking during my teen years, and didn't get sober until my late 30s. Initially, my psychological, emotional, and spiritual development were closer to that of a 16 year old than to someone who was 40. It took a number of years—with many kinds of help and substantial personal growth—for me to make up for my lost years.

Generally, an addict's relationships have been skewed as others have turned themselves into codependent pretzels in attempts to "help" their now "crazy" addicted family member, friend, or significant other. Significant emotional and psychological damage is incurred either in living with an addict, or in being raised by one. The dysfunctional homeostasis of these relationships will need to unwind and re-orient towards health, and each impacted individual will need to be restored to normal development, in order to achieve the optimal outcomes for the addict, the family members, and the family as a whole. The process of bio-psycho-social-spiritual healing may entail the use of many different therapeutic approaches over an extended period of time. Sustained healing for those willing to do the work will require commitment on the part of all participating family members to show up and do their own recovery work. Family Recovery Therapy is a model that elegantly and effectively guides all family members, individually and collectively, through a complex maze of modalities, approaches and therapies, while dealing with any resistance encountered in the process. The aim of FRT is to restore normal development and to achieve optimal health for each individual and each affected relationship.

Not a small task! However, addiction recovery is the very healing process needed. If an addict or a codependent admits powerlessness over their respective addiction, sincerely asks for guidance, and takes in the support that is offered, a successful outcome can be achieved. Millions have trod this path.

I believe that Murray Bowen offers an elegant, comprehensive, and easy-to-follow theory of family systems, although there are many other approaches to family therapy that can be used successfully as well. Below, I will review several major aspects of Bowen's work and explain how each relates to the work of the FRT therapist in intervening and guiding the impaired, addicted family through the first year of sobriety. The FRT therapist supports each family member's quest to achieve their optimal level of differentiation, encouraging each of them to slowly replace their feeling-based reactions with more rationally-based choices.

Differentiation of Self

As Bowen explained, each of us is driven by both our thoughts and our feelings. One's level of differentiation refers to the capacity of an individual to separate their feelings from their thoughts and to base their behavior on thinking rather than feeling. Those who are "highly differentiated" base their actions on rational thought, and those who are "poorly differentiated" tend to base their actions on feelings. Bowen points out that there are very few individuals who can *always* base their actions on rational thinking and not be swayed or overwhelmed by their feelings.

Addicted/codependent family systems exhibit various levels of differentiation, but the vast majority of families that are significantly impacted by addiction and codependency, over time, become poorly differentiated. Family members react to the ubiquitous craziness in their lives, and their behavior is prompted more often by emotion than by rational thought as they attempt to navigate the drama and incoherence of a family system in upheaval.

The good news is that Family Recovery Therapy works, and my experience is that the individuals who complete the initial year of treatment are well on their way towards restoring their underlying differentiation potential—if they continue to do the work of recovery, to stabilize their lives, and to grow. Of course, this process may take years, especially if the addiction or codependency started in the teen years, had a long course, or existed in prior generations of their family of origin.

The addict, including this author, has a diseased brain that craves its "medicine," the substance or behavior that can temporarily reduce our pain or give us pleasure. Craving dictates our choices, and these powerful feelings of desire, want, and need affect our actions. Of course, our behavior negatively impacts our attempts to have successful relationships and jobs, and significantly affects other aspects of our lives. The result is that we can feel disorganized and dysregulated, and can be unhappy. Because of our dysphoric mood, we futilely try to "get it together," and because of our diseased brain, we are unable to use our prefrontal cortex to rationally think our way out of our addiction or our bad feelings. We become more and more desperate—and use more and more of our substance—as we attempt to make the pain go away, but things get worse. Hopefully we become willing to reach out for and accept help. (An addict's willingness to accept help can often be delayed by a codependent who continues to enable the addiction in an attempt to try to reduce the codependent's own pain.)

In the process of pursuing relief from our feelings and seeking our substance, our healthy development is sidelined. We cannot fully benefit from any wisdom we might garner from life's positive experiences, which would lead to our healthy development—which leads to more bad feelings, and increased desire to numb ourselves in a never-ending downward spiral. In recovery, with the elimination of addictive substances, the addict slowly regains physical and emotional stability. As recovery continues, the addict begins to develop healthier relationships with healthier people and to return to a pre-addiction level of differentiation, or to attain an even a higher level of differentiation than experienced earlier. Slowly, the addict's healing brain and new environment offer him the opportunity to begin to think rationally, to use guidance, and to make sane decisions that lead to renewed self-confidence and hope.

As we have seen, the codependent is, of course, also impacted by addiction. Perhaps, before connecting with an addict, the soon-to-become codependent was a fairly differentiated individual, whose actions were based for the most part on rational thinking. But as the loved one slowly succumbs to addiction, the codependent becomes upset, and naturally tries to "help" the addict. As we know, only the addict can make the decision to choose help. Thus begins the codependent's downward spiral: the codependent offers help, the help does not work, more help is offered, more resistance is encountered, etc. Slowly, the codependent begins to experience fear, loss, confusion, anger, and hopelessness as the relationship deteriorates. The codependent begins to lose the capacity to differentiate feeling from thinking, and makes the majority of their decisions based on feelings.

Here, again, is Stephanie Brown's perspective on codependency (from a conversation with her, referenced in Chapter 2):

> Unhealthy codependency is developing an addictive emotional attachment to another person. The addict has an addictive emotional attachment to alcohol or substances or to being out of control in some way. The codependent develops exactly the same out-of-control emotional investment and attachment to a person. The center of the self of the codependent becomes invested in being able to control somebody else, which is never successful from a recovery frame. The codependent then deepens that intense attachment, abandoning the self to become invested in that attachment or bond to another [personal communication, 2021].

Trying to make an addict change, trying to help them, significantly impacts the codependent over time, as the codependent loses their ability to pursue their own lives, goals, and dreams. Years, and then decades, of this process render the codependent, as Bowen would say, "poorly differentiated," and as Al-Anon would say, "insane." The solution, FRT treatment, establishes goals for the codependent that are very similar to those of the addict. Just as the addict must let go of their attachment to their medicine, the codependent must let go of their attachment to the addict—and then must move their focus away from the addict. They must redirect their energy to their own development: regain sanity, reach their differentiation baseline or beyond, and develop a healthy lifestyle and healthy relationships to support their ongoing recovery.

It's very simple. One might imagine that a codependent could easily think, "Hey, this person has a disease, is an addict, and is resisting help—I'm out of here." No brainer—return to healthy differentiation.

But it's not easy. It takes time for the codependent's neuronal networks to shift, just as it does for an addict. The prior homeostasis, the previous "way things have always been," will change and be replaced by a healthier, steady state over time, as treatment, education, and practicing new behaviors help family members establish new ways of thinking and behaving.

The FRT therapist may spend 50 or 60 minutes a week in therapy with the codependent or addict. However, that still leaves 167 hours a week when even the most motivated addict or codependent will be immersed in their prior homeostasis, in the unconscious dynamics which pull them to "stay the same." More than just an hour or two of psychotherapy will be required to disrupt this homeostasis and establish healthy patterns of interacting. This is why FRT recommends that codependents attend social support groups where they can benefit from the group's reinforcement of recovery messages. 12-Step and other free programs are widely available and offer a comprehensive process for achieving the bio-psycho-social-spiritual recovery required for a return to full health.

There are many types of social support and mutual aid groups in existence, but the 12-Step groups are the most available of free support groups, and provide perhaps 90 percent of the long-established options. From a bird's-eye view, the 12-Step recovery process can be seen psychologically as an amalgam of multiple psychotherapeutic approaches: cognitive-behavioral, Rogerian, existential, transpersonal, relational, and psychodynamic; as well as providing experience in group therapy. Over time, the 12-Step process effectively addresses many of the bio-psycho-social-spiritual maladies that affect those whose development has been sidelined by addiction and codependency. (Hence the worldwide explosion of various 12-Step programs for many dozens of mankind's ills.)

Triangles

Each of us faces a dilemma. How do we develop a self that is fully differentiated and capable of making rational decisions despite the influence of others, and how do we form close, loving emotional attachments with others—where we drop into our heart, let go of the ego, and merge into loving oneness—without at the same time losing our ability to rationally act on our own behalf?

Once again, from Goldenberg et al. (p. 197):

> Bowen's theory assumes that an instinctively rooted life force in every human propels the developing child to grow up to be an emotionally separate person, able to think, feel, and act as an individual. At the same time, Bowen proposes that a corresponding life force, also instinctively rooted, propels the child and family to remain emotionally connected.

Conflict naturally arises when we enter into a relationship. One person, at a particular time, may want to be emotionally close, while the other, at the same time, may want to be alone, separate. Healthy people in healthy relationships make room for these differences, participating in an endless cycle of closeness/distance, trusting that it will balance out. However, even in the best of cases, conflict can arise, which leads to tension.

Almost by definition, addiction and codependency create stress that upsets a stable dyad, and the natural tendency is to bring others into the relationship to ease the tension. Addictive/codependent family systems are naturally prone to conflict, and unhealthy triangulation is common. For example, parents of a young adult addict can be at odds about how to manage their child. The mother wants to buy groceries and pay their son's rent; the father wants to withdraw financial support. The mother then turns to her own mother for emotional support and confirmation that she is doing "the right thing." The son-mother-grandmother triangle provides stability, but also fosters the son's addiction. One task of the FRT therapist is to help de-triangulate family systems that undermine recovery.

A codependent wife may triangulate others into her relationship with her addicted husband—for example, her mother-in-law. Her mother-in-law may then turn to another family member, perhaps her own brother, for help and support. A series of triangles may form in a family, even extending to multiple generations, as each person tries to reduce stress and "fix the problem" that can only be truly addressed by the addict. An addicted family's level of differentiation drops as the situation deteriorates.

In interpersonal conflicts, it is not unusual for individuals to adopt stances that can involve acting defeated, blaming, or taking charge. Steve Karpman, M.D., formalized these roles as Victim, Persecutor, and Rescuer (1968). He termed the dynamic interplay of the positions as "The Drama Triangle" and referred to the interactions as "games."

Proponents of Transactional Analysis, and later, psychotherapists in general, adopted these terms to describe unhealthy communication patterns. In dysfunctional systems—including codependent, enmeshed, or poorly differentiated

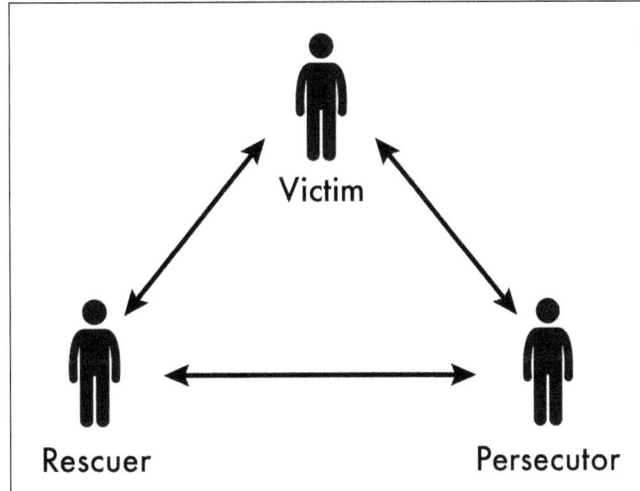

Figure 5.3 *The Drama Triangle.* The roles of Victim, Persecutor, and Rescuer in the Drama Triangle, with arrows indicating that people can rapidly switch from one role to another, even in the same conversation.

families—it is common for family members to adopt these roles in their interactions with each other. Family members may switch roles, and can often move quickly in and out of roles, as the dynamics in the relationships shift. Most individuals will be defensive if their "games" are pointed out. Family counseling can raise each family member's awareness of their behavior to the point that they can take personal responsibility for their actions and refrain from enacting any of the three roles. Each individual can learn to identify his or her own triggers, become aware of their responses, and consciously shift from an emotional to a rational reaction. Family members come to realize they are 100 percent responsible for their own attitudes, behavior, and lives, and can choose to simply stop playing a game. Below is a more detailed description of the behaviors common to each role. This description has been adapted from the writings of Claudia Black and Sharon Wegscheider-Cruze.

Victim:

There are two types of victims:

Pathetic Victim—"Poor me. I don't know how this happened."
Angry Victim—Pretends to be powerful, yet at same time denies responsibility. "Look what you've done to me."

- Takes little responsibility for actions or feelings.
- Discounts their capabilities: "There is nothing I can do." "I am not strong enough." "Everyone is against me."
- Places the majority of responsibility for success and failure on others.
- Complains about all the reasons why something cannot be done. Often plays the "yes-but game." When you suggest a change, they will say, "yes that is a good idea, but it won't work for me."
- Uses blame and guilt to manipulate others into doing what they want.
- Associates with people they can blame for their sorry state of affairs.
- Connects with people who will listen to their woes (rescuers).
- Predominant feelings: helplessness and hopelessness.

Persecutor:

- Plays the bad guy.
- Acts largely out of anger and rage.
- By criticizing, demeaning, and discounting others, the persecutor keeps the other two positions in motion—the victim abdicates responsibility for what is wrong, and the rescuer tries in vain to fix it.
- Maintains control by playing off the helplessness of the victim or the guilt of the rescuer. These ploys contribute to the persecutor's control, which generates a feeling of omnipotence.
- Criticizes others without giving guidance on how to improve. Tends to remind others of their past mistakes.
- Predominant feeling: anger.

Rescuer:

- Discounts the ability of others to solve their own problems.
- The proverbial knight in shining armor, selflessly puts their needs aside to come to the aid of others.
- Feeds information to victims that they want to hear, such as, "You know it's not your fault." Or, "Things will get better, just you wait and see."
- Has few boundaries, presumes that others simply cannot survive without them.
- Believes, often subconsciously, they are a saint/martyr, acting unselfishly for another's good. This lofty position can create a high, which can make the rescuer position addictive, and all-encompassing.
- Sends this message to others: "You are inept. You cannot take care of yourself. You are not good enough. Therefore, I will be in charge. I will take care of you."
- Sees themselves as a rescuer-martyr and then ends up as a victim-martyr.
- Predominant feeling: guilt.

One solution for the addicted family—borrowing a concept from Bowen—is to triangulate *recovery* into the family system. This means that recovery, the new words and behaviors learned in therapy and in group meetings, plays the role of the rational adult that interrupts the dysfunctional family pattern. This change is a positive shift away from the prior dysfunctional patterns. The FRT therapist guides each family member away from engaging in dysfunctional addictive/codependent interactions or in playing unhealthy roles, towards differentiation and adopting healthy behavior patterns, which in turn leads to a saner, more functional family.

The Nuclear Family Emotional System

As noted above, Goldenberg et al. describe Bowen's concept of a nuclear family emotional system:

> Bowen (1978) contends that people choose mates with equivalent levels of differentiation to their own. According to Bowen, the resulting **nuclear family emotional system** will be unstable and will seek various ways to reduce tension and maintain stability. The greater the nuclear family's fusion, the greater will be the likelihood of anxiety and potential instability, and the greater will be the family's propensity to seek resolution through fighting, distancing, the impaired or compromised functioning of one partner, or banding together over concern for a child [Kerr, 1981].

I believe there is a higher probability for addiction to develop in poorly differentiated families because substance use can become the "medicine" to handle the pain of dysfunctional enmeshment that characterizes these families. However, it is also true that addiction will lower the level of differentiation in families. Family members, propelled by fear for their loved one, draw in closer to the addict and try to fix or rescue him. Of course, these efforts are almost always fruitless, and family members get further entangled. They do not understand that trying to fix the addict is a nearly impossible mission. It is the job of the FRT therapist to help codependent family members refrain from their efforts to rescue the addict because these very actions can prevent the addict from taking responsibility for the consequences of his own behavior. The FRT therapist educates codependent family members and guides them to stop enabling the addict, which often precipitates the crisis that causes the addict to hurt enough to finally reach out for help. It is only when codependents learn to recognize their own enabling behavior, and understand its consequences, that they can be encouraged to act more rationally.

The FRT therapist is trained in psychodynamic therapy and family systems, and assesses the overall level of differentiation when choosing interventions. In the early stages of Family Recovery Therapy, individuals are often quite unaware of their behavior or their level of enmeshment. They may not recognize that they blame or rescue either the addict, or other family members. For instance, the father of a 30-year-old addict may be scared his son is going to be stranded somewhere, and insist on paying for his gas and his cell phone. The mother may blame her husband for rescuing their son, and for spending money that was allocated for another purpose. Both parents may blame their son for his addictive behavior, and feel angry and victimized, because they really do not understand addiction. Interventions by the FRT therapist at this stage must begin with psychoeducation, because the system, albeit dysfunctional, is balanced, and sudden disruption may derail the nascent recovery process. The parents need to understand how their behavior is enabling their son's addiction. They need to learn to handle their anxiety and anger without rescuing or blaming, and to understand what to say and do differently to manage the situation. Later in the therapy process, after the mother-son-father dynamics have been explored, and after the parents have received support and guidance from both therapy and their support groups to set boundaries, the FRT therapist can be more directive in guiding the parents to stop enabling their son.

The Family Projection Process

There are various ways unstable families, including all poorly differentiated families, seek to decrease tension. One means of doing this is through a "family projection process," which occurs when the anxiety or emotional conflicts of a parent unconsciously get transferred onto a child, who then becomes the focus of attention. Generally, it is the least-differentiated child in the family with whom this process gets played out.

Bowen elegantly describes the unconscious dynamics that thwart differentiation among family members and thus set up the next generation to achieve a similar level of differentiation. Of course, using drugs to medicate the stress that naturally develops in these unstable family systems can be a tempting means of coping, although this further dysregulates the family. Addiction affects not only the user, but the entire family, and we know that some form of addiction impacts nearly half of all families in the United States.

Lack of differentiation in the family, aggravated by the family projection process, can contribute to the development of addiction. In his book, *In the Realm of Hungry Ghosts* (2010), Gabor Maté talks about his work with "down and out" addicts in Vancouver, Canada. Many of his adult clients who were neglected, unloved, and parentless as children—products, no doubt, of poorly differentiated families and possibly targets of a family projection process—became hypersensitive, and turned to substance abuse to ease their ever-present vulnerability to small stressors.

The strain of addiction and codependency can further diminish differentiation in an already enmeshed family. With increased emotional fusion of family members, there is a higher likelihood of a family projection process occurring. A mother who is worried about her husband's addiction may triangulate her child into the drama. This can reduce anxiety in the family system as a whole, and stabilize the family, but it can impede the growth and development of the child.

An FRT therapist can support the differentiation process in a family that has become enmeshed as the result of addiction. In fact, one of the often-overlooked benefits of addiction treatment is that a comprehensive systemic approach can enable the addict and the codependents to develop healthier lives than would have been the case had addiction not entered the picture. FRT can provide a sustainable path to growth, development, and healthy differentiation.

Emotional Cutoff

In general, healthy children come from healthy parents, who, in turn, came from healthy parents, and so on. However, addiction interrupts and skews healthy development.

In a poorly differentiated family system, where the pre-existing levels of differentiation and closeness may already be compromised, codependency and addiction move the relationships to a point of even greater emotional fusion. Sometimes a family member tries to escape the family fusion and conflict by physically moving away or emotionally distancing to the point of only very superficial, if any, contact. Bowen points out that these attempts at "emotional cutoff" leave family conflict unresolved.

The FRT therapist guides the members of the addicted/codependent family system into recovery and slowly repairs relationships, whenever possible. Through their participation in FRT and social support groups, family members learn how to create healthy boundaries, and it can become safe to resolve old issues. There are situations, however, in which an addict, codependent, or other family member chooses to decline treatment, despite the efforts of the therapist and the recovering family members to make room for the person to get help and heal. This individual may choose to disconnect from the family and to cut off communication. While the goal of the FRT therapist is, of course, to move all family members towards healing the broken system, this is not always possible. The FRT therapist can only work with the family members who are willing to participate in the recovery process. Those family members who do engage in therapy can heal and grow, both as individuals and as a family, albeit an incomplete one. As recovery continues, there is always hope that the resistant family member will, at some point, choose to reconnect with the family and engage in the recovery process.

This chapter speaks to a critical flaw in the current paradigm of addiction treatment—the failure to address the *family system* that enables addiction. In addition, the needs of family members are often overlooked in current addiction treatment. Bowen's work illuminates the interconnectedness of family members and the interplay of dynamics among them, thereby highlighting the inevitable impact of the family members and the addict on each other.

Part Two

Practice

Chapter 6

Introduction to Case Studies

When I was developing the FRT model, at times I felt like Lewis and Clark—traveling through uncharted territory. I have made numerous wrong turns, committed many clinical errors, and been baffled by the results of some of my decisions. I have also been guided and helped by others whose work has formed a strong foundation for this approach: Stephanie Brown, Ph.D., who formulated a family-systems based developmental model of addiction recovery (*The Alcoholic Family in Recovery: A Developmental Model*, Brown & Lewis, 1999); Brad Reedy, Ph.D., founder and director of Evoke Therapy; Timmen Cermak, M.D., addiction psychiatrist; Kevin McCauley, M.D., addiction physician; and Murray Bowen, M.D., psychiatrist, who formulated an invaluable perspective on family systems. In the end, I feel confident about what I have learned, and this knowledge has formed the foundation of the FRT Principles. The FRT model and the 14 Principles comprise a new and different approach—different enough from what is currently being practiced by perhaps over 95 percent of addiction treatment providers for me to call it a "new paradigm."

Part Two of this book includes a series of case studies. In order to provide a perspective from which to understand the cases that follow, I first present a general overview of how I work with a family.

Thinking systemically from the beginning is core to this approach. The client is not the person calling, but the *system* surrounding the caller. Beginning with the first phone call, I'm assessing "who else," besides the caller, are key players. I want to corral the key people from the start, in order to prevent the splitting, projection, and coalition-building that usually characterize the dysfunctional homeostasis of an addictive family system.

While my work is grounded in all of the Principles, I view Principle 12 as particularly useful in understanding the unfolding process of working with a family from the beginning of treatment:

FRT Principle 12
All members of the family seeking treatment must be fully informed of, and understand, the therapeutic goals, as well as understand and agree to the treatment plan, which includes specific recommendations for different stages of treatment.

Principle 12 unfolds in three stages: first, joining with the family and laying a foundation for the possibility of our working together; second, educating the family about treatment, which includes informing them about my approach and referring them to my books and website for more information; and third, engaging the family in treatment, introducing them to the Treatment Agreement, and getting their consent to the agreement.

The first stage, joining with the family, occurs in the initial sessions, during which I instill hope and reassure the family members that treatment can help their situation. The FRT model works most effectively if everyone capable of benefiting from recovery comes together at the outset. Early in the process, if I am working with the family of a young adult, I say something like, "My hope, a year from now, is to see a young adult addict with a year of continuous sobriety, who has been employed in a developmentally appropriate, honorable, full-time job for most of that year, who is successfully launched 'from the nest,' and to see a family system relieved of stress, happy, and functioning normally." That is the goal. The parents may simply want the drug problem to go away, but we need to broaden the frame of reference, both to reduce the risk of relapse, and to address their child's lost development, as well as to give the family hope that we can use this process for even greater healing.

Engaging a prospective family in a process that leads to health and recovery is a delicate process. Typically, the family has been surviving in the milieu of addiction and codependency for a long time. The FRT therapist must slowly draw the family into recovery, and allow space for their ambivalence and fear, then gradually encourage them to take the next step toward positive change.

We know what needs to happen, but we also must be well aware of our clients' resistance. We need to honor their fear and discomfort at the prospect of facing their situation, making significant changes, and embracing the unknown. If we encounter resistance, fear, uncertainty, or objections, we address these directly, but we are always heading towards the goal. We are always doing the difficult work of advocating this treatment model (Family Recovery Therapy) while going only as fast as the family members are able to move, and dealing with the resistance as it comes up. It can take weeks or months of slowly working with the family members before they fully understand the problem, because of their fear, denial and rationalization—the homeostasis in which they live. But we must not shirk from the hard work of laying out the complete program, in general terms. When working with a substance-using teen or young adult, FRT will require the parents' participation; when a spouse or parent is the substance user, other adult family members will need to participate. The family members will need to understand their role in creating the current crisis—how their decisions were in part responsible for the situation, and how they have enabled the years of substance use or out-of-control behavior—and the necessity for them to modify their behavior, going forward.

Family members during this early stage are likely to be confused and overwhelmed. Anxious to find help for the addict, they may have looked at addiction resources on the Internet, and become perplexed by the variety of treatment options available.

A YouTube video entitled *Rehab* (Oliver, 2018), in which the comedian, John Oliver, describes the current state of addiction treatment, is an excellent resource for a family at this stage of treatment. While humorous, the video accurately depicts the chaos, corruption, and inadequacy that plague much of the treatment industry. The current rash of terrible addiction treatment programs in America is, in part, a result of enforcement of the Mental Health Parity and Addiction Equity Act of 2008, which mandated that health insurance companies must treat addiction on a par with any other medical disorder—which then encouraged a slew of inadequate, money-driven, "Addiction Treatment" programs to pop up. (Although it is vital that governments recognize that addiction is a treatable disease, not surprisingly, there are always opportunists.) The 19-minute John Oliver video is an eye-opener, and will be helpful as we educate the family about treatment options and the questions they need to ask treatment providers. *(Note: I recommend that you pause here and watch the video. You can Google "Rehab John Oliver" or check the reference list [Oliver, 2018]. The video accurately summarizes the mess we are currently in and highlights the urgent need for a new addiction treatment model, as laid out in this book.)* It is crucial to explain to the family how FRT both differs from other treatment options, and offers a much higher probability of sustained success than other approaches.

During the second stage of treatment—informing the family about therapeutic goals and the treatment process—I speak in general terms about what the Treatment Agreement entails. I do this only after I am reasonably certain that they are "on board," and ready to follow the treatment plan—otherwise, I continue to answer their questions and give them time to accept their problem and ask for help. It is important to understand that this process could take weeks, months, or even possibly never happen. If a family member does not agree to the treatment plan, I will work with the other committed individuals. My goal is to help them let go of their hopeless attachment to rescuing the active addict, and to encourage them to disengage from the resistant family member, so they can focus on their own recovery process.

If the family members are on board, I go down the list of treatment provisions. I let the family know that we may need to place their loved one in a detox facility or Residential Treatment Center (RTC) for a short period, after which he will join our scripted step-down program, an Intensive Outpatient Program (IOP), which may include his residing in a sober living environment (SLE). I tell them that every family member will need to attend some kind of group for support, a local "social support and mutual aid group." I also explain that there will be a specific plan in place in case of relapse, that drug testing will be part of the process, and that regular individual and family therapy is part of the treatment plan.

Usually, family members who are focused on their loved one's life will easily agree to the general treatment provisions. Getting the buy-in of the family members at this point is essential, because later, they may balk at some stipulation—participating in family therapy, or attending social support and mutual aid groups, or supporting the addict's going to a detox center if a relapse occurs. However, this model requires that each family member acknowledge their role in the family dysfunction and be willing to do the work to support everyone's recovery.

Early in my work with teens and young adults, my fear of holding the parents to their agreement to attend social support groups led to failed cases. A parent would say, "Hey, I didn't know I agreed to go to meetings. I'm not comfortable doing that." Parents would not attend social support groups, and I would try to hold the treatment process together—which is usually not possible without the parents' full participation. Their resistance, not unexpectedly, often led to their child's resumption of addictive behaviors and the family's backsliding to the prior homeostasis.

It is in stage three, engaging the family in treatment, that I introduce the Addiction/Codependency Family Treatment Agreement and its specifics (see Appendix E). In a family session, I explain the different parts of the Treatment Agreement in detail. By this stage, the codependent family members can understand the wisdom of this agreement as well as the role they will play in the recovery process and the specific work they will need to do. The need for them to comply and do their work will make sense to them, especially when they see their loved one's treatment unfold in real time, and they understand that their treatment, the treatment of the family, will parallel the treatment of their addicted loved one. If the addict has been in residential treatment, I work directly with the residential program staff to coordinate their discharge plan with the recommendations of our Treatment Agreement, as well as to facilitate a seamless transition for the addict from residential to outpatient treatment.

Below is a very brief summary of the initial steps the FRT therapist follows, starting with the therapist's first contact with the concerned family member and continuing through the first several sessions. The summary should be viewed as a general guide, since every situation is different, every therapist has their own style, and it is important for a therapist to be flexible and respond appropriately to each particular situation.

Preparation for returning the initial call from the client:

- Have genogram handy (see Figure 6.1). A genogram is a diagram similar to a family tree that depicts the members of a family and indicates their relationships with one another (McGoldrick et al., 2020).
- Note the "presenting problem" on the genogram (this is often mentioned in the caller's initial voicemail message and may need to be referenced later).
- Wonder, "Who else is concerned about this problem?"
- Wonder, "Who are the enablers?"
- Be ready to plant the seed, "I work with the family system."

Initial phone call to the caller, typically one of the enablers:

Chapter 6. Introduction to Case Studies

- Goal: if a "fit," get them into the office ASAP—see this as a possible emergency! This could be a "hitting bottom" moment for someone in the family system, and this opportunity could pass—schedule an initial session as soon as possible.
- Introduce self.
- Listen for a short while.
- If they are calling about an addicted family member, ask about any "adverse consequences" from the person's substance use.
- When it is clear that they are interested in coming to a session, say, "Who else is concerned?" It is best to get everyone who is concerned to attend the initial session, even by speakerphone, if geographic considerations make it impossible to attend in person.
- Schedule session, tell them the fee, and let them know that they will be signing an Informed Consent form before starting the session.
- If available, send them a web link to a description of your qualifications. Mine can be found at LarryFritzlan.com.
- Keep the call fairly short. If the client has a problem, we may be able to help: the aim is to get them into the office. I have discovered that spending a lot of time on this initial call often results in cancelled sessions, perhaps because I have given the caller too much information and overwhelmed them.

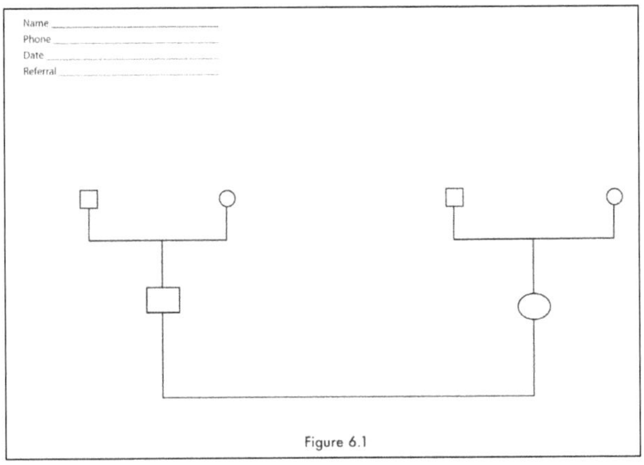

Figure 6.1 *Genogram Form.*

Initial Sessions with enabling codependents:

- Have them sign the Informed Consent form before beginning the session.
- "Join with them." Be Rogerian—be compassionate, show unconditional positive regard, be non-judgmental, congruent (Rogers, 1995).
- Think clinically: assess, evaluate, diagnose.
- I usually start out with something like this, "What's going on, how can I help you?"
- Let them know that I'm an FRT therapist, that I work with families where addiction and codependency are present, that I work from a family systems perspective, and that my client is the family system.
- Perhaps plan an additional session or sessions with the enabling codependents to get this "enabling subsystem" engaged and on board.
- Let them know that soon I'd like to meet with all of them, including the

addict, but, when we meet, I will meet first with the addict alone, and then with all of the family members together.

First meeting with both the addict and the enabling codependents:

- In this session, I will first meet with the addict alone to reassure him that "I have his back," and that I am interested in the welfare of the whole family. I let him know that I need his help in order to help the family get healthy. I make it very clear that this is not a process of "ganging up on the addict."

Meeting all of them together:

- Review what you have heard from each person, answer questions, and make recommendations.
- It is vital that the FRT therapist be authoritative and take charge of the session, quickly interrupting any re-enactment of family drama and slowly allowing them to hear the reality of their situation from a professional, while also holding a positive and structured container. (I will typically say, near the beginning, "this will be a 50 minute session.")

The role of the FRT therapist shifts and changes as treatment unfolds, which is demonstrated in the case studies that follow.

A number of FRT Principles inform the therapeutic process and contribute to a successful outcome. I reference some of the 14 Principles specifically in the case studies, as well as providing commentary on how I use the FRT model in each case. Of course, the cases that follow are not real cases. Each is a composite of many cases that I've drawn from to demonstrate the FRT model. The characters do not refer to any individual or family I have treated; confidentiality is always respected. It is my hope that these examples, which include an array of individuals exhibiting a variety of addictive and codependent characteristics, will guide you in assessing the clients you encounter in your work as an FRT therapist.

Chapter 7

Case Study—Young Adult

"I think my son has a problem with drugs. We need help." This was the message that Ellen, the mother of a 19-year-old, left on my voicemail. She had been referred to me by a local psychologist who'd heard I'd had some successful outcomes working with families in situations like hers.

I returned the call and spoke with Ellen, who seemed quite anxious. I asked her to explain what was going on. She began, "I was referred to you because I understand you work with young adults who have problems with drugs. My ex-husband found a bag of pills in our son's car two days ago. We found out that they are fentanyl. Our son, Peter, has been acting strangely recently, much more up and down than usual, and we are concerned he might be using drugs."

"Fentanyl is an opioid, a highly addictive drug." I said, "Does he have a history of using narcotics or any other drugs?"

The mother replied, "Yes, and I think he has been using more drugs lately. We know that Peter started smoking pot in his sophomore year in high school and had been hanging out with a group of friends that we think are pretty heavy drug users."

"OK," I said, "Perhaps I can help. I specialize in working with families who are impacted by substance abuse, and clearly you may have a problem with your son. I wonder who else is concerned?"

Ellen replied, "His father and his older brother are worried, too." I was proceeding with Ellen, as I do with any new caller, in keeping with Principle 14:

FRT Principle 14
Typically, a member of the enabling subsystem contacts the treatment provider. It is vital that the provider begin to engage the caller in the Family Recovery Therapy treatment model during this first contact.

I also learned from Ellen that she and her ex-husband, Tom, had divorced when Peter was 12, and that Peter lived part-time in each household. Ellen, Peter's mother, was now single, and Peter's dad had a new wife. I needed both of the biological parents to get involved. While stepparents can play an important role in family dynamics, they typically have neither the legal nor the emotional leverage of the biological parents. Ellen repeated that Peter's older brother, Ed, was also concerned.

"I think it will work best," I suggested, "if you, your ex-husband, and your concerned older son meet with me together so that we can explore this more fully and you can help me get a better picture of the situation. Would they be willing to come in?"

She said she thought they would, and I offered her a few times I was available to meet with them.

I have heard this kind of story many times and wanted to help Ellen, to let her know that this is the work I do, and to answer any questions she might have. But my primary goal in the phone call was to invite her and any other concerned family members to come in for a session in which we could explore the situation in more depth. I was already thinking systemically, and wanted all of the key players to participate in the treatment process from the very beginning.

I knew that the family could easily call a number from a slick TV commercial, advertising "1-800-Addiction-Help-Now," and dispatch the "problem" to some random treatment center to fix. An important part of my job would be to help the parents understand and trust my Family Recovery Therapy (FRT) treatment model.

In the first session, I met with the biological parents, Ellen and Tom, and their older son, Ed. I reviewed what Ellen had told me in our phone conversation. Tom and Ed supplied some additional details. Then I introduced the concept of family systems treatment. "Your now-adult son, Peter," I said, looking at the parents, "is 100% responsible for making the decision to start and continue to use drugs, but you, the family members, are also 100% responsible for how you respond to his use. To get to the bottom of this, we are best served if everyone is willing to participate in and support the recovery process."

"Could you tell us about how you work, what the next steps would be?" Tom, the father, asked. "Sure," I said. "The first thing is to get a good picture of the problem, for me to learn the nature of your son's condition. After another session or two with you and Ellen, I'd like to have a session where first I meet alone with Peter, and then with all of you, so I can thoroughly assess what is happening. I will have a better idea of the extent of your son's substance use, the impact it has on his life, the family dynamics, and what action might be appropriate. It's important to understand that drug abuse, including addiction, often happens within a family system, and that, possibly, in some ways, it has been enabled by you."

I explained, "In general, if we find addiction is the correct diagnosis, and you choose to work with me, Family Recovery Therapy proceeds by enlisting the whole family in a process that will require everyone's participation. There will be specific agreements I will need each of you to accept as we continue through the recovery process. And," I added, "let me explain what I mean by recovery. If there has been ongoing substance abuse, your son's natural development, his maturation process, has been interrupted, and what we are aiming for, in addition to stopping the drug problem, is restoration of his lost development. Furthermore, if you have been focused on your son's drug use instead of on yourselves, your own lives have also been impacted, perhaps significantly."

"But," I said, "we are only at the beginning phase, and I'd like to suggest that we set up another session for me to get more information, and then for us to meet again, and include Peter, so we can all look at the facts."

I *didn't* tell them that, if they work with me, they will be part of an intensive outpatient program that will require them to devote two to three hours each week to some sort of brain-rewiring work, and I didn't tell them that there will be setbacks along the way, and that their child could have brief relapses, or that addiction is a powerful disease and their child could die, regardless of what they do.

"Let me tell you a little more about how I work," I continued. "I work with substance use issues from a family systems perspective. There are many factors that go into our behavior and the choices we make. Most of us are strongly influenced by the people around us. There are the current interactions at play, but there are also long-term unconscious dynamics that affect our behavior. I work with the family system and with all of the family members to get a deeper understanding of the problem and to come up with a long-term solution."

This kind of interview is not easy. The family naturally wants the doctor to "fix this" and have the problem go away. Their wish colludes with the treatment industry's desire to "get heads on beds," and creates a world in which many parents send their kids to multiple treatment programs until remission is achieved, or they run out of money, or their kid has a long course of addiction, and perhaps even dies.

We, the FRT therapists, can't do much about the parents' wish for a simple fix, and we can't immediately fix unethical treatment programs that are willing to take the case and a family's money. We must, however, be truthful and stand by our principles and our approach, and support the treatment plan, even if we lose a paying client. In fact, resistant parents that I have seen for only a session or two often return after some more bad things have happened and they are ready to roll up their sleeves and follow our guidance. I often get cases where the family members have tried other approaches and are finally willing to be part of a comprehensive, family-based, treatment process.

"Let me be honest with you," I said. "From what you have told me, I believe that your son has a multi-year attachment to drugs, and I suspect that we may only be seeing the tip of the iceberg. We know that he is probably using opioids, that he has a lifestyle and a social life embedded with substance users, and that supporting him to achieve a substance-free lifestyle will be a long-term project. And," I added, "this is what I have been doing for most of the last 25 years, with many successes. Of course, I've also met with families who've chosen not to engage in this process.

"I have a recommendation for you," I said. "There's a book I'd like you to read. It's about a family with a teenaged daughter who got into drugs and alcohol when she was 15 or 16. The mother consulted with a therapist who works like I do and included the family in treatment. The book is by both the mother and the daughter, and was written many years later. There was a painful hitting bottom experience which led to recovery, and the book has a happy ending. It will be very helpful for you to read this. It describes a path towards recovery that I think might be similar to yours. The book is called *The Lost Years: Surviving a Mother and Daughter's Worst Nightmare*. Kristina Wandzilak and Constance Curry (2006) are the authors." (Over the twenty-plus years that I've been working as a therapist, I have given away close to 400 copies of this book.)

After two sessions with the parents (I'd included their older son, Ed, only in the first meeting), I was clear that they understood and supported my general approach. My next step was for them to come back in with Peter. I knew treatment would entail working with the conscious and unconscious dynamics within the family—the family system that affected Peter—as well as with the individual family members. When the parents and Peter arrived for the next session, I asked first to see Peter alone. I do this to reassure the potential addict that I'm not there just on behalf of the parents, that I'm an ally of the whole family system, that he has every right to speak up and advocate for himself, and that he can trust that I will support his needs as well as those of the other family members. I immediately liked Peter. He was present, he had his own life, he "sort of had" a part-time job, but mostly he was hanging out with his drug-using friends, and basically thought what he was doing was fine, regardless of his parents' view. Yes, the parents found his stash, yes, he had been using drugs for a while, but he did not think he had a problem. I told him his parents had already told me pretty much everything he had mentioned: the pot use in high school, the drug-using friends, the poor school performance, and the impact his drug use had had on his moods around home. I asked him if there was anything that he wanted me to keep confidential and not disclose to his parents. He agreed that I could share everything he had told me. In his mind, it was his parents who had the problem, but he was willing to stay in the room and let me bring his parents into the conversation.

Then I brought in the parents. My first meeting with the addict and the codependent family members is pivotal. For the first time, the family is together with a professional who is hearing all the facts of the situation and listening to everyone's opinions and concerns. I began by asking each person's verbal permission to disclose what they had told me—they agreed. Then, looking at everyone, I said, "I am honored to help with some of your concerns." Looking at Peter, I continued, "I'd like to review what I was told by your parents and brother when I met with them. Peter, you don't deny that you have been doing drugs, but you don't see it as a problem—and you don't deny that the drugs that your father found in your car belong to you."

I went on, looking at the parents, "And, Tom and Ellen, you've been aware of changes in Peter's behavior for nearly four years. You've noticed that he is often unusually tired, and that sometimes he might even seem intoxicated. At other times, he seems sort of giddy, excited, and rambling in his speech. And you said that you know about his past drug use. You told me that he was a good student until his senior year, which is when you became aware that he was smoking pot and hanging around a different group of friends—and that his grades slipped to the point where he almost did not graduate. He did manage to graduate, and now he is working part-time at an auto parts shop. Did I get all this right?" I asked, and they nodded.

I said all of this slowly—the family members, together, were hearing a new reality—their situation, as perceived by a professional, someone outside the family system. I wanted all of it to settle in. My allusions to denial and to the existence of a problem—for all of them, and for the system as a whole—could be disconcerting, but I wanted to set the stage for the interventions to follow.

Peter's father spoke first. "I think that pretty well describes the situation. But what do we do now?" I replied, "That's what we are here to talk about. First, to get agreement from all of you about the facts of the current situation, then to look at what it all means, and what makes sense going forward."

Let's step back for a moment and imagine that the family, instead of calling me, had called an interventionist. Let's imagine that the interventionist was informed enough to know that a "surprise intervention" often backfires and is not advised, so they choose to do a "systemic intervention." In a systemic intervention, an interventionist gathers the concerned family members, with the addict present, and encourages the family members to express their concern for the addict's wellbeing. The interventionist's goal would be to get the addict to agree to go to residential treatment, and he or she would be highly motivated to get the addict to board a plane headed to a treatment center that day, or the next day at the latest. The interventionist would discuss the role that the "system" played in the family and probably recommend that the codependents attend a support group such as Al-Anon. If Peter had agreed to go to rehab, the interventionist might make some phone calls confirming his placement, and perhaps offer a few follow-up calls, but basically, the interventionist would step back and turn the case over to the treatment center. In truth, most interventionists would collude with the premise that "the addict is the problem," ship the addict off, and bow out, letting the treatment program take over the case, and leaving the family members to deal with whatever the treatment center suggested. In contrast to this process, the FRT therapist, as described in this book, does the job of the systemic interventionist—meeting with the family and the addict, finding and arranging admission of the addict into an appropriate residential program, if residential treatment is warranted—but continues "hands-on" involvement with the family, and with all treatment providers, going forward through at least the first year of continuous sobriety. Other providers involved in the recovery process can include staff at detox centers and residential treatment centers, medical doctors, psychiatrists, and sober living home managers.

It turned out that Peter, over the previous two years, had shown several signs of addiction, including dropping grades, altered sleep habits, episodes of depression, and periods of unusual elation. According to his parents, Peter had exhibited these behaviors since his senior year of high school. The parents had crossed the line from parenting to codependency when they started to believe that lectures and yelling could somehow get Peter to stop escalating his drug use—they were in denial of the role they played in exacerbating his behavior. Rationalizing that his substance use was "typical teen experimentation" further supported their denial of a deeper problem. And now Peter was no longer a minor. Peter's parents needed to move from a "parent-child" relationship to an "adult-adult" relationship with Peter to support their now-adult son's development, and to give him the freedom and autonomy to become his own person.

I was at a delicate juncture with Peter's parents. The art of psychotherapy in family addiction treatment is to describe the significance of the process that lies ahead without scaring or overwhelming the family members—to educate, to inform, to deal with the resistance, to slowly help the family members emerge from their denial, and to move forward gradually enough to keep them engaged in therapy.

Over the next three weeks, I met individually with Peter, his father, mother, and older brother. Each of them, like the four blind men describing an elephant, painted a very different picture of the family's dynamics, the differing parenting styles, and the consequences of Peter's growing up in two different homes. In the meantime, Peter continued using drugs and coming to sessions, while I gathered more information, answered the parents' questions, and sought the optimal placement for Peter. Peter had agreed to drug testing, but at one point, he tried to fake his urine test by substituting a bottle of someone else's urine.

It was now becoming more obvious to Peter, to his family, and to me, that Peter was behaving like someone with a serious drug problem. In addition to fentanyl, he had been using heroin, cocaine, amphetamines, and Xanax; engaging in binge drinking, and vaping pot and nicotine. By now, Peter was coming to accept that he may have crossed a line and could benefit from some help. And, importantly, he was beginning to realize how financially dependent he was on his parents, and that he would have to abide by their decisions, or walk out and support himself—and being on his own was not a prospect he was prepared to consider. His parents began both to accept that Peter needed treatment, and to recognize their untenable predicament if they continued to house and support their son and allow the status quo to continue. They knew his drug use could get much worse—and that they were enabling it.

When I met with the parents alone, I said, "I think this is an important perspective for you to consider. Peter is an adult, and yet he is fully dependent on you for housing, food, money, use of a car, and cell phone. Imagine that we have a conversation with him where he is given a choice between continuing to get your support—which would entail his getting some sort of treatment that he would have to agree to accept—or no longer getting your support; that you, his parents, would tell him that he would be on his own."

The parents were nearing a tipping point. With my guidance and support, they were gaining the courage to grasp their role and the need to follow my recommendations.

This point is essential. It is at the core of Family Recovery Therapy: unless the codependent enablers can both recognize the problem and understand their role in *perpetuating and enabling the addiction*, and be willing to trust "powers other than themselves"—in this case, the FRT therapist, the social support groups, and other parents—a positive systemic outcome is highly unlikely. In fact, I cannot think of a successful case where the family as a whole "recovered" without each family member agreeing to follow my recommendations and doing the individual work necessary to grow and resume normal development. Let me refer you to Principle 2, which is foundational to understanding the dynamics of an addictive family system:

FRT Principle 2
Effective treatment of addiction usually involves treatment of codependents, because codependents enable addiction. Codependency is a chronic relationship pattern that has profound mental and physical consequences and is characterized by an obsessive focus on other people. Codependents may need lifelong recovery support, which can take many forms.

Working with a young adult addict has a unique risk. A young adult addict is balanced between dependency *both* on parental support *and* on drugs and a drug-using peer culture. If the parents, embedded in codependency, try to fix their young adult child's addiction by implementing more rules, threats, promises, etc., the young adult may simply distance themselves from the parents and move, full-time, into a drug-using culture—at which point the parents could lose any leverage to facilitate the addict's choosing treatment. At that juncture, the codependent parents are powerless to influence the young adult's choices. Many of the homeless people on our streets are, sadly, individuals who got into drugs at a young age, and lived in families who did not receive this kind of treatment, and were not able to make it in the world.

It would be many months before Peter realized the impact of the change in his "codependent parents." The parents were letting go, accepting that Peter was an adult and that he needed to take responsibility for his own life. The parents were moving from a "parent-child" relationship with Peter to an "adult-adult" relationship with him. Their history of treating him as a child when he was no longer a child was part of the reason he was still behaving like a child.

Our work had laid the foundation. The facts were on the table, including Peter's extensive use of various drugs. The parents had come to understand their role, not only in failing to catch and treat the problem earlier, but also in supplying financial support—a cell phone, use of a car, and room and board—which had enabled Peter's drug-using lifestyle to continue. They saw the problem and were ready to accept the guidance offered by a family systems therapist. This would require them to do their own recovery work as Peter did his, and would entail supporting Peter's attending residential treatment.

And Peter, while naturally resistant, had at this point accepted the inevitability of what could happen. He had known friends who had gone to rehab. Over the previous weeks, he had become savvy enough to recognize that he was on a slippery slope with drug use, that it could become even more of a problem, and that, without his parents' support, he was on a path towards becoming homeless.

I told the family, Peter included, that I thought the next step would be for Peter to go to a residential wilderness treatment program. Peter understood that, if he wanted his family's support, he would need to cooperate with treatment. This meant he would need to agree to "go away" to treatment. He had no clue what this really entailed, except for stories he had heard of others who had been "sent away to rehabs." And I gave them the links to some YouTube videos about addiction to look at when they got home (see Appendix F). Addiction and addiction treatment are very complex issues, and it is important to get as much information as possible.

But what I had in mind was different from simply dispatching Peter to a treatment program. Sending a teen or dependent young adult, or anyone, for that matter, to rehab and expecting it to "fix the problem" is naive and usually unsuccessful. Most of us are deeply embedded—consciously and unconsciously—in the homeostasis of our lives: our work, peer culture, extended family, and friends. The "time out" in a "spin dry" treatment program, followed by discharge right back into the previous culture of drug-using friends and an unchanged enabling codependent family system, is contraindicated. Drug use in these situations usually resumes quickly, in spite of the family's hopes and the treatment program's assurances to the contrary.

Instead, under my guidance, the family and Peter would continue to follow the comprehensive, multi-part, family systems-based treatment plan that I had described to them earlier in general terms: therapy with the parents while Peter was away; then, once Peter returned and was residing in a sober living environment, the plan going forward would include family therapy, individual therapy for Peter, drug testing, a specific relapse plan, Peter getting a full time job, and participation by every family member in social support groups. Throughout treatment, I would monitor every family member for mental health and physical issues, and coordinate treatment with any other involved providers or adjunctive services. In short, as summarized in FRT Principle 5 below, I would continue to guide the treatment process and support Peter and his family members in developing fulfilling lives:

FRT Principle 5
As the treatment team leader, the FRT therapist guides the family throughout the continuum of care and collaborates with all supportive therapeutic services, which may include other treatment providers, interventionists, treatment programs, physicians, and any other adjunctive services.

At this point in my career, I had worked with wilderness programs for many years. When teens or young adults do their recovery work in the wilderness, away from the influence of cell phones, texting, and social media, I find that their treatment, as part of FRT, is usually successful. Over time, I have been able to educate these programs about my FRT approach and to coordinate treatment effectively with them. When I initially worked with residential treatment programs, the staff had behaved in ways consistent with the current treatment paradigm: they would thank me for the referral, take over the case, do their job, and then make the best referrals they could at the point of discharge, as they had been doing for years. They had never worked with a dedicated FRT therapist who insisted on being part of the process on a weekly basis. These residential programs assumed that, after they admitted the client, the referring therapist, perhaps after a single consultation, did not have any further role. The residential program did not understand that my client, who was only *temporarily* their client, would be returning to our family-based, intensive outpatient program when he was discharged—barring unforeseen events or psychological or medical issues that would necessitate his referral to another provider. Until I was able to develop a working relationship with the staff at these programs, I was not copied on the emails that were sent to the parents, updating them on their child's initial progress, or on the emails containing the parents' homework—the staff did not understand that I was continuing to meet with the parents. Nor did they initially grasp that I was treating "the system," which meant I needed to integrate their program with mine to consult with the field therapist, and participate in the weekly calls between the field therapist and the parents, and that I would work each week with the parents on the assignments they'd been given either by the treatment program or by me.

I have had nearly a 100 percent success rate using this approach when I have worked with healthy and motivated parents who want to have a healthy relationship with their child. Teens ages 17 and under may need an additional placement after a time at a wilderness program, such as a therapeutic boarding school. In these cases, especially with younger teens, I have often discharged the family, because it may be years before their child will return home, if ever, and the family often needs a different kind of support going forward. In some cases, the parents have re-engaged me at a later time to coordinate the "returning home process."

The day arrived for Peter to fly to the wilderness program. He was met at the airport by the program staff and transported to the field office for an intake appointment, a medical exam, and an opportunity to collect equipment and clothing—and then transported directly to the field. The staff emailed updates to his parents and me throughout the day, until Peter departed for the field. I had already talked to Peter's wilderness program therapist and had given her a summary both of the systemic dynamics of the family and the particular concerns I had about both Peter and his family.

The program staff immediately put the parents to work, requesting they each write an "Impact Letter" that included not only a statement of their love and support for Peter, but also a frank description, from their perspective, of his problematic behavior. I scheduled a meeting with the parents to discuss what they had written, and made some suggestions to keep their letters factual and remove any blame. We scheduled the first conference call with the field therapist to take place after she had had a session with Peter, and had observed his behavior in the field when he interacted with others in his group. The field staff, who were in intimate contact with

Peter, 24 hours a day, also provided their observations and assessment to the field therapist.

This would set the tone for the next seven to ten weeks—a weekly meeting with the family, a weekly conference call with the parents and the field therapist, and weekly scripted letters back and forth between Peter and his parents. Early on, Peter wrote a "Letter of Accountability," taking responsibility for his actions, which he listed in detail. This dovetailed nicely with the letter the parents had written to him with their perspective on his actions. Writing the letters slowed things down and prevented everyone's emotions, projections, and defenses from obfuscating their communication, and allowed time for thoughtful reflection by all of them. Peter would initially read his parents' Impact Letter in a group setting, allowing other members of his group to get an accurate picture of who he actually was—as opposed to what his ego presented. Peter also got to know his peers' stories, which allowed him to better understand them, as they all worked together building camp, hiking, doing their assignments—and coming together multiple times a day for process groups or to play games.

An extended residential stay, properly guided, gives the addict time not only to detox from drugs (and from texting and social media) and to get healthy, but also to reflect on his life, his dreams, and future plans. The addict in this setting is often receptive to education about addiction and to treatment recommendations. By week three or four, the staff, who had been watching Peter, agreed with me that an intensive, family-based outpatient program for addiction would be the appropriate next step, and had told Peter in general terms what that would look like. He had picked up from his peers that, following his stay in the wilderness program, there would be some sort of aftercare plan that he would be expected to follow. And it was recommended that he not move back home with his parents, but instead move to some sort of sober, supportive living environment.

His wilderness therapist and I had been discussing how best to present the aftercare plan and Treatment Agreement to Peter, and to get his acceptance. The plan had been presented to him in general terms, and perhaps two-thirds of the way through the program, he was shown a copy of our Treatment Agreement (see Appendix E), which he discussed with his therapist. After I consulted with the field therapist, and gave Peter some time to digest the plan, I arranged to have a satellite phone call with Peter in the field, to discuss the details. That call went well. I had a good connection with Peter, and we went over each part of the agreement, making sure that he understood and agreed to each point. At the end of the call, Peter was excited at the idea of coming back to California and starting a new life, getting support both to reunite with his family and friends, and to move forward on a healthy path—and to address his substance use problem.

This "consent to the agreement" process is vital. It would be easy for Peter, who was looking forward to coming back to California, to agree to almost anything while he was still in the field. At the point when Peter returned and the "rubber hit the road," he would have already talked about the agreement in detail, and agreed to each very specific and non-negotiable point of the agreement.

Understanding the concept of a "container" is vital to this process. The container that Peter existed in prior to the parents' call to me was wide open. He was basically free to roam widely, hang out with whomever, use drugs, and comply with very loose expectations from his parents. In the wilderness program, his container was very tight. There, he was expected to comply with a strict schedule, complete multiple chores, master the complexities of packing and organizing his pack, and set up his shelter and bedding. Peter attended many meetings with staff, therapist, and groups, and was expected to accomplish many challenges and chores—one of which was for him to learn how to build a fire from materials found on the ground. Mastering this skill typically takes many weeks to accomplish.

The container Peter would return to at home would be very small compared to his life before the wilderness program. Nearly every hour, initially, would be structured around his SLE, new job, individual, family, and group therapy, 12-Step meetings, meetings with a sponsor, and drug testing. Slowly, as he matured and recovered, he would become self-sufficient and independent, and no longer need so much external guidance—but that would require diligence, patience, and most of all, time, not unlike learning to make a fire with sticks.

Back in California, I had been meeting with the parents weekly. We had discussed Peter's progress and the letters to and from Peter. We had also explored each parent's experience of going to social support group meetings. Both parents were resistant to attending the groups at first, but they began to understand that they were learning more about their codependency, the deadly nature of addiction, and parenting. At this point, I helped them understand that attending support groups, in addition to reinforcing their personal growth, would also model what we expected Peter to do when he returned from the wilderness program. (Later, many weeks after Peter had returned, he told me, "Hey, it's crazy to see my parents working on their own stuff, they have always been all up in mine, and they aren't so crazy anymore.")

My work with Peter's family followed the guidelines presented in Principle 4:

FRT Principle 4
During the first year of treatment, the FRT therapist monitors, assesses, and guides the family in an integrated treatment process, which addresses biological, psychological, social, and spiritual recovery.

The time came for Peter to come back, and my anxiety rose, because this is a dangerous point in treatment—where treatment can easily become derailed. I can think of three cases where the parents' noncompliance with the "transition plan" sabotaged treatment. In one case, the mother insisted that she "must" have her son spend "just one night" with her before he moved into the sober living environment (SLE). Shortly after arriving home, her son went looking for drugs in his car. The parents had thoroughly cleaned out his car, but had not thought to look behind the ashtray. Their son looked behind the ashtray, found some opioids he'd stashed there, took them, and got high. He did go to the sober living environment the next day, with everyone knowing that he had relapsed, because they drug test every new client. His relapse became a topic of conversation at the SLE, and he became defensive and resisted the norms of the sober house, which stipulated that his months of being sober in rehab no longer counted since he had just relapsed—and that he had to become a newcomer all over again. The relapse set off a chain of events with the result that he moved back home, continued to use drugs, and the family dropped out of treatment.

In another case, the parents insisted their son go from the wilderness directly to a "big deal" birthday party and then spend a few days at home before moving into the SLE. He did not relapse, but the events re-established the codependent relationship between the son and his mother, and her codependency undermined the recovery process. The son moved home, and the family dropped out of treatment.

In a third case, the parents insisted that their young adult son go directly from the airport to a wedding—where the father promptly offered his son a glass of wine! This last situation occurred when I was still developing my family recovery model. Looking back, I could have predicted that the parents' refusal to attend social support groups while their son was in residential treatment foretold a codependent system that would resist systemic addiction treatment. Today, I describe my model to prospective clients. If they are not interested in following it, I will respectfully let them go—hoping that I have offered them some insight that might, after the next crisis, lead them to try treatment again, this time with a deeper understanding of their role, and with more commitment to the treatment process. The co-occurring disease of codependency can be lethal for the addict, and the codependents' denial and unwillingness to grasp this can predictably lead to failed treatment. I sometimes wonder if codependency kills more people than addiction.

Kevin McCauley, M.D., in his "Return to Flight" program (McCauley, 2007), describes a very comprehensive addiction treatment program for military and commercial pilots (see Appendix D). McCauley references the FAA-funded substance abuse program for impaired pilots, the Human Intervention and Motivation Study (HIMS), which coordinates identification, treatment, and return to flight for pilots with substance issues (www.himsprogram.com). McCauley, in his description of effective addiction treatment, highlights this critical step-down transition in the treatment process and emphasizes the addict's vulnerability when transferring from a residential program to an outpatient program and a sober living environment. McCauley explains that recovering addicts are unconsciously programmed to return to the prior homeostasis—using drugs—upon leaving the treatment facility, and he recommends that "the van from the treatment program drive the addict directly to the sober living home without stopping anywhere." I had already discussed Peter's transfer from residential treatment to the SLE with both Peter and his parents, and had coordinated his transfer with the manager of the sober living home.

When Peter left the wilderness program, he was put on a plane to fly home. His parents and I had arranged for him to go directly from the airport to my office, where he would reconnect with his parents and we would sign the Treatment Agreement. This was a joyful moment—Peter had a big grin on his face, looked great, had gained weight, and was proud and delighted about his weeks of adventure and countless personal growth experiences.

After the joyful greetings and hugs, I asked everyone to let me briefly speak about what was next. "I'd like all of you to sign the Treatment Agreement." We accomplished this quickly, since I had already talked at length about the agreement with each of them. I also asked Peter to sign a release of information giving me permission to introduce him to some young people I knew in AA.

"Now, I'd like to set up our next meetings." I told Peter that I'd see him the next morning, and I would meet with the whole family the day after. And then I said, "It's important to understand that you are all in treatment and that I will be giving you some direct suggestions. What I want you to do after this session is not to talk to each other."

I let that sit with them for a moment, and they all looked at me like I was crazy. I laughed and said, "Seriously, we will meet in two days, and then, going forward, I don't want you to talk to each other." I went on, "I'd like to save all of that for our sessions. For the next couple of weeks, as each of you continues to adjust to this new lifestyle, to attend your meetings and get on with your life, I'd like to keep the important conversations inside this room. I will be in touch with Peter every day and will let you know if I have any concerns. And, of course, you are free to check in with me if you have any questions." I got all of them to agree to this and ended the session.

Peter's parents drove him from my office directly to the sober living environment (SLE), and left him with his new housemates to get settled. His housemates had arranged for Peter to go with them to an AA meeting that night, where I had additional young men with solid recovery standing by to greet him, and then his housemates accompanied him back to the SLE for a house meeting.

Because treatment is integrated with 12-Step recovery work, as stated in FRT Principle 6, my understanding of the 12 Steps was invaluable in working with Peter's family:

FRT Principle 6
The FRT therapist must be well-versed in the 12 Steps and have a thorough understanding and appreciation for the fundamental role that mutual aid programs play in recovery from codependency and addiction.

During my session with Peter on the day after he arrived, I asked him about the SLE, his housemates, and the AA meeting he had attended. He had, as planned, gone with several SLE housemates to the AA meeting, and been introduced there to other recovering young adults. Peter said he had raised his hand at the meeting and introduced himself when they asked for newcomers. When the AA meeting ended, a number of friendly folks approached Peter, offered him encouragement, and gave him their phone numbers. He reported that the meeting was okay, and he planned to attend another meeting that night. Good news!

Treatment and the AA meetings would build a foundation for Peter's ongoing sobriety. He was learning that his prefrontal cortex, by itself, would not be able to resist the cravings of his midbrain. Hopefully he would come to understand that AA meetings were his "medicine," and that these meetings would override not only his midbrain's craving, but also the pressure from drug-using friends to "have just one drink or drug." He would face enormous challenges—his unconscious drives and cravings would clash with the recovery messages from his 12-Step fellowship, his wilderness education, and therapy. In my experience, most young addicts will relapse without a tightly structured recovery program.

I urged Peter to keep in mind what he had learned in treatment about "relapse prevention." I discussed the role of a sponsor, who would help him work his way through the 12 Steps. We reviewed again his out-of-control behavior when he was using. He could now see that some of the crazy things he'd done were signs of his addiction. We also talked about the road ahead, the family therapy, the recovery work, and the expectation that he get a job. He was still stoked about being back in California. He was agreeable to the plan he and his field therapist had discussed during previous weeks, and that we had talked about several weeks earlier and reviewed again with his parents on the day he returned from his wilderness program. We spoke about drug testing, which provides valuable support in recovery, as stated in FRT Principle 11:

FRT Principle 11
Regular drug testing is a powerful tool and will be used in addiction treatment.

I explained to Peter that relapse is always possible, and that drug testing would be an added "tool" to remind him there would be immediate consequences if he did relapse. He understood that if he relapsed, he would need to go to a detox facility for 72 hours, change his sobriety date (he was sober over two months at that point), and admit his relapse to his family, his SLE housemates, and at group level at his AA meetings. I was aware that he might relapse at some point, but kept this information to myself in that moment—I didn't want to rain on his homecoming parade. (I had already mentioned to his parents the possibility that he might relapse.)

I told Peter I wanted to drug test him that day. At this point, Peter was eager to show that he was clean, and he readily went to the bathroom to provide a urine sample (I discuss drug testing in more depth in Chapter 14).

We also talked about Peter getting a job. It is not unusual for young adults who abuse drugs to start using as early as middle school, and later to exhibit predictable developmental delays—emotionally, psychologically, and socially. Starting an entry-level job can be somewhat anxiety-producing for the young adult addict, especially when his previous job history has been spotty, at best. The FRT therapist understands this and will walk the client through the process. Over the years, I have placed nearly all of my young adult clients into developmentally appropriate, honorable, entry-level, full-time jobs. I have found that these kinds of jobs—coffee shops like Peet's and Starbucks, grocery stores such as Whole Foods—provide a safe and sane initial job experience. These employers tend to have stable management. They provide training and set reasonably high expectations, but also understand that their new hire may be embarking on their first-ever paid job.

In the county where I work, the process of applying for a job usually entails going to a job location, talking to a manager about the hiring process, and then completing an online or in-person application. Some of my clients have been so frightened at the prospect of working that, to normalize the process, I drive them around to various locations so they can simply observe people their age at work. Having a job is part of the treatment structure, along with the SLE living experience and attending social support groups, all of which move the young client towards normal development and adulthood. In fact, I often observe that young adult addicts, by the time they have one year of sobriety—having completed the 12 Steps, been steadily employed for nearly a year, attended many dozens of therapy sessions, and lived with sober people—are more mature and stable than many of their peers who have experienced a year or two of college. The "treatment"—showing up for work consistently and living a sober life with peers—comes close to what every parent wants for their kid: a successful launch out of the nest to living on their own and developing normally.

The task of an FRT therapist is so much more than simply doing drug treatment! In essence, we are treating each member of a family system who is willing to address both the current issues at play and the unconscious dynamics that inform their systemic homeostasis—which are often influenced by the parents' own childhood experiences.

As much as we want to think that the residential treatment program has "fixed" the addict, we need to remember that the addict has returned to his previous "treatment"—the powerful influences that have comprised his environment for his whole life. Two months of residential "brain washing" cannot compete with 19 years of previous influences: family, friends, peer culture, and society. We want to create an environment—a container—where the addict's individual development can resume. The prior homeostasis could be re-established in an instant if, for instance, a codependent parent was to resume behaving the same way he or she did prior to the addict's treatment. Something as simple as a parent saying, "Don't call your friends," to a young adult struggling for self-agency could elicit an oppositional reaction from the young person, with both parties quickly returning to the well-worn emotional paths that existed in the past. The old reactions could erase any new norms that recovery had installed. A "fuck you" from the addict, followed by a call to an old drug-using friend, could obliterate any recovery that had been achieved and start a cascade of events—leading the family right back to the prior homeostasis: an out-of-control, drug using/codependent family system. As mentioned earlier, I have had cases where the willful, treatment-resistant codependent has sabotaged the addict's fragile recovery and refused to address their role in the problem.

In the family session that took place two days after Peter's return from the wilderness program, I was met with a very different family than I'd been with ten weeks earlier. The residential treatment, the many letters, therapy sessions, and 12-Step meetings had set the stage for this particular meeting. Everyone was relaxed, and the mood was hopeful, but I was well aware of the long path in front of us. Each family member was glad that the presenting problem was "fixed." After a few minutes of joyful conversation about the significant changes Peter and his parents had made, I reminded them of the work ahead. "I'd like to use an analogy here," I said. "You have all signed an agreement which lays out the course of treatment. We are looking at a future in which Peter has a year of continuous sobriety, and you have all completed the 12 Steps in your support groups. I'd like you to imagine we are all playing baseball and the goal is to go around the bases and get to home base. From my perspective, you have hit the ball well and made it to first base. Congratulations! And, now, let's do the ongoing work to get to second base, and third, and eventually to home base; let's keep the eye on the ball and reach the goal we all agreed to."

I explained, "You are each individually practicing new skills and working towards building better relationships—the prior 'crisis' has passed, but we are in a 'guarded prognosis' phase, and we are headed towards developing functional relationships, based on healthy behaviors grounded in recovery principles." I went on, "There will be plenty of time—like, the rest of your lives—to get together and have fun. But for now," I said, looking at Peter's parents, "we want Peter, with your support, to focus on his 'recovery medicine,' his personal therapy, the social support groups, his sober peers, his job, working the 12 Steps with his sponsor, and family therapy, all of which will support rewiring his brain into that of a healthy and normally developing young adult." Again looking at the parents, I continued, "And we want the family system to address some of its, perhaps decades-long, relationship patterns, as you do your own work in family therapy and in your support groups."

Then I brought up the "no talk" suggestion again. "For the next few weeks I'd like you to not talk to Peter. I want him to focus on his new treatment and for you to save your thoughts for our next family session. In a few weeks, you can plan more social time, when you can get together, but even then, I'd like you to stick to 'shoulder to shoulder' activities like hikes or movies where there is little possibility of revisiting past events or prior dysfunctional communication patterns." Then I said, "This may sound dopey, but you will have to trust me. Share new, present-time experiences together, with minimal eye contact."

This cannot be stressed enough—the FRT therapist actively and authoritatively guides the family system through the process of adopting new behaviors. The "bottom" the family experienced and the unanticipated adjustments that occurred during the crisis phase have passed; the happiness that each of them feels now could easily trick any of them to "forget" where they have been and accept the present situation as the "new normal." This is why it is essential that all family members understand from the very start that they will be involved in an ongoing recovery process, and that treatment will unfold as spelled out in the Treatment Agreement.

As Stephanie Brown and Virginia Lewis describe in their book, *The Alcoholic Family in Recovery: A Developmental Model* (1999, p.19): "This finding—the need for family systems collapse—is central to our whole theory of recovery. It is the collapse of the family structures and defense mechanisms that protected and maintained the drinking that clears the ground for the transformative process of recovery." It is essential that family members grasp that recovery entails *a radical transformation.*

The therapist is also prone to "forgetting" the presenting problem, the systemic and individual conditions that informed the treatment plan. Step One, in both AA and Al-Anon, shapes the foundation of the recovery work: "We admitted we were powerless over alcohol—that our lives had become unmanageable."

The concept of powerlessness can be extended beyond alcohol and applied to many other problems or situations—including the family system, other people, and obsessive thinking. Each person regularly reviewing his or her "bottom" will help everyone involved, including the FRT therapist, remain alert to the arc of treatment.

We expect the addict to get a 12-Step sponsor with whom he will typically have daily contact, and who will guide him in "working the Steps." His 12-Step sponsor, his recovering peers, the manager of his SLE, his boss at work, and I will continue to nudge Peter toward a new way of thinking and behaving. At this point, there is nothing substantial his parents can offer beyond love, support, and modeling their commitment to their own work. But there is a whole lot they can do to disrupt, even sabotage, the treatment. Driven by the unconscious pull of the prior homeostasis and their own personal needs, they could tug Peter away from the "education" he is getting from his new support system, and pull him back into their prior drama—"the way it's always been." The enablers and the addict will forget, over and over, and may be lured by memories of the past, and I will remind them, over and over, as I guide them forward in therapy and recovery. This is an essential role for the FRT therapist—like a coach who continually prompts a baseball player to use his new, more effective, batting stance.

The codependents agreed to get sponsors and work the 12 Steps in Al-Anon. Their challenge is to "keep the focus on themselves"—and support Peter in doing the same. I encouraged them to keep in mind the Serenity Prayer: God, grant me the serenity to accept the things I cannot change. (Such as Peter, who now has his own separate, and more developmentally appropriate support and guidance.)

The courage to change the things I can. (Which is only themselves—to let go of their natural parental desire to take care of their "troubled child," and to recognize that he is now getting appropriate guidance from others to facilitate his development—and for them to honestly face the Herculean task of focusing on themselves.)

And the wisdom to know the difference. (Which is very challenging—the members of an enmeshed, fused, codependent family system were naturally thrown into turmoil by the crisis caused by addiction, and were driven to reduce their anxiety by trying to change others.)

This was the work that would unfold, week by week, going forward. There would be many things to talk about in the family sessions, including Peter's job, his SLE experience, and everyone's individual 12-Step work—as well as their ongoing lives. After a few weeks, the treatment would begin to feel more routine, but there are always surprises that pop up.

For example, two months after he had arrived home, Peter brought up in an individual session his wish to "try some controlled drug use." Of course he wanted to! Addicts *always* have cravings—caused by unconscious memories of pleasure or instant pain relief—that morph into fantasies of substance use. (In my early recovery, for instance, a billboard advertising Budweiser would elicit a powerful memory of the pleasure of the first sip, and I would suddenly realize that momentary bliss was just around the corner. To this day, I still periodically experience that craving, which now is quite fleeting, because I'm still taking my "medicine"—going to social support groups and checking in with my mentor.)

An addict's vulnerability to relapse is ever-present in the mind of the FRT therapist. An addict's midbrain is always subject to thoughts of drug use and cravings, which can override his prefrontal cortex—if the addict lets them prevail over what he has learned about preventing relapse. Thinking about using is common for all addicts, but I took Peter's words seriously. We talked about the fact that these thoughts are normal among all addicts, as well as about the consequences of acting on them and actually relapsing.

Two days later, Peter mentioned that some of his old friends were returning home from college and planning a party that evening. I was concerned. I reminded him that he had agreed to abide by a Treatment Agreement stipulation, "staying away from using friends for 90 days," and that he had only been in treatment with me for 60 days.

Peter listened to me and agreed that he would not go to the party, but just "hang out" with his friends. I asked if these friends had problems with drug and alcohol use or were solid friends who could support his sobriety and recovery. He assured me that they were "Okay," but, somehow, I did not totally believe him.

I was apprehensive, and decided to contact Peter's parents and express my concern; I asked them not to mention to Peter the information he had shared with me. I had already told both Peter and his parents that I would share with the parents any information I learned in regard to possible drug use or failure to adhere to the Treatment Agreement.

This is tricky. We want the client in the room to feel that they can trust us—the therapist—that what they say will be kept confidential; but we must remember that we are treating the family system, not an individual, and must think carefully about what we reveal to other family members. I had let everyone in the family know, early on, that drug use or the concern about drug use would not be kept confidential. I include the following in my Informed Consent form, and have each family member sign the form:

> In family therapy, or when different family members are seen individually, confidentiality does not apply between family members. We will use our best clinical judgment when revealing such information.

The following day, I heard from one of Peter's friends that Peter had relapsed. I later learned that Peter had, in fact, gone to the party. At the party, he did some "controlled" drug use that did not work out the way he had hoped—once he started, he lost the ability to stop, and he used a lot more than he had originally intended.

I see two possible explanations for this relapse: either Peter *had planned to use* before the party, and had decided not to talk about it—either to me, to his sponsor, or at his meetings, where he could get the support he needed for his cravings; *or he really intended to stay sober* and hang out with his friends, but his prefrontal cortex was simply unable, at that time, despite his recovery support, to override the craving that he experienced when he was surrounded by substance-using friends.

After hearing that Peter had relapsed, I called Peter, and he did not deny it—instead, he did his best to let me know that it was not a big deal. I reminded him of our agreement—a relapse would require a trip to the local detox facility for 72 hours. Peter first tried to talk me out of his going to detox, and then tried to persuade me to let him postpone going.

"I've only been working at my new Starbucks job for a month, and I'm scheduled to work for the next four days. I'll go on my days off." I was firm and said that we had an agreement and he needed to adhere to it. I advised Peter that he should let his parents know what had happened, and told him that I was going to call his parents if he refused to go to detox. He replied that he would "think about it"—in other words, he was refusing to agree to go. I called Peter's father and explained the situation. The father, as a result of our work together and his attendance at social support groups, had a new perspective about the fallacy of trying to change Peter. He called Peter and said the following, "Keep your agreement with Larry; bring the car home and let us drive you to detox, or I will turn off your cell phone and take the car away." There was no lecture, no judgment, just a simple statement of the consequences. Within hours, Peter was in detox, having called his boss and explained the situation.

The next day, I visited Peter in the detox facility. He was contrite and sober and realized, as a result of his experience, how powerful his addiction was.

This event is illustrative of the power of the "surround" that the addict lives in. We are an affiliative species and have powerful drives to conform to group norms—which is why, as FRT therapists, we are always including social influences beyond the individual and the family in our clinical thinking.

At that party, Peter had quickly succumbed to his craving and consumed a large amount of multiple substances. He understood, at a deeper level, how powerless he was to control his midbrain, and how his midbrain derailed his ability to think and make wise decisions.

Incidents like this, correctly addressed, are among the most important and valuable turning points in addiction treatment. Young adults in recovery (or adults whose addiction begins in their teen years) are typically immature, because regular drug use has delayed their critical emotional, psychological, and social development during these formative years. They do not yet have the mental wherewithal to grasp the deep, personal experience of the ego's loss of control, of "hitting bottom" and "admitting powerlessness." These are cognitive concepts that recovering young adults do not fully understand, unlike an older adult with late-onset addiction, who can better comprehend the reality of lack of control.

For Peter, this relapse was significant. He seemed to understand how insane his thinking had been and how unmanageable his behavior had become, but he hadn't realized how upsetting the ensuing consequences would feel. He was now able—perhaps for the first time—to personally experience craving, loss of control, and adverse consequences in real time, and with a brain that was relatively intact after four months of sobriety, education, therapy, and a happy, fun, sober life.

Peter's parents were rattled, but I explained my thinking about relapse, and we all quickly "got back on the recovery bus." Peter had a new sobriety date, which was humbling, but which supported his new awareness. He had to become a "newcomer" all over again, raising his hand at his meetings when they ask for "newcomers in their first 30 days of sobriety." He had to, with the help of his sponsor, start the Steps over again, beginning with Step One, "We admitted we were powerless over alcohol—that our lives had become unmanageable"—something that now had much more meaning to him. And, we reset the calendar. Completion of the treatment agreement, as stated, requires "one year of continuous sobriety."

Peter's relapse had been a vital part of the treatment process. After his relapse, Peter stayed on track with treatment and with his recovery program, and maintained his sobriety going forward as he successfully navigated the challenges of life: emotional ups and downs, school, job, dating, and family relationships.

Many of my successful young adult cases include relapses. As upsetting and painful as these are, I understand and welcome them, since we have immediate and concrete consequences in place. The addict is often putting the most important piece of recovery in place with a relapse—acknowledging to themselves that they can't control, by themselves, their midbrain's insistent craving, and that they need regular contact with their sober peers. This is the primary purpose of social support and mutual aid groups: to remind us, one day at a time, that we have a chronic, relapsing brain disorder—a disease. Recovering addicts who understand this know they need to stay close to their meetings and bring their cravings-to-use feelings to their therapist, sponsor, and these groups, because every addict is vulnerable to looking for a quick, simple chemical solution when faced with life's endless complex challenges. Having cravings is, by definition, what this brain disease is all about. The addict needs regular reminders of their condition, so they won't "forget"—and suddenly find that their prefrontal cortex was unable to resist the power of their midbrain's craving—and relapse.

And Peter's parents, the codependents, had many "codependent relapses" during that first year. They had been Peter's parents for twenty years, and naturally offered suggestions and guidance to their child for the issues he faced as he struggled with his life, his job, and his relationships—issues they had always had something to say about. But they had also agreed, on paper, to no longer "parent" in the same way. Peter was my "expert" at catching his parents' "slips." During family sessions, I often asked Peter if he had noticed his parents having any codependent relapses, and he was quick to point them out. Every normal teen or young adult strives for independence from their parents and naturally resents any lack of trust the parents exhibit by telling their now-adult child how to run his life.

In a normally developing family, parents naturally transition from a parent-child stance with their child to an adult-adult relationship. In the course of normal development, a young adult individuates, and the parents come to accept that their child is growing into an adult—and step back with pride and let their offspring guide their own lives. However, when addiction is present, it is not uncommon for this process to evoke heightened and long-term conflict. The FRT therapist repeatedly guides the parents to put their focus, not on the addict, but on their own personal process—and not to get sidetracked by the past.

Also, it is not unusual for an addicted/codependent family system to be part of an extended family system that includes other addicts and codependents. Often there is a multigenerational history of enmeshment and poorly differentiated relationships, including problems such as addiction, physical, emotional, or sexual abuse, mental illness, divorce, and broken families. Family Recovery Therapy provided Peter and his parents an opportunity to look at and learn from these patterns in more distant family members.

After the first year, how recovery proceeds varies from family to family. When I survey my work using the FRT model, I realize that nearly all of the addicts I have worked with have been successful in putting their addiction into remission, but not all of their parents have chosen to continue a growth-oriented lifestyle of differentiating themselves from the unconscious homeostasis of their families of origin.

The process, the treatment, the ups and downs of Peter and his family's therapy, were all part of the path I had anticipated. As we approached graduation from treatment, one year of continuous sobriety and completion of the 12 Steps by every family member in treatment, we all began to wonder, "What's next?" I was comfortable with Peter's situation. By this time, some of his friends were also in recovery, and his other friends accepted and supported Peter's recovery—although one had overdosed and died. Peter had an active AA program and enjoyed his meetings, and he assured us that he would continue his 12-Step participation. He had been steadily employed at Starbucks and had been promoted from barista to assistant manager, with benefits and increased pay.

I wondered about the parents' commitment to continuing to attend social support groups after we terminated, but knew that what they had learned had set the stage for Peter's ongoing personal development. I was confident that the whole family system had changed to the extent that Peter would be able to take care of himself in spite of his parents' occasional and natural attempts to try to control his behavior. Peter was solidly on his own feet and would be able to tolerate his parents' slips without being knocked off his path into adulthood.

As of this writing, nearly six years after the family's discharge from treatment, Peter is in college. He has had a number of jobs along the way. He has stopped and started college a few times, but he is currently seriously engaged in his senior year. Peter is planning on becoming a registered nurse, which came as a surprise both to him and his family. He still attends two or three AA meetings each week and sees himself as an "addict in recovery," with five years of continuous sobriety. And, based on his age (24), I would not be surprised if he were to relapse again, because he is still young and still has a diseased brain. Relapse is simply part of this disorder. But, with his parents' loving involvement, the comprehensive 12-Step process, and therapy, his brain and his life have largely been restored to health, and he has attained normal development for his age. He is now a self-supporting adult. If he relapses at this point, he will likely return fairly quickly to his 12-Step meetings. We see this process of relapsing, and then returning to meetings, occurring over and over again. Addiction is a chronic, relapsing disorder. Of course, it is possible that if Peter relapses, he will begin a downward spiral of addiction, hit a bottom, and then either return to recovery—or even drink and use and die an early death. But, because of the work we all did, Peter's chances of putting his disease into sustained remission have been greatly improved. Had his mother not called and set treatment in motion, Peter could have become one of the sad statistics that we all read about.

CHAPTER 8

Case Study—Spouse

"My husband is an alcoholic and I need help." The female caller sounded distressed. A colleague had recently told me that he had given my name to a woman who was concerned about her husband's alcohol use. As the caller, Jennifer, described her concerns to me over the phone, I started to fill in a genogram, which provides a visual snapshot of the family system. Jennifer reported that she was "fighting" with her husband, Bill, and that she thought he had a problem with alcohol and drugs. Their 15-year-old son, Vincent, had taken on some of the roles neglected by her husband. I explained that I am an FRT therapist and I work with the whole family, but I would like to begin by seeing her. I scheduled an appointment to meet with her the next day. (The FRT therapist, as I see it, is a first responder in the crisis of addiction, and I always schedule an appointment with a concerned caller as soon as possible.)

FRT Principle 14
Typically, a member of the enabling subsystem contacts the treatment provider. It is vital that the provider begin to engage the caller in the Family Recovery Therapy treatment model during this first contact.

FRT Principle 3
In Family Recovery Therapy, the client in treatment is the family system that suffers from both addiction and codependency.

The FRT therapist, from the very start, keeps in mind the systemic approach.

When Jennifer came in the next day, it was apparent that she was quite troubled. She talked about leaving her marriage, the distressing emotional communication between herself, her son, and her husband, the emotional abuse among all of them, and the daily fights between herself, her husband, and her son. And she talked about finding drugs in her husband's car and blurted out that she "had had it."

I let her know how I worked and suggested she consider getting the book I co-authored with Avis Rumney, *My Addicted Spouse* (2017a). I told her a little about my practice and briefly mentioned my focus on addiction and codependency, and my approach of working systemically with the family. Meanwhile, I focused on establishing a therapeutic relationship with her, listening compassionately and attuning to her emotional state. I explained that "recovery" is a slow but direct path to help her stabilize, and that there are clear guidelines to follow. I asked her if she was familiar with any of the social support and mutual aid groups where she could connect with individuals in situations similar to hers. She was not aware of them, but seemed open to hearing my suggestions about checking them out.

These groups comprise a critical adjunct to the work of therapy. The FRT therapist coordinates the work of social support and mutual aid groups with therapy, as a kind of adjunctive "group therapy" being done with another "clinician"—the recovering individuals the client encounters in these groups. The members of the addictive/codependent family, to sustain growth and recovery, will eventually transition out of clinical treatment into long-term involvement with these support groups. We introduce clients to these groups as soon as it is appropriate and they are ready. We know that codependency can be a chronic condition. Principle 8 speaks to the codependent's need for support beyond the first year of recovery:

FRT Principle 8
Since addiction and the codependency that enables it are chronic conditions, it is recommended that the addict and codependents develop ongoing support beyond the first year of continuous sobriety.

FRT therapists are well-versed in the workings of social support groups, as noted in Principle 7:

FRT Principle 7
The FRT therapist, who is a state-licensed medical or mental health professional, must be knowledgeable and experienced in many paths to growth and recovery. Ideally, the therapist is engaged in a personal recovery practice, whether 12-Step or other, in which capacity, the therapist stands shoulder-to-shoulder with the family members.

At our next session, Jennifer seemed a little less anxious than initially, but she still sounded pretty hopeless about her marriage and was very concerned about the impact of the stressful home situation on her son. She reported more incidents of her husband's drinking and of fights at home. I asked her if she had been to any meetings, and she said she hadn't.

She cancelled our appointments for the next few weeks, and eventually texted me that she "couldn't afford" the sessions. She had a good job but had taken off the last few months to care for an ailing family member. I told her that it was important for her to stick with therapy and that I would see her "pro bono" for a while. I did not hesitate to offer her this, because I wanted to rule out the role of resistance in her cancellations. It turned out that it was a little of both—finances and resistance. She came in for a couple of sessions, pro bono, which reassured me that it wasn't only her resistance keeping her from coming in, and said she would be able to start paying when she returned to work in a few weeks.

The following week, Jennifer seemed somewhat reserved. She finally told me that she had not gone to any meetings.

In keeping with Principle 4, the FRT therapist, in essence, acts as "a treatment program" run by one person:

FRT Principle 4
During the first year of treatment, the FRT therapist monitors, assesses, and guides the family in an integrated treatment process, which addresses biological, psychological, social, and spiritual recovery.

I understood that Jennifer was conflicted about attending support groups. On the one hand, she wanted to change, and on the other, she was afraid of the unknown. I reviewed her commitment and desire to go forward, and then got out a copy of the Al-Anon schedule and asked her to choose which meetings she would like to go to. She picked three. I asked her if she would be willing to text me after each meeting and let me know how it went. She eagerly agreed, welcoming my support. The next morning, knowing that she had planned to attend a meeting that day, I texted her to let her know that I was looking forward to her text. She replied, "thank you," and that led to a series of texts that resulted in her getting to all three of the meetings she had planned to attend, and deepening her commitment to the support group recovery process.

During one of our initial sessions, when I explained that my approach is systemic and that I work with the whole family, I let Jennifer know that, if she felt it was appropriate, she was welcome to invite her son or husband to come in for a session, just to let me know ahead of time. For our third session, she alerted me that she was bringing in her 15-year-old son, Vincent. She had explained to him that she was "seeing a counselor to talk about the conflict at home." They arrived with a fresh story of the previous day's fight between Vincent and his father. I introduced the subject of his father's drinking, and first Jennifer, then Vincent, launched into a description of a family system full of drama. In their reports, all three of them engaged in endless, ineffective behavior and cycled through the interchangeable roles of victim, rescuer, and persecutor, known as the Karpman Drama Triangle (Karpman, 1968) (see Figure 5.3).

I reflected on my own family when I was growing up. I so wished that my siblings and I could have talked with a trusted professional. Having such a person listen to a description of our situation, and explain what was going on, would have gone a long way toward helping us dis-identify from the repetitive crises. A therapist could have helped us understand that there was simply mental illness present in my family. This kind of guidance can help family members develop compassion for the sufferer—in my family, as in Jennifer's, everyone was suffering—and learn coping skills to avoid the drama and move forward with their individual lives and development.

Eventually, Jennifer began to work again, and started going to more, and different, Al-Anon meetings. She was beginning to "get it." She showed up to therapy sessions, sat on the edge of her seat, and asked rapid-fire questions. She wanted to know what would happen in the future, but, over and over again, I brought her back to the present day, and I reminded her simply to follow suggestions and "trust the process." Jennifer related that her husband was curious and somewhat annoyed at her coming to see me, and at her interrupting the normal routine at home by going out in the evenings to "those meetings." When Jennifer mentioned that he had asked questions about what she talked about "in those sessions," I reminded her that her husband, Bill, "was welcome to come in, too."

I received a text from Jennifer saying, "Bill would like to come see you, alone, would that be OK?" Because I work with everyone in the family, I replied that it was fine, and I asked her to have him call me to set up a session. It is not unusual for a spouse in this situation to ask to come in. Since his wife had been seeing me for many weeks, and he probably was thinking that at least some of what was discussed was about him, he wanted a chance to tell his side of the story.

Bill called me the next day to schedule an appointment. He arrived on time and presented himself as one would expect for a successful banker. He was tall, somewhat slim, well dressed, and had a worried look on his face. I naturally slipped into my familiar Rogerian mode, and was accepting, empathic, and received his words with unconditional positive regard. I wanted him to feel safe and to be able to trust me. I explained that I was a family systems therapist and pointed to a three-generation mobile that hung in the corner of my office. I explained that I saw my role as helping facilitate improvement of each member of the family as well as the family as a whole. I looked at him and said, "How can I help you?"

He agreed that there had been a lot of discord in the family, that they had a teenaged son who was "a pain in the ass," and who "always wants to fight with me." He also said that he and his wife had lots of fights, and that there was little intimacy between them. I asked if he could imagine a happier scenario, a family that got along better. He was not sure, and replied that the problems had been going on for a long time, and he didn't foresee the others changing enough to make that happen.

I was curious and asked Bill if he would be willing to give me an example of one of the conflicts at home. He reported that there had been a recent situation where his son had been disrespectful and had refused to respond to some simple requests. The discord had nearly escalated into a physical fight between him and his son. The part he left out, which Jennifer and Vincent had described at an earlier session that they attended together, was that he was very intoxicated at the time.

I was aware that Bill's wife had labeled him "an alcoholic," but I needed to remain open to the possibility that alcohol was only a side issue, and that there were many other explanations for their discord—not all substance abusers meet the medical diagnosis of addiction. I needed to know a lot more before considering the possibility of addiction.

At one point, I asked Bill, "If Jennifer were in the room, what do you think she might say her concerns are?" "She thinks I have a drinking problem," he said.

I asked, "Do you think there is any merit in her concern?" "Not really," he replied. "I like to drink, but I keep it under control. I think she makes too big of a deal about it. It's not a problem." That was enough. Alcohol and his drinking had entered the conversation, and I did not pursue it. My hope would be to get Bill and his wife together in the room, where a more balanced discussion could occur. I asked him if he would be willing to come to a session with his wife. He agreed, and we set up a session for the two of them to come in together. Bill and I spent the rest of the session discussing what was good about his marriage. I came to understand, with him, that he wanted to keep his family together and would be willing to engage in couples' therapy to explore and seek resolution for some of the issues that stood in the way of a better relationship.

During the next session, when they both came in, I reminded them that I'm a licensed marriage therapist and that my goal was to learn more about what was working in their relationship and what was problematic, and, over time, to help them work things out for the better, if that was possible.

Jennifer wanted to focus on Bill's drinking—she said it was central to their conflicts. But I was aware that Bill was the "gatekeeper," the one who might feel unsafe and walk out the door, prematurely ending the work. I made the decision to give him a little more power and let him talk at length about the conflicts from his perspective, making sure he was heard and validated. I knew the substance-use issue would come up, but I also wanted to solidify his trust in me and in the therapy.

(This approach, siding with the addict's denial as a tactic to engage them in therapy, is something that I had warned Jennifer about previously. I knew she might be upset and think that we were "wasting the session," but my goal was to establish a therapeutic alliance with Bill.)

Jennifer agreed with Bill that she was often upset and that they would engage in loud fights that they both knew upset their son. Eventually, when she had the floor, Jennifer expressed her fear that Bill had a drinking problem. I asked her to give me an example of when it had been an issue, but before she spoke, I explained that many people like to drink, and not all of them have a problem with it. I was purposely colluding with Bill at this point to soften what I knew would eventually emerge.

If he was an alcoholic, I knew he would be defensive, and I wanted him, for the moment, to be able to keep his denial intact. I knew the only way he would get to a deeper understanding of his problem would be for it to happen on his own terms. And I wanted to keep him safe—for the sake of the therapeutic alliance.

Jennifer gave examples of several situations in which it appeared to me that Bill could not control his substance use. I suggested that "there might be other reasons for this behavior," again supporting Bill. I wanted Jennifer to have me hear her story with Bill present, but I also did not want to trigger him and have him bolt from therapy.

"Jennifer," I said, looking directly at her, knowing that Bill was hearing me, "Bill is the world's leading authority on his experience, and he may not see his drinking as a problem. But I'd like to offer some simple definitions of what problematic substance use looks like. There are four simple criteria, all of which need to be present for someone to have a problem with substances. They are: loss of control, craving, adverse consequences, and chronicity—that the problem has been going on for a while."

It was nearing the end of the session, and I said that I'd like to make a suggestion. "What I'd like the two of you to do is to come back next week and discuss this situation further. And, I'd like the two of you to not make changes in your behavior this week, keep doing what you have always done, and simply notice what happens, then come back next week so that we can discuss what the week was like." Bill, seeming relieved, agreed. Jennifer seemed somewhat upset that I had not been more direct with Bill's "problem." I suggested that she keep going to her support groups and keep learning about how she loses her serenity when she is with Bill, and reminded her to focus on herself instead of on her husband's behavior.

Reflecting on the session after they left, I felt it was a success. They had agreed to come back, and by giving them information about addiction, I had planted the seeds. There was no way that I could tell if Bill had taken seriously the words I had used—loss of control, craving, adverse consequences, and chronicity—but it was possible that he had heard information that might ultimately be critical to his realizing he had a problem with drinking—if, in fact, he did.

In my mind, we were now in the middle of a systemic intervention. In crisis situations, my intervention colleagues perform systemic interventions in the space of a couple of days—they get the codependent family members on board and sometimes can even get the addict to begin treatment. However, an FRT therapist can take the time to slow the process down. This pace permits the family members in their current homeostasis to integrate the information, and it allows the situation to evolve without provoking even more disruption. After all, the dysfunctional situation has existed for a long time and recovery, if it happens, will unfold one day at a time.

At the next couples' session, we discussed what they had learned over the previous week, during which I had suggested that they simply observe—and not try to change—their patterns. It became apparent that Bill's drinking was problematic. He had been quite intoxicated on a number of occasions. He did not deny it: "Yes, I guess I did drink a little too much, I don't think I'll do that again," was his typical response. During that session, I asked Bill if he would be willing to come in for another individual session with me, and he agreed.

When I met with Bill alone, I asked him if he ever wondered if he might have a drinking or drug problem. I was not surprised when he said he didn't think so. I also inquired if he would be open to my asking some questions about his drinking. I explained that I had a few standard clinical testing instruments that inform professionals about whether or not a client has a problem with drugs or alcohol. Depending on the situation, I use the Alcohol Use Disorders Identification Test, or AUDIT (Babor et al., 2001), the Michigan Alcoholism Screening Test, known as the MAST

(Selzer, 1971), and AA's Twelve Questions (Alcoholics Anonymous World Services, 2018b) (see Appendix G). I told Bill that these tests are not definitive, but that they may provide some useful information that can illuminate a discussion about substance use.

Bill agreed to my asking him the questions from two of these testing instruments. The results clearly showed Bill that there might be reason for concern. I explained again that these questionnaires were simply guides, but that they might indicate a possible problem. At this point, I reassured Bill that there might not be an issue that needed any sort of addiction treatment. "But," I said, "I would like to give you a little more information to consider." I explained that he could diagnose himself if he was curious. I suggested, if he was willing, to try some controlled drinking. He said that he would be open to that. "Here is what I'd like you to do," I said. "Before you drink, make a decision about how many drinks you will have. It's fine if you want to drink a lot, just try to make that decision before you start. See if you can stick with your decision. If you can stick with the decision you made beforehand, it is a good sign that you can control your usage. And, if you are okay with this, maybe pick one day to not drink." He reassured me, as the session ended, that it was OK for me to share what we had discussed with his wife the following week during my individual session with her.

A few weeks later, during the next couples' session, I reviewed what Bill and I had discussed during our previous meeting regarding testing instruments and his decision to see if he could stick with an agreement he made with himself to limit his drinking to a pre-determined number of drinks, and possibly, to take a day off from drinking. He seemed somewhat hesitant, and I moved on, again not confronting his denial. I imagined that, if he had a problem, he would not like to share it with either Jennifer or me, but I had put the conversation into the room and between them, if only briefly. I would let him stew with that issue, which could cause him to feel deeply conflicted, perhaps not even consciously. It would be premature for me to confront Bill's process at this point.

Jennifer came in for an individual session. She acted like she had in previous sessions—she was expressive, sitting on the edge of her seat, talking and asking questions in a rapid and pressured way. Her codependency was in full flower: she reported that Bill's drinking was still a big problem, that she did not think he would change, that he was still drinking with his drinking buddies, and that she was wondering whether to stay in the marriage. I reminded her to "trust the process," and shifted the focus to her recovery, what meetings she had been to, and what she had been learning about herself.

It had taken many years for the members of this family to evolve to this point of homeostasis, which was held in place by unconscious forces, and I was well aware that many steps were needed to get this family back on a path of normal development. Chronicity is a hallmark of addiction and of codependency, as described in FRT Principles 1 and 2:

FRT Principle 1
Addiction is a chronic, relapsing, treatable medical disease with profound mental and physical consequences. Addicts will need long-term, possibly lifelong, recovery support, which can take many forms.

FRT Principle 2
Effective treatment of addiction usually involves treatment of codependents, because codependents enable addiction. Codependency is a chronic relationship pattern that has profound mental and physical consequences and is characterized by an obsessive focus on other people. Codependents may need lifelong recovery support, which can take many forms.

Throughout the treatment process, the FRT therapist needs both to observe what is happening currently, and also to return to and remind the clients that, if there is active addiction and codependency present, these are serious, but treatable concerns—and that there is a well-worn path to healing.

Jennifer was witnessing glimmers of this path in the support groups where she heard the stories of others who had been in even worse places than she was, but who had, over time, been able to do the work to get back to happiness for themselves, even if not in their marriages. And I reminded her that I felt that my work with Bill was going well, even if it did not seem like it to her. After all, their process was unfolding in real time at home, and between them—there were fewer arguments and disruptions as she focused on herself and did not get involved in Bill's attempts to modify his behavior. And, there was not the sudden and disruptive change that can shake up a family when an addict is sent to rehab with the family hoping for a "major shift" that will "fix things." Bill, at some point, might see the wisdom of addiction treatment, but it was clear right now that he would be resistant, and if pressured, he might consent, but might have serious reservations which could undermine his treatment and eventually lead him to resume drinking.

"It is important," I said, "to fully understand that we really don't know what your husband will ultimately do, but you are now more aware of how you are changing and that your personal progress is very much in your control. You need to, as is often said, 'trust the process' and keep doing your own personal work."

Murray Bowen often talked about how two people in a stressed relationship may triangulate in a third entity in order to reduce tension. The addict may triangulate their addiction into the dynamic to help relieve stress. The codependent may triangulate in another family member, such as a child, for instance. In Jennifer's family, her son had been triangulated into the stressed marital relationship to provide relief for the marital dyad. The goal in Family Recovery Therapy is to help the addict and the codependent accept another, different, "third entity," which consists of the recovery community and the treatment process. Optimally, both the addict and the codependent will develop trust in the support and healing offered by both the FRT therapist and the mutual aid groups. These sources will guide them both along the path to interrupt the downward spiral of addiction and codependency, and move the family forward on a path toward restoration of normal development.

Because social support groups are a vital component of Family Recovery Therapy, and 12-Step groups are widespread, it is essential that the FRT therapist be knowledgeable about the culture and process of 12-Step recovery, even if the therapist is not specifically involved in these groups. Principles 6 and 7 speak to the FRT therapist's need to be familiar with 12-Step recovery and with other paths to personal growth:

FRT Principle 6
The FRT therapist must be well-versed in the 12 Steps and have a thorough understanding and appreciation for the fundamental role that mutual aid programs play in recovery from codependency and addiction.

FRT Principle 7
The FRT therapist, who is a state-licensed medical or mental health professional, must be knowledgeable and experienced in many paths to growth and recovery. Ideally, the therapist is engaged in a personal recovery practice, whether 12-Step or other, in which capacity, the therapist stands shoulder-to-shoulder with the family members.

I met with Bill individually again. He was beginning to "get it." The information about addiction had landed. When I asked Bill how he was doing, he was quiet for a moment. Then he started to complain about the "problem teen" at home and the ways his wife was pressuring him to change. When it felt appropriate, I brought up the topic of his looking at his drinking and reminded him of our earlier discussion. Bill said that, for the most part, he was able to stay within the limits he set for himself, but noticed that there were times he was unable to. I asked if he would be willing to give me a little history of problems that had occurred in his life that may have been caused by his drinking and drug use. I was somewhat surprised at his willingness to reveal a list of situations in which his substance use had resulted in bad consequences. Bill described a period he had used amphetamines to make him "better at work," and also relayed a number of alcohol-related problems that had occurred in high school and college.

I asked him if he thought any drug- or alcohol-related situations in his adult life might have impacted his relationships with his wife or son. This is a question that the FRT therapist must be mindful not to ask until it is clear that the client will answer "yes." Asking this too early in the process may elicit defensiveness from the client. The substance-using client, we must remember, has most likely been asking themselves this question for a long time, and simultaneously using the defenses of denial and rationalization to avoid answering it in the affirmative, either because they don't understand the problem, or they don't know how to get the help they need. If we have done our work, if we have educated the addict about the fact that addiction is a disorder of an organ, the brain, and explained that there is a simple fix, if they are willing to choose it; they may start to wonder, themselves, about addressing the problem.

I did not push the discussion any further. Bill had admitted to another person, me, that possibly he had a substance-use problem. I imagined that he might be frightened at that moment. I wanted to give him a little space to integrate this new reality into his ego. After a period of silence, I let him know that, if he did have an issue with substance use, there were some options to consider if he wanted to address it. I asked him if he would like to hear what some people who have had trouble controlling their substance use have done to get help. I was not surprised when he said; "I'm not interested in doing anything right now." But his demeanor suggested he was open to hearing my ideas.

"Okay, let me say a little about it, in case you ever become interested." He nodded yes. I described why some people get into trouble with drugs. Their "loss of control" could be attributed to a number of factors, including pain, even unconscious pain, from childhood, and that these individuals self-medicate to numb discomfort. Some people develop problems with substances when they lack guidance to limit their use, and they often respond to a course of cognitive-behavior therapy. Others suffer from depression or anxiety and use substances to manage their moods. And, I mentioned again that there are those who have the medical disease of addiction and cannot control their drug use.

As I described to Bill the reasons some people use substances to cope, I was aware that we can never really know what is going on in another person's mind. Sometimes the therapist's goal is purely to maintain a relationship with the client, and that can mean simply respecting their pace and not moving them forward in the process too quickly. I said to Bill, "This is useful information, and it's good that you know that there are simple ways to address a substance problem, if you ever want to consider doing something about it."

I thought back to when I learned I needed help to deal with my alcoholism. In my case, I was told by a professional that I had a substance-using problem, and that I could get help, but another eight months elapsed before my ego succumbed to reality and I realized that the way I was "controlling" my alcohol use was not working. It was then that I asked for help.

I knew that there was a possibility that if I offered Bill too much information, he might distance from counseling, and continue drinking, something that unfortunately happens far too often. It is the clinician's acceptance that he cannot control the outcome that keeps his countertransference (and codependency) in check. The therapist must refrain from pressuring the addict—who naturally will distrust anyone who discredits his choices. I felt that Bill knew that I respected his decisions and empathized with his position, and that I was ready to listen if he ever wanted to discuss any of it. I let Bill know again that I was available to talk. As it turned out, I did not see him again for many weeks.

Jennifer had continued going to support groups, and even developed connections with a few women there. The focus of my work with her gradually shifted to helping her accept her new recovery lifestyle and what she was learning about herself. She had asked a woman to be her sponsor, and began to call her regularly. Jennifer moved from fearing the chaos of a dysfunctional and depressing home life to living one day at a time, finding hope, and trusting that a better future was unfolding, regardless of Bill's drinking. She always had a story or two of his antics, but she was no longer automatically stepping into the drama he created. At one point, she told Bill that she was "no longer interested in talking to him if he had been drinking." Bill, predictably, had a tantrum, which started a fight, and resulted in a momentary return to the prior, emotionally fused, chaotic homeostasis. But the fight resolved quickly when Jennifer stopped responding to Bill's barbs and instead said she was going to a meeting.

Jennifer was no longer willing to enable their prior "intimacy." The alcoholic, typically incapable of the true intimacy of sharing authentic feelings, often views a couple's dramatic arguments and fights as a form of emotional connection. Jennifer's decision to disengage from that dynamic, and her refusal to participate in any form of uncomfortable emotional connection with Bill when he was intoxicated, left Bill with space to consider his own behavior. He saw his wife's progress in recovery as a threat to their connection. She was regaining her equilibrium, becoming happier, and spending more time at meetings and on the phone with other recovering women that she had befriended.

I have heard the following story at a number of social support meetings that I have attended:

> My drinking was not a problem, oh, maybe a little bit, but then my spouse started attending those damn meetings. She would no longer fight with me, she would go out at night to meetings, and she'd be on the phone laughing with someone. The next thing I knew, I was in recovery!

As time passed, both Bill and Jennifer could see the writing on the wall. Their marriage, to be successful, would require *both* of them to change. The prior homeostasis was no longer working for Jennifer, or for their marriage.

Again, I often reflect on my own family's experience, which is pertinent here. When I was 18 years old, my mother, after attending only a few Al-Anon meetings, had an epiphany, confronted my alcoholic father and told him he had to stop drinking or she would divorce him. Neither of my parents was getting any support to consider other options. My father, unable to stop drinking, left home. My mother, devastated, divorced him. Some years later, my father died as a result of his addiction. Poorly planned interventions can fail because they do not provide sufficient support for the family to change and establish new norms, which is a process that takes time. This is the wisdom of Family Recovery Therapy—the slow, clinical approach that honors *all* family members and guides them forward at a pace that is sustainable. This optimizes the possibility that the addict can maintain sobriety and that each family member can get support to change—to heal their codependency.

Jennifer, six months into our work, and solidly ensconced in her support group, again wanted to talk about what the future would look like. In the past, when she brought up this topic, I always brought her back to the present day, and said something like, "Remember, you need to stay in the present, to live one day at a time, and to trust me and the recovery process. You have been to enough meetings to have heard stories of those who have been in your shoes, and how their lives improved, slowly, over time, sometimes taking years." She had also heard stories of those in her shoes who had separated from their addict spouses, and had even sought divorce and started new lives. And she had heard stories of couples who had separated, and after years apart, had reconciled, rejoined their families, and pursued healthy lives together.

This time, when Jennifer brought up the topic of the future, I gave her space to talk about her thoughts. It was clearly an option for her to move out, and to take their 15-year-old son with her. She talked about the possibility, if she moved out, that Bill might eventually choose to change and get help, and they could reconcile—she didn't think he really wanted to destroy the family. She had finally reached a point where she could make a more informed decision, a decision I had suggested in previous sessions that she postpone. She had developed a fledgling support system that could help her if she did decide to move out. I expressed my concern, as I had earlier, that if she did not yet have her feet solidly on the ground, or had insufficient support, a decision to leave Bill now might simply provoke another crisis—one where she would not actually leave him, which would only escalate the drama, solidify her codependency, and reaffirm Bill's need to drink.

A few days after my session with Jennifer, Bill, perhaps intuiting his wife's thinking, called me and asked if he could come in and see me. He was clearly in a dour mood when he arrived and promptly announced that he "thought he had a problem with drinking."

At this point, I needed to empathize with Bill and be curious about what he meant. It would be tempting to think he was ready for "rehab," and for all that addiction treatment could entail, but it is important to understand that "having a problem with drinking" could mean any number of things to Bill. He could be self-medicating to relieve discomfort, and I needed to make room for him to fully explore and thoroughly understand what he was thinking and feeling before I began to consider making recommendations.

Stepping back briefly, I'd like to compare this moment, months into Family Recovery Therapy, with the chaos that existed in the family when Jennifer first called me. Bill had received significant information about drinking and family relationships from his sessions with me, and he had had time to reflect on what he had learned. Jennifer had changed her behavior, and, for the most part, had stepped out of the alcoholic drama triangle game and distanced herself from Bill's drinking behavior. They had both made important progress.

I'd also like to compare this process to what a "surprise-model interventionist" might have done if Jennifer had instead called them and asked for help. The interventionist would have arrived at the home, met with Jennifer, gathered information from her, perhaps invited a few other family members to join them, and then set up a meeting that included Bill. In the meeting, everyone would describe the impact of Bill's drinking on them. The interventionist would suggest that Bill enter residential treatment for his "alcoholism," and, perhaps, that Jennifer attend Al-Anon to get support for herself. This kind of approach would have been risky if Bill were still in denial and resistant to the pressure to go into treatment, but went along with the plan. While this kind of intervention might be successful, it posed the danger that Bill might leave treatment early, resume drinking, and create even more discord in the family.

To succeed in making transformative changes in our lives, the prospect of a fundamentally different future needs to be considered thoroughly and approached carefully, with a clear understanding both of the process involved and of the support needed to make the shift. Change usually happens by degrees. The addict, whose denial has been intact for many years, needs to go through a learning process over time, to become ready to accept the reality of his addiction—his loss of control, adverse consequences, and dire circumstances—before he is likely to consider treatment. The FRT therapist, from the beginning, slowly works with only the family members who are willing to change, the enabling codependents, and guides them to alter their behavior and to focus on themselves. In this way, the family system can shift in ways that may allow the addict to awaken to his problem.

The addict, with dawning awareness of the extent of their problem, will typically try to control their substance use, only to discover, as they grasp their powerlessness, that they need outside help.

When Bill had acknowledged in a therapy session a couple of months earlier that his drinking had been problematic, he clearly had begun to develop a deeper understanding, despite his denial, of the difficulty his drinking was causing. Certainly, two months earlier, he had not been ready to acknowledge his loss of control. Now, however, he was not only saying he had a problem, but also seemed ready to look at it more closely. He asked, "Do you think I should go to a program?" "Yes, obviously," I thought, but did not say that, yet. I didn't see an imminent crisis, and wanted to slow him down and let him get more information—I didn't want him to take a flight into a "fantasy recovery" only to change his mind a moment later.

"What makes you think you have a problem?" I asked. "Well, I've been thinking about what you told me about alcoholism, the loss of control and the crazy shit happening, and I think I have finally admitted to myself that there is something I need to look at. I think I need to get into some sort of program or something."

This next stage—providing a relatively uninformed, frightened addict with a detailed, concrete plan of action—may best be described through the lens of salesmanship. The "customer" (Bill) is "in the market" for our "product" (addiction treatment). We can mention the "benefits" of our product—better health, renewed harmony in their marriage and family, improved performance at work, and so on. But before we can "make the sale," we need to explore the person's resistance and be sure they are ready. Our job is to be attuned to the client and to assess the degree to which they are prepared to move forward. The client may need more time to "think about it," to ask more questions, or to try some more controlled drinking, before they are ready to sign up. It is only when we are convinced that *they are ready to accept help* that we begin to inform them about what addiction treatment looks like.

At this point, I was clear that I needed to offer Bill some options—I knew that he needed effective help, but first I wanted to know what he was thinking. I asked him what he thought he needed. "I don't know, but I'd like to hear about the choices."

I thought back to how I'd begun recovery. When I had sought help with my addiction, four decades earlier, my situation was very different from Bill's. I was frightened, and realized that I could not control my drinking on my own, and I needed help. I made a few calls, found a support group, showed up at a group meeting, and followed the suggestions I heard there. It was some years later before I sought mental health assistance to begin to heal my past and restore the development that had been derailed by growing up in an alcoholic home and becoming an addict. I was not going to recommend that route—simply attending support groups—to Bill. I knew I had been lucky. While this route works for many people, there are others who go to a few support group meetings and continue drinking, thinking, "well, that didn't work, these people are crazy."

Any treatment options I would suggest to Bill would be comprehensive, grounded in the 14 Principles, and would include his family. Treatment could start with a residential program, followed by a long-term intensive outpatient approach. Or, it could start as outpatient, assuming he was stable enough for that to be successful. Residential stabilization would certainly be recommended if outpatient treatment did not provide sufficient support.

Adding residential treatment to our outpatient, year-long plan can ground the addict in recovery and get them off to a solid start. But there are some downsides to this: residential treatment is often costly, and it would require Bill to be away from his job and family (see Appendix H). To my mind, the real work would be done, long-term, in his home environment, with his family, friends, work, and local support groups. Sometimes starting treatment at home, as vulnerable as the addict may be, is the best way to build a good recovery foundation. At other times, especially if the addict's health is badly depleted or they can't stop drinking, a stint in a residential program is indicated. As noted in Principle 4, The FRT therapist assesses the addict and the family, evaluates treatment options, and guides the recovery process by making recommendations appropriate for the specific situation:

FRT Principle 4
During the first year of treatment, the FRT therapist monitors, assesses, and guides the family in an integrated treatment process, which addresses biological, psychological, social, and spiritual recovery.

The individual session with Bill had covered a lot of ground. He had admitted he had a problem and wanted to know about treatment. He asked, "Okay, what does treatment look like, what do I have to do?" He might be ready to embark on the healing process his wife had already begun. I offered hope as I described the general format of treatment. I explained to Bill that addiction has consequences that impact the biological, psychological, social, and spiritual aspects of both the individual and the family, and that a treatment program needs to address each of these. I said that our FRT program would initially require him to commit "a few hours a day" to his recovery process, which I commented, "is much less time each day than what you lose to your alcoholism when intoxication and hangovers are factored in." I explained that our intensive outpatient treatment program included education, individual and family counseling, attending social support groups, and drug testing. I further explained that his time commitment would decrease somewhat as treatment progressed, and that the program continued until he had a year of continuous sobriety. I also said that if residential treatment were part of the plan, a residential program would recommend a step down to an intensive outpatient program, such as my FRT program.

I clarified that my approach is family-systems-based, and that Jennifer and his son would be expected to be part of the program. And I told Bill that if this form of treatment did not work, if he was unable to stay sober in an outpatient program, then a residential program would be recommended. I also gave him a list of YouTube videos that would give him another view of addiction and treatment that I thought was appropriate for him to look at (see Appendix F).

I suggested that we set up a session with his wife to discuss a possible treatment plan, and I scheduled the joint session as soon as I could. At the end of a joint session, I would want them to fully understand the "purchase" they were considering—to have answers to all their questions, and to be prepared to "sign on the dotted line." If we, ourselves, remember making a major purchase—a car or a house—we can recall riding an emotional rollercoaster while preparing to sign documents. The car salesman, realtor, or loan officer led us through a process that made signing the detailed documents almost an afterthought—and yet, the "devil is in the details." Spelling out the details with Bill and Jennifer was critical. Both of them must understand and agree to each of the terms, because down the road they might resist and test boundaries if their fear of change emerged—they might push back and question or try to negotiate specific agreements.

I started the couples' session with a review of where we had been: How frightened Jennifer had been at our early meetings, her slow acceptance that she was living with a problem drinker, and her gradual shift in attention to caring for herself, while letting Bill get a clearer understanding of his own issues. I reported that Bill had slowly come to understand that he did have a problem and that he had decided to get help for it. I asked Bill if he had told Jennifer about what we had talked about in our previous meeting—about his acceptance of his alcoholism and the options for treatment. Bill replied that he had not talked with her about realizing he had a problem. "Would you be willing," I asked, "to share some of what we talked about yesterday, and what you are thinking?"

Slowly, Bill turned to Jennifer as he responded. "Yes. I think I need help with my drinking problem. I met with Larry yesterday, and we talked about some of the options, some of the things I can do to get help." Part of me was internally jumping up and down with joy, and another part knew that this was a radical shift in the couple's homeostasis, and that almost anything could cause either one of them to say something that would upset this fragile opening. They were anxious, and again, like a good salesman, I took control and did what I could do to normalize this moment and the feelings they were having, and to help guide each of them towards the goal. They both seemed to want this "shiny new car"—a vehicle that was clearly going to meet their needs far more effectively and joyfully than the one they were currently "driving"—but they harbored many fears and concerns.

I reviewed where we had been, what was happening right now, and what I thought needed to happen next, based on what they had told me. I explained that Bill's long history of alcohol use had become problematic, that Jennifer's concern had slowly drawn her into a codependent relationship with Bill, and this had evolved into a marriage and a family in crisis. I said that now they could seriously consider embarking on a path that would lead them to a better future. They were quiet and seemed open to my next thoughts. I knew, as the salesman, that there were a large number of details that they would both need to agree to if I were to accept them into my program, details that they, at this moment, might object to. I stopped speaking, and asked each of them if they had any questions at this point. I needed to stay neutral, to be ready to let each buyer consider their willingness to move forward, to give them space, if needed, and to continue to address their resistance and not pressure them.

There were two possible outcomes: either they would agree to "think about it," which would lead to their "buying the car," or, they would want to "think about it for a while." The FRT therapist, going with what develops, will work with either option, letting the process unfold, working with the resistance, but keeping intact the therapeutic relationship with the clients.

This is often the moment when an interventionist, a drug program, an addiction call center, or a drug counselor will take advantage of the addict's vulnerability and push the sale, resulting in a conflicted and ambivalent customer with misgivings, who starts treatment feeling pressured and not fully committed. I think AA's first three Steps clearly explain what an FRT therapist wants the addict (and codependent) to understand and accept. In those three Steps, in essence, the addict accepts that they have an alcohol problem and they understand that there is a process of recovery which is available to them, if they are willing to ask for help, follow directions, and trust the process. And the codependent similarly understands that they cannot fix the alcoholic, that they, too, need to ask for help, follow the guidance they receive, and let the recovery process unfold.

Once I became confident that Bill and Jennifer wanted help, like the couple who want the new vehicle, I said, "Great, let's review what we're talking about."

The FRT therapist, from the first phone contact, has been building the foundation of the treatment model—and, trusting the model. Both Bill and Jennifer had heard me mention, in general terms, that "addiction is a family systems problem," that there is a "well-worn path to healing," that the path involves "drug and codependency counseling, psychotherapy, drug testing, the use of 'social support groups' for both the addict and the codependent," and that the treatment process "supports the addict through the first year of continuous sobriety."

They seemed to be with me, so far, and I began to fill in more details. The goal at this point is to spell out the rationale for each point in the Treatment Agreement. In this way, when we get to the specifics, they will already have heard and understood the overarching reasoning—not unlike a car buyer understanding the details of a car's warranty.

Picturing the exact sequence of events that occur in purchasing a car may be helpful in understanding this moment. You are witnessing your client and his family standing inside a dealership, thinking about taking possession of a shiny new car, imagining wonderful scenarios of driving it around, parking it at home, etc. However, they still have to go into that room, the inner office, with a salesman, and sign a bunch of documents, many of which they may not fully understand, before they can drive the new car off the lot. Obviously, starting addiction treatment may not be as much fun as buying a car, but the salesman—or FRT therapist—does not want the deal to fall apart in the document-signing process, so he will clearly review the details, and say something like I said to Bill and Jennifer:

> The program requires the addict and the codependent each initially to commit a few hours a day to the recovery process. It includes education, counseling, reading, attending social support groups, drug testing, and possibly other elements. And, if this does not work, if Bill is unable to stay sober in an outpatient program, then I would recommend a residential program. This is a family-systems-based approach, and Jennifer is expected to participate in the program—and either of you may also be referred for additional support, if needed. Your time commitment will decrease somewhat as time goes on, and the program continues until Bill has a year of continuous sobriety.

I then said, "Do you have any questions?" I wanted to address their concerns now. I wanted assurance that we would not get bogged down in any of the specifics later. From using this approach successfully with many dozens of families, I had learned that this model works, that progress in the early days and weeks can bring relief and hope to painful lives. I wanted them to fully understand and willingly agree to all parts of the treatment plan. And I knew that refusal to agree with *any* of the agreement's points portended possible failure and a break in the connection between us, as well as the very real possibility of relapse and loss of healing for the whole family.

If I sense clients are ready to initiate Family Recovery Therapy, I bring out the Treatment Agreement (Appendix E) and read it slowly, one line at a time, explaining anything that is unclear, answering any questions, and getting their consent. Bill and Jennifer seemed ready to go forward.

I explained that there are three parts of the agreement: one for the addict, one for the codependent, and one for the family system. And then I read them the Treatment Agreement. "This is the 'Addiction/Codependency Family Treatment Agreement' and the following are treatment recommendations."

Looking at Bill, I said, "this is the *Treatment for the Addict*:"

1. *Addict agrees to stop all substance use, detox, and, if appropriate, move into a sober living environment.*

"Let me explain this." I continued, "Many addicts are so impaired that they need to be medically detoxed to get the support they need to be safe. Bill, how much have you had to drink in the last few days? Do you think you could stop now, or do you think you need to go to a detox facility?" I had a sense, from previous sessions, that he would not need a detox facility, and expected him to say that, but I had planted the seed in case he relapsed in the future and did need that help. Detox after a relapse is often a medically-recommended escalation of treatment which can help focus an addict's attention on the chronic and relapsing nature of addiction. He said that he did not need detox, that he could stop drinking on his own.

Then I brought up the "move into a sober living environment" clause of the agreement. I explained that living in a sober living environment (SLE) is standard protocol for those who are unable to stay in remission while living in their current, often stressful, home environment. Looking at Jennifer, I said, "This is a particularly challenging time in every addict's recovery, and you need to understand that Bill, in order to be successful, will need a lot of support, and you will need to focus on your program to optimize his chances of remaining sober." I asked Bill if he thought he would benefit from moving into a local, supportive living environment for the initial stage. He said, "No, I would like to stay at home."

"Okay," I said, "just know this is an option, if you are not able to stay sober at home."

2. *Individual and Family Therapy.*

I explained that each week I would work with all three components of the program, the addict, the codependent, and the family. This would include daily in-person or phone sessions with the addict for the first week or two, until I was assured that he was engaged and comfortable with his social support groups. The frequency of our sessions would decrease over time, but at a minimum would continue weekly until a year of continuous sobriety and completion of the 12 Steps were achieved. Bill and Jennifer both nodded their consent to this part of the agreement.

3. Addict agrees to attend 12-Step meetings, get a sponsor, work the Steps, go to 90 meetings in 90 days, and then continue to go to regular meetings until graduation from the program.

"No surprise here," I said. I had mentioned more than once that "the program would require a few hours a day," and would include "some sort of support group, probably 12-Step." I told Bill that AA was the most available support group, with over 300 meetings a week in our county, most of them within 15 minutes of his home. I explained that recovery is "a day at a time," and that regular meetings would not only support his staying sober for that day, but help him address the problems resulting from his many years of dependence on alcohol. I stopped and asked Bill if he had any questions. He didn't.

I explained that, in order to "work the 12 Steps" he would need to get a "sponsor," someone like a peer-counselor, who had been sober for some period of time, at least a few years, and who had experience in working the Steps. I let him know that, in a fashion, he had already done the first three Steps: he had acknowledged his drinking problem, his inability to abstain from alcohol; he had learned that there was a path towards wellness; and he was in the process of signing an agreement to follow that path.

4. Addict agrees to frequent, random drug testing.

There were two reasons for this stipulation, I explained. One was to let him know that knowledge of any substance use on his part would be shared with his family and me. The other was to give him one more tool to help the part of him that wanted to stay in remission, even though there was another part of him, his midbrain, that would regularly create cravings that could lead to relapse, and drug testing might just be the tool that prevents a relapse.

Bill nodded in agreement.

5. Addict agrees to get a developmentally appropriate, honorable, entry-level, full-time job.

I laughed out loud, because I already knew that he had succeeded at keeping a job, and only briefly described the rationale for this requirement. "In some cases, an addict has not been able to keep his job, or his job isn't compatible with recovery. These folks need to get work where they will learn to be responsible and accountable, and build their self-esteem as part of their recovery."

6. Addict agrees to stay away from "using friends" for 90 days.

"I'm not talking about you attending occasional social situations with non-addicts," I elaborated. "I'm talking about hanging out with those with whom you regularly drank in the past and who may themselves have a problem with alcohol—people who might not be supportive of your decision to get help." I described that, in my case, when I got sober, my former drinking buddies fell into two categories: those who previously drank a lot, but who then became very supportive of my sobriety and drank moderately or not at all when they were with me, and those who drank heavily and typically had no use for someone who would no longer be one of their drinking buddies.

Bill nodded his acceptance.

7. Addict agrees to go to a detox facility if they relapse.

I explained that relapses are basically telling us that this level of treatment is insufficient to sustain remission, and that we need to temporarily escalate treatment. 72 hours in detox not only gives the addict a safe place to become medically stable, but also offers a time-out to reflect on loss of control and the reality of addiction. Bill nodded that he understood what I was talking about. Perhaps as many as half of my clients have had at least one relapse during the first year of treatment. Their subsequent stay in a detox facility was, for them, the last nail in the coffin of their substance use, and led them to recommit to the process of recovery. At the detox center, witnessing other addicts in worse shape than they were and who were struggling to get sober, gave them the boost to embark on sobriety with renewed commitment.

8. Failure to succeed in this Intensive Outpatient Program (IOP) will result in a referral to a Residential Treatment Program.

"We have talked about this before," I said. "Some people really do need to enter a residential treatment program, and I will make that recommendation if this outpatient program is not sufficient." Again, I asked Bill and Jennifer if they had any questions. Both of them seemed to take in my explanations of the stipulations of the Treatment Agreement, and to understand the rationale behind them.

9. Referral to other 12-Step programs may be made if the need arises.

"We know," I said, looking at both of them, "that the addict's brain's craving and need to get its 'hit' can sometimes also be drawn to gambling, sex, spending, food, and other forms of compulsive behavior. If I see the need to address anything that arises as we move forward, I may make that referral as well."

I turned my attention to Jennifer. "This is the part of the Treatment Agreement that specifically pertains to you." I continued reading.

Treatment for the Codependents:

1. Individual and Family Therapy.

I reviewed what I had said to Bill about therapy. And I added that I would continue to have weekly individual sessions with her for the time being.

2. Codependent agrees to attend a minimum of two Al-Anon meetings each week, get a sponsor, and work the 12 Steps.

Jennifer nodded. She already attended multiple meetings each week and had started to work with a sponsor.

3. Codependent agrees to remain abstinent from substances during the initial two months of treatment.

I had not mentioned this to Bill in my orientation to the program, but Jennifer had heard this point weeks earlier when she first asked me about the details of the program. She agreed.

4. Referral to other 12-Step programs may be made if the need arises.

I had already mentioned this a few minutes earlier in talking about the stipulations of the Treatment Agreement for the addict. I said to Jennifer, "Sometimes, codependents turn to using unhealthy behaviors as a way to cope." She nodded in understanding. (There are codependents who later discover their alcohol use is a problem, and who then seek recovery for substance use.)

Looking at both Bill and Jennifer, I explained that the third component of the agreement described treatment for the addictive/codependent family system—not only for them, but for their son.

Treatment for the Family System:

1. Family Therapy.

Pointing to the three-generation family mobile hanging from the ceiling in a corner of my office, I said, "I'm looking at the larger family system as I guide this treatment. Addiction and codependency skew the relationship dynamics of all the family members, perhaps for generations. My plan is to continue to periodically bring your son, Vincent, into this process, because he has certainly been affected by the dynamics in your family." They both nodded.

I read points 2 and 3 together:

2. Family agrees to attend, together, three Al-Anon meetings in the first 90 days of treatment (meeting to be chosen by the FRT therapist). (Arrive 10 minutes early, stay 10 minutes afterward.)

3. Family agrees to attend, together, three AA meetings in the first 90 days of treatment (meeting to be chosen by the FRT therapist). (Arrive 10 minutes early, stay 10 minutes afterward.)

I spoke to both Bill and Jennifer. "While each of you will have your own individual course of recovery, designed specifically around your needs and your issues, it is vital that you understand each other's programs as well. Attending meetings of the other's program will give you some insight into your partner and his or her recovery, and will enable you to better support one another's recovery process." Bill would attend three Al-Anon meetings with Jennifer; Jennifer would join Bill at three AA meetings. I added that their son, Vincent, would not be expected to join Bill and Jennifer at their meetings, but that there were Alateen meetings for kids his age that would be helpful for him to attend.

Jennifer was already familiar with the concept of arriving early and staying after meetings, and had been doing that with her Al-Anon meetings for some time. I turned to Bill and described, "There is an opportunity before and after a meeting for 'fellowship.' It is a time to talk informally with other recovering people, to connect with other people in your shoes. Sometimes people go out for coffee after meetings, which strengthens their sense of community."

Graduation:

The Intensive Phase ends after all adult family members reach these milestones:

1. *Addict: One year of continuous sobriety and completion of the 12 Steps.*
2. *Codependent: Completion of the 12 Steps.*

I asked them if they had any questions. They both looked a little overwhelmed—we had covered a lot of information. But they also both seemed relieved: here was a plan with very specific directions for each of them that would guide them forward. They said they didn't have any questions. I handed them the Treatment Agreement for both of them to sign, and made a copy of the signed document for each of them. I congratulated them for their courage to step up and commit to this valuable, life-changing process.

We were ready to begin the daily individual and family work. I had anticipated that we might successfully complete the Treatment Agreement today, and had already confirmed that there was a nearby AA meeting. I knew an AA member who would be attending. "Okay, Bill, I'm wondering if you would be willing to start now, and to get to a meeting tonight. If you give me permission to contact him, I have a friend who will be there and would be glad to welcome you to the group."

I was aware that, to maintain some self-agency, Bill might resist and say that he "wanted to start tomorrow," and I was, at this point, fine with that if we "could have a brief phone conversation tomorrow." He chose to go to the meeting the next day, and to talk with me on the phone afterwards. I scheduled a session with him for the day after that.

"One more thing," I said, "I'd like you guys to not talk to each other." I expected they would be surprised, and I laughed. "What I mean is to not get into any serious discussions about anything important, and to save those conversations for our therapy sessions." I added, "Of course, you have to communicate with each other. But, at this stage, we are embarking on a journey that will result in the two of you building a new, healthier relationship, and I'd rather each of you, for now, keep the focus on your own individual life, and on your own program and therapy work. We will have time in our couples' sessions to deal with whatever issues may come up."

The goal at this point was to have Bill, for one day, neither drink nor use substances, and for him to attend one social support meeting that day as well. He would then have a session with me the next day, to process his experience at the meeting. And I would set the stage for him to repeat it, one more day, one day at a time. I explained that I wanted to see him or talk with him on the phone every day for the next week, to support him and answer any questions he might have. I scheduled sessions around his job and had phone sessions with him on weekends. I let Bill know that, after the first two to four weeks, we would cut back to two individual sessions a week, while continuing with a weekly couples' session with his wife. I told him we would maintain a similar schedule through the first three months of treatment, and then review our progress to date—and that, if I had any concerns, I might request more frequent meetings. I explained to Bill that our session frequency would slowly decrease as his commitment to his recovery group deepened. I reiterated that at the point when he'd had one year of continuous sobriety, he would have the option of terminating our work together and would depend on his meetings for support going forward.

If we could maintain the initial momentum, I knew we would establish a strong foundation for the ongoing "trudge" work. For Bill and Jennifer, hope and stability were beginning to return to their home life. Their son, Vincent, perhaps sensing that his parents no longer needed to be "cared for," began to expand his activities outside of the home. He became more like a typical teen. I had met Vincent early on, when I was beginning to work with Jennifer, and I wanted to understand more about how he was faring. A few weeks into our work together, I asked Bill and Jennifer to bring Vincent in with them for a session.

With Vincent in the room, I reviewed what his parents had taken on—the format and rationale of the treatment program, and the treatment commitments each of them had agreed to follow. I wondered out loud if he was aware of any changes around the house.

"My dad isn't drinking, and my parents aren't fighting anymore," Vincent said. "How is that for you?" I asked. "It's really good they're getting along, and my dad not getting drunk is great." I probed a little further, asking Vincent how these changes affected him. Vincent replied briefly, "I guess it's better."

I asked Vincent about the Alateen meetings he was going to. He replied, "They're okay. There're some kids I sorta like."

I nodded in acknowledgment. I told Vincent that I would have occasional meetings like this, that included him and his parents, throughout the first year of his father's sobriety, and that he was welcome to come to any other sessions if he had any concerns. I added that I knew he had been impacted by "all of this," and that I expected that he would have some things he'd want to talk about at some point. I said he was welcome to contact me and that I might even ask him to come in by himself. He seemed to appreciate these suggestions.

By the time Bill achieved the three-month milestone, their family was considerably more stable and seemed to have settled into a solid routine of recovery work. There was much to talk about. I reminded them that I was wearing two hats—I was both a licensed mental health professional trained in marriage and family systems, and I was a certified drug counselor. I said that in much of our early therapy, I was working primarily as a drug counselor, but that in time I would move more into the psychotherapist role as we explored their relationship, past and present, and the embedded dynamics and emotional history they had each brought to their marriage from their families of origin.

Bill had grown up in a home with a distant, possibly alcoholic, father and a very anxious mother. He had had very little experience of emotional connection and closeness. That later became a focus of our work. He also was unhappy with his job and his career choice, and began to wonder about his options. Jennifer also had come from a troubled home. Her parents fought a lot and she had been the "peacemaker." She'd thought it was her job to act as an intermediary between her parents, and between her siblings and parents. As treatment unfolded, it became apparent that Bill and Jennifer each had "holes" in their development. Each of them brought up examples of basic life lessons that they had missed. Jennifer labeled herself as a "busybody." Wherever she worked, she interceded in the affairs of her co-workers, thinking that they needed help and she should intervene. Bill had missed out on having a healthy, functioning relationship with his first authority figure, his father. He perpetually felt inadequate and didn't think he had the right to advocate for himself in the jobs he had held. Consequently, Bill often ended up not liking his work, even though he had slowly advanced to a position of authority in his job.

Bill and Jennifer were actively working with their respective sponsors in navigating the 12 Steps. They talked about their progress, both with each other at home, and in session with me. It was heartwarming to witness the shift as each of them, with their sponsor's guidance, made amends for harm they had caused. Each took responsibility for how they—even with the best intentions—had hurt the other. Making amends brought them closer. At one point, Bill, Jennifer, and Vincent went on vacation together. Family vacations had formerly been unpleasant and fraught with tension and discord—Bill's drinking would provoke Jennifer, who would start to criticize Bill, and they would end up arguing. However, each member of the family returned from this vacation reporting that "it went well" and "it was a lot of fun."

About ten months into Bill's first year of sobriety, I brought up with Bill and Jennifer the subject of graduation and terminating the family's work. I reminded them that termination was, of course, contingent on Bill's continuing to maintain sobriety, and on Bill and Jennifer each separately completing the 12 Steps. I explained that we would end the formal treatment as set out in the Treatment Agreement, but they were welcome to continue working with me in any way they found helpful.

I have witnessed a wide range of scenarios with the termination process. There have been families that stayed in treatment beyond the year of sobriety because they had not completed the Steps. I have had families who completed the year of treatment, but chose to continue individual or family work. And, of course, I have had families who have chosen to stop therapy before completion, for numerous reasons. However, over the years, I have honed my ability to broadly conceptualize the trajectory of the disease and the arc of recovery. I have experienced very few premature terminations, especially as I have become more skilled at communicating with clients at the outset of treatment the possible roadblocks they may encounter in the first year. Sometimes clients who have terminated prematurely return, years later, to work on specific issues. I tell the families I work with that I'm like the family doctor—I'm always available to consult with any family member, or the family as a whole, if they wish to return.

Many clients, after a course of therapy, continue to actively engage in improving their lives and building healthier families. Nearly all of them continue to attend support groups to further their development. Those who do not continue on a path of recovery with the assistance of groups, nonetheless recognize, and are grateful, that they have climbed out of a potential death spiral and created happier, healthier lives. It is a great joy for me to run into folks I've had the privilege of working with at the local Home Depot or Starbucks, and to be greeted by their smiles of recognition and witness their apparent happiness and engagement in life.

As an FRT therapist, I often think that I have the best possible job: working with families that have been wounded by addiction and codependency, and guiding them towards health and renewed development. With this comprehensive approach, we address many of a family's biological, psychological, social, and spiritual issues and establish a solid foundation for the next generation to go forward and create a healthy future.

Chapter 9

Case Study—Parent

A caller left a brief message and a phone number on my voicemail. When I returned the call, a woman answered the phone. She sounded anxious, just as she had in her message. "I was referred to you by one of your colleagues," she began. "I understand you work with families where there's someone with an alcohol problem." She paused, then blurted, "I'm concerned about my father."

"Yes," I said. "I do work with families with substance use problems. Tell me a little more about what is going on."

Sue, the caller, told me that her father, Robert, had had a drink or two in the evening, sometimes more, "for as long as I can remember." But since his wife—Sue's mother—passed away fifteen months earlier, Sue said, "I believe he has been drinking more than usual. In the evening when we speak, he often slurs his words and sometimes gets angry. A couple of months ago, when we were leaving a restaurant after we'd had dinner and he'd had more than few drinks, he fell down, tore his jacket, and broke his arm."

"Who else is concerned about your father?" I asked. "My two sisters," replied Sue.

I explained to Sue that I work with the family when there's a possible alcohol problem, that family members can be affected, and I begin by meeting with any of the concerned family members. Principle 14 speaks to this process:

FRT Principle 14
Typically, a member of the enabling subsystem contacts the treatment provider. It is vital that the provider begin to engage the caller in the Family Recovery Therapy treatment model during this first contact.

I asked Sue whether her two sisters would be willing to come in with her for a session. She assured me that they would, and we scheduled a time to meet. Meeting with all the concerned others at the very beginning of therapy, and keeping the focus on the family system, is in keeping with FRT Principle 3:

FRT Principle 3
In Family Recovery Therapy (FRT), the client in treatment is the family system that suffers from both addiction and codependency.

From the very beginning, I look for the key players in the family system. This is a critical step. The addicted family members most likely have been concerned for some time. Bringing all of the key participants together at the outset of treatment, I find, greatly increases the chances of uniting the "enabling subsystem" around the "problem," which, from the codependents' perspective, is typically, "how to fix the addict." During the initial phone call, I press this point of wanting concerned others' participation in the first meeting, and will include distant family members in the initial session on a speakerphone or conference call, if necessary. I may postpone the initial session until all the concerned others can attend so as to avoid splitting and coalition-building. This is critical, since codependents who are left out of the process during the initial stages may see the meeting as just another bit of drama, and will often unconsciously resist, blame those "stirring up trouble," and ultimately undermine treatment. The result will be that the addict is confronted with conflicting messages, as some of the enablers continue to rescue, failing to see their part in perpetuating this family disease. The addict, of course, will distance himself from those who may confront his defenses, and continue relationships with the untreated, surreptitiously enabling codependents who will avoid talking about "the problem."

After I got off the phone, I wondered if Robert, Sue's father, was using alcohol to medicate his grief. The loss of a loved one is almost always traumatic, but, with support, the majority of people come to a place of resolution within six months or so. For some people, though, the loss is too much to resolve, and they don't heal. Instead, they remain emotionally dysregulated and are unable to manage their moods and emotions. They may self-medicate with substances, and even become suicidal.

At my first meeting with the three sisters, after we introduced ourselves and settled in our seats, I asked them, one by one, to give me some background on "the problem." At this point, I was simply a concerned therapist—empathic, congruent, and aligned with them around their common concern: their father's drinking.

Sue was distressed as she talked about the night her father had fallen when he was leaving a restaurant. She had immediately taken him to the emergency room; he was clearly intoxicated. At the emergency room, her father had admitted that "maybe he had had a little too much to drink," but he shrugged it off as insignificant. Sue added that her father often refused to agree not to drive after drinking, claiming that he was "fine."

As Sue continued to relay to me her concerns about her father, I understood that her father had returned to most of the activities he had pursued before his wife's death—he had resumed his life-long passion for golf with friends, and he came to daytime family gatherings, showing up in a good mood and enjoying playing with his grandchildren. It was evident that there were close and loving connections in the family. Also, Sue did not think her father seemed sad or depressed, so I ruled out my concern that he was using alcohol to medicate his grief. I learned from Sue that her father had exhibited signs of a severe alcohol-use disorder earlier in his life. She reluctantly told me about a number of times that he'd been intoxicated when she was growing up, and mentioned that he had had a DUI when she was in grade school. But Sue reported that her father had always been able to "get back on track" after these episodes. I was beginning to think that Robert had been a functioning alcoholic for many years, and that his alcoholism was progressing. His family was starting to come out of denial as his symptoms became harder to ignore.

From Sue's sisters, Angie and Carol, I learned more about their father's past use of alcohol. They described that, since they were children, their father had had episodes of binge drinking. Their mother had complained about his alcohol use, and the two parents would occasionally have loud fights, but nothing seemed to change. Sometimes, their father would proclaim that he had "stopped drinking," and he would stop for a while—for a few months, even as long as a year. But inevitably, he would drink again, at first moderately, but slowly his intake would increase, and eventually there would be an incident when he was clearly intoxicated and behaved badly. When they'd been children, the three girls had felt embarrassed by their father's drinking and his drunken, loud behavior, especially in front of their friends. I explained to Sue, Angie, and Carol that the symptoms of addiction include loss of control, adverse consequences, craving, and the substance use continuing for a long time. The three of them glanced at each other and nodded, acknowledging that their father seemed to fit all of these criteria.

I wondered if they were ready to hear about the role they had played in this family disease. Some codependents are so impaired and poorly differentiated that I need to "collude" with the projection process—seeing the alcoholic as "the only problem"—for some time before they can begin to see their role in the situation and be willing to personally engage in the recovery process. I sensed that these three women would understand the concept of codependency. "I'm wondering," I mused out loud, "if you may have enabled your father in any way?"

"I think I have," said Angie. "For years I have been with him, sometimes having a few drinks with him, and even watching him drink to excess, and I've never said anything."

Sue added, "I guess I have as well. His drinking has been the elephant in the room for so long that I no longer let him come over to our home in the evenings, but I've never told him why, which is because he will get intoxicated and become embarrassing." Carol nodded in agreement.

"Addiction," I said, "alcoholism, in this case, is best seen as a problem that affects the whole family, and the family members often unwittingly, and perhaps unconsciously, play along with 'the way things have always been.' Enabling and codependency are interchangeable terms that we often use for the behavior of family members who are close to an addict." I then asked them if they would like to hear "what can be done about the problem." As I expected, they said "yes," and I continued.

"I see the treatment of addiction through the lens of both family systems and addiction treatment. Addiction is a potentially fatal brain disease that, without intervention and treatment, is progressive—it always gets worse. Treatment is pretty straightforward. The enablers agree to get help to understand and change the roles they play, and, ultimately, to stop enabling, which could shift the dynamics of the family—sometimes even causing a welcome crisis, which may be a 'hitting bottom' moment. For the addict, this shift in the homeostasis, away from 'the way things have always been,' can lead him to begin to acknowledge his problem, and then to become willing to follow some simple suggestions to address it. Actually, addiction treatment is quite simple and straightforward, but each step can be challenging because it requires facing reality. Treatment almost always starts like this, what we are doing right now: meeting, talking about the problem, and becoming willing to take the next step. We are actually at the very beginning of what is often called a family system intervention."

I then talked to the three of them about family dynamics and how drinking and enabling behavior can become normalized by tacit understandings that are accepted by everyone. "The three of you, in your father's mind, are fine with his drinking. You have, in essence, given him the message for decades that his excessive and problematic dependence on the daily intake of alcohol is 'fine.' Yes, you have 'mentioned' your concern about his drinking, but he has ignored your concerns. You have failed to get his attention in a meaningful way."

I continued, "Your role—your going along with his drinking, and your failure to break through his denial—is typical. Most people think that someone like your father would simply use common sense and adjust his drinking, but it is important to understand that, by definition, addiction is a brain disorder that renders the victim unable to change their behavior, unable to stop by themselves. The addict actually views substances as the 'medicine' that soothes them. Addressing the codependent mindset, the unconscious support of the alcoholism, is fundamental to successful treatment. If the enablers refuse to look at their role in perpetuating the disease, and fail to change themselves, successful resolution becomes much more difficult—in fact, it might not even be possible.

"Treatment for alcoholism," I went on, "is based on the alcoholic getting support to not drink, one day at a time. As we proceed, treatment also includes addressing the impact of the disease on the alcoholic and on the family members, and doing the work to repair the damage. For the alcoholic, after the acute initial stage, support consists of regularly attending social support and mutual aid groups with other recovering alcoholics who help each other to not drink—one day at a time. There is a very similar avenue of group support for the enabling codependents that helps them to understand the disease of addiction and to stop enabling. Alcoholics Anonymous is the most available support group for alcoholics, and Al-Anon and Co-dependents Anonymous are the most available support groups for family members of alcoholics." I gave them a list of the local Al-Anon meetings and suggested they attend a few meetings before our next session. "In fact," I said, "it is recommended that you attend six different Al-Anon meetings, soon, if you can. At first, the meetings may seem strange. You will hear people sharing openly about alcoholism and addiction, and speaking frankly about their lives in relation to their 'qualifier,' the alcoholic."

I continued, "Families suffering with addiction typically have 'no talk rules' about actually speaking out loud about what is happening. Acknowledging that 'not talking' has been the norm is part of the recovery process.

"I suggest that you arrive before the meeting starts—it's like a movie, you don't want to miss the beginning. Grab a seat in the middle, get a cup of tea, and take a look at the literature table. During the meeting, they may ask if anyone is new to the meeting. Introduce yourself by your first name. This might seem scary, but remember that everyone in the room has been in your shoes at one point and will understand. We typically recommend that you get to six different meetings, because they are all slightly different and some may feel more comfortable to you than others. Regardless, they are all offering the same message of help and support.

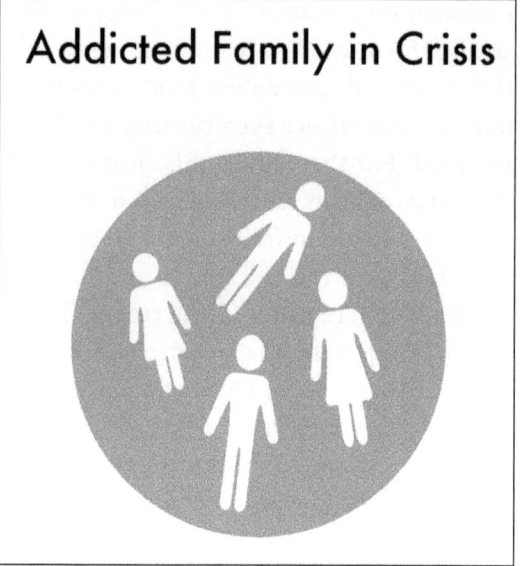

Figure 9.1 *Addicted Family in Crisis.*

"I think these diagrams might be helpful," I suggested. I showed the sisters four diagrams (Figures 9.1–9.4) which illustrate possible trajectories of addiction/codependent treatment.

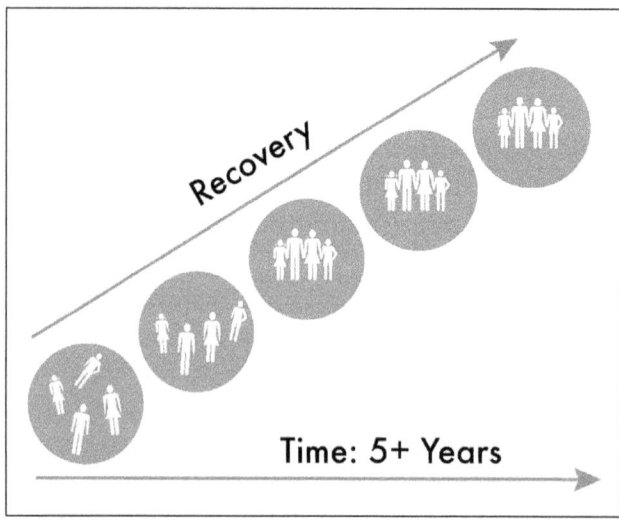

Figure 9.2 *Addiction Treatment—Optimal Outcome.*

"This diagram [see above] represents a family system suffering from addiction and codependency, probably not unlike what you are experiencing now."

I explained, "This one [see diagram left] shows a family in which the addict and codependent family members go through a recovery process, do the work required, and, over time, are able to achieve healthy development and functioning. The family goes from a point of crisis and instability, to gradually developing more stability, and then becomes a cohesive family that continues on a path of recovery and restoration of normal development."

I continued, "And this one [see diagram right] depicts an outcome which is unfortunately all too frequent today, given the drawbacks inherent in the current model of addiction treatment. Addiction providers today typically view the addict as 'the problem' and do not understand the complex dynamics of the family system, or between the addict and other individuals or communities. When the role of the enabling codependents is not directly addressed, 50 percent of addicts will relapse within the first year after treatment, most likely returning to a family in crisis."

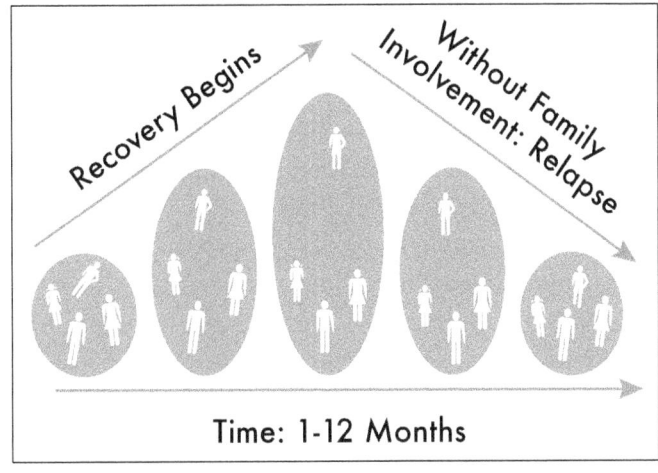

Figure 9.3 *Addiction Treatment—Common Outcome.*

I pointed to the fourth diagram (see below). "And this diagram represents a situation that can occur. Sometimes, one family member seeks help and gets into recovery. That individual develops a healthy life, while the resistant or untreated family members do not. The result is that the family splits apart. The recovering individual—addict or codependent—moves on, and the rest of the family continues to suffer."

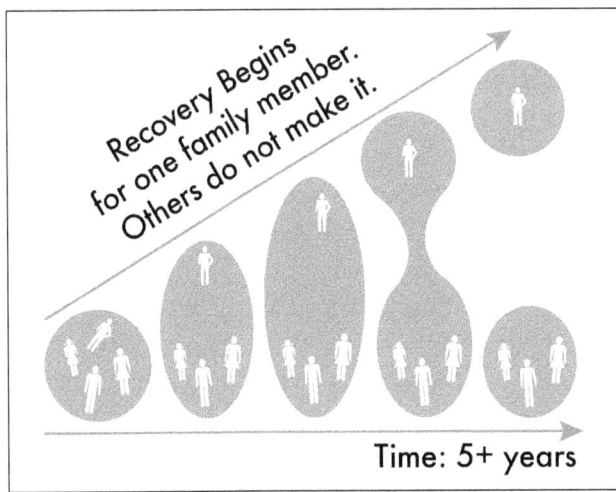

Figure 9.4 *Addiction Treatment—Partial Family Recovery.*

The three sisters were quiet. They appeared thoughtful as they looked over the diagrams I showed them. I asked if they had any questions, but no one did. I ended the session and set up another meeting for a week later. I reminded them to give me a call if "anything comes up."

By the time of our next session, each of the three sisters had attended some Al-Anon meetings. They reported on their experience of the meetings and what they had learned about themselves from going. Each sister had been a little shocked to hear stories similar to their own from other people in the room, and was surprised to learn that other people actually had found ways to manage their situations—and, that they no longer were continually worried about their substance-abusing relative.

I reminded them that I had no idea if Robert had a serious problem, but it was clear that they thought he did. "Regardless of what Robert does, you can get support to take care of yourselves and to reinforce the understanding that you can't get your father to change, but that you can stop enabling him and stop colluding with his denial. What he does about his drinking will be up to him." The sad reality is that in some cases, especially if this disorder is not addressed early, some individuals will never recover and will die early deaths (see Appendix I).

During our weekly sessions, I asked the sisters to check in about their relationship with their father and what, if anything, had changed. Sue reported that she had told her father she was no longer willing to talk to him if he had been drinking—which was new behavior for her, and a stance that angered Robert. Sue had calmly told her father, "Dad, I love you, but I feel uncomfortable when you have been drinking. You sometimes don't make sense and sometimes get angry for no reason." Perfect! Sue was only taking care of herself, but Robert got a not-so-subtle message about how his drinking had become a problem in his relationship with his daughter.

In our sessions, I also asked the sisters to report what they were learning in the Al-Anon meetings. They talked about having "aha" moments as each of them discovered how they had been impacted by growing up with an unavailable, often unloving, and sometimes abusive father, as well as with a stressed-out, anxious, controlling, and codependent mother.

We continued to talk about addiction and codependency, and the role each of the sisters played in allowing their father's disease to persist. I reminded them that I saw the current work with them as therapy for codependency. Later, hopefully, we would bring their father into the process and deal with the possibility of alcoholism.

I had been working with Sue, Carol, and Angie for six weeks, and they had been to multiple Al-Anon meetings. They were at a point where I believed they were ready to let their father know that they had been meeting with me to discuss their concerns about his drinking. A few days later, Sue called me and reported that her father was annoyed that people "were talking about him" and that he was "not interested in talking to anyone." I was not surprised at his reaction.

"This response is common," I told them, "and we need to respect his resistance and stick with what we are doing." I continued to meet with Sue and her two sisters, and only briefly talked about their father. I focused on them and their codependency, and their newfound awareness that the only person they could actually change was themselves. They deepened their understanding of the disease of addiction and of their powerlessness to change their father.

I reminded them that their father might choose to address his disorder—and, he might not; that alcoholism kills, but the most effective approach to helping him was exactly what we were doing. I was optimistic. I also pointed out that at least they were getting help to look at the impact on them of growing up in an alcoholic family and getting guidance to rebuild themselves into healthier individuals, so they would not pass this family legacy on to the next generation.

A few weeks later, Sue called me to say that her father had agreed to come in for a session with his daughters. When the four of them arrived, I asked Robert to meet with me alone for a few minutes.

As I described in previous case studies, I like to meet with the "problem person" alone the first time they come in. I wanted to see Robert outside the family system to establish a relationship with him, which is why I asked him to come into my office first, while his daughters remained in the waiting room. I let him know that I was a family systems therapist and was focused on the wellness of everyone in the family, and that his daughters had contacted me because of some concerns that included him. "I understand that you lost your wife a while ago, you are retired, you like to play golf," I hesitated for a moment, "and that your daughters have some concerns about your drinking. I don't know if your drinking is a real problem, but I think it would be good to help alleviate their concerns." Robert agreed that he "sometimes drank too much" but that his daughters' concerns were unwarranted, and he felt that his drinking was "normal." Then I brought in his three daughters. For the first time in their lives, the alcoholic and the codependents in the family were in a room together with a licensed family therapist.

My goal for this session was simple: get all of them to agree to come back and continue this recovery process. I had alerted the sisters that this session would not be confrontational. I wanted to be direct, but not so direct as to lose the connection with Robert. I did not know the extent of Robert's substance dependence, the level of his denial, or his willingness to hear anything I said. I started out by focusing on his daughters' concerns. "Robert," I said, "perhaps you don't have anything to be worried about, but I appreciate you coming in to answer your daughters' questions. I know you love your daughters, and they have some concerns, and perhaps you can help me help them." (I was making him my partner in helping address his daughters' concerns—something that he seemed happy to do.)

I asked each of the three daughters to talk about their experiences, their reactions, their thoughts about what it had been like growing up in a home with their father's drinking, as well as the impact of his more recent behavior—and for them to keep the focus only on their experience, not to bring their father's role into that conversation. It is easy for codependents to blame the alcoholic, but I wanted to avoid putting Robert on the defensive. I simply wanted him to hear what his daughters had experienced. If they spoke about him, I knew that he could become defensive and ashamed, and then he would be unavailable to hear how their lives had been disrupted. If they only talked about their experience, it made it possible for him to feel safe, and at the same time, able to understand what they had experienced. The sisters repeated the stories they had told me in their earlier sessions, and Robert seemed to be able to listen.

It was time to end the session and I asked Robert if he might be willing to come back by himself "to help me understand his daughters' struggles." He agreed, and I sighed quietly to myself and scheduled the next session. Success!

The next day I got a call from Sue. She was agitated and wondered what the session had been about. "Why didn't you confront him about his drinking?" she demanded. I smiled to myself and asked her to describe the core message of the Al-Anon meetings and the *Serenity Prayer*. After a moment she said, "Oh right, I can't change anyone."

"Bingo," I said, "I think the session went very well. Your father felt comfortable enough to come and see me by himself, and this is how an FRT therapist works—slowly, one step at a time. We are still in a critical, early stage. My goal is to guide you, your sisters, and your father, if you are all willing, towards recovery, and you will have to trust me." I reminded her again that neither she nor I could control the outcome. "Your father may cancel the next session and drink himself to death, but the best thing you can do to help him is to keep showing up and keep getting help for yourself, because you will be better off, regardless of what ultimately happens to your father. As I've said, Family Recovery Therapy addresses recovery for both the addict and the codependents, and you will have a treatment process very similar to his, if he enters treatment."

My words to Sue were grounded in Principle 2:

FRT Principle 2
Effective treatment of addiction usually involves treatment of codependents, because codependents enable addiction. Codependency is a chronic relationship pattern that has profound mental and physical consequences and is characterized by an obsessive focus on other people. Codependents may need lifelong recovery support, which can take many forms.

Robert came in for his individual session. After some chit-chat to put him at ease, I asked him how it had been to sit with his daughters and hear some of the things they had experienced. "Well," he said, "it pains me to hear what they have been going through."

"I'm curious," I said, "do you think that any of the upsets your daughters talked about have anything to do with your drinking?" "Maybe," he said, "but I don't think I have a problem."

I saw a crack in the denial when he said "maybe," but I also heard, and wanted to protect, his defenses with that last part of his statement. "Perhaps you don't," I said, "but I'm wondering if you might be willing to let me do an assessment of your drinking, just to rule out any problems?"

"What do you mean, assessment?" he asked. I replied, "Here is what I'm thinking, Robert. Your daughters are concerned about your drinking, and a simple assessment—answering some specific questions—would reveal whether or not you have an issue that might be good to talk about. Some people can drink and not get into trouble, some people may drink a little too much and need to rein it in, and some people have something that needs to be addressed." I went on, "Modern medicine is now coming to understand that some people's brains are wired in such a way that drinking can cause problems—it's actually a medical condition. I'm wondering if you would be willing to take a few verbal tests to just rule out such a problem. Would you be willing to come in for a session and let me check that out?" He agreed, and we set up another one-on-one session for the following week.

Getting Robert to "yes" required gaining his trust. Based on this session and the previous one, I sensed that he trusted me and that he would be willing to come in for a testing session. I have worked with some families for months before getting to a point where I felt confident asking this question. I did not want to get a "no" answer, nor did I want to miss an opportunity. By using the terms "medical condition" and "rule it out," I was using language similar to what doctors use, in order to put his mind more at ease.

Addiction can be a hard thing to nail down. From the outside, we can often see symptoms of addiction, but an addict in denial is sometimes the last person to know that they have a problem. Fortunately, over the years, the stigma of having a substance problem has somewhat diminished in the public at large. But at an individual level, the addict's ego defends against the main hallmark of addiction—loss of control—in order to protect the illusion of control. I viewed the testing instruments as simply more information, and grist for the mill for each family member to learn more about their situation and to chip away at the entire family's ego defenses.

I primarily use two testing instruments: The Alcohol Use Disorders Identification Test, known as the AUDIT (Babor et al., 2001) and the Michigan Alcohol Screening Test, or MAST (Selzer, 1971). Sometimes I also use AA's Twelve Questions (Alcoholics Anonymous World Services, 2018b), but in this case, I chose to use only the first two (see Appendix G). These tests are self-reports and ask the person a number of questions regarding their quantity and frequency of use, the consequences of use on various aspects of their life, and whether there have been incidents of loss of control.

I said to Robert at our next appointment, before bringing out the tests, "One of the hallmarks of someone who does have a problem with substances is to deny or minimize their use, so be mindful of a tendency to do that when you are considering your response to each question. If you do find yourself wanting to alter the reality of your alcohol use, just note that as an indicator of a potential problem."

I read the instructions and asked Robert to respond to each question, marking his answers. We went through the two tests. When we finished, I added up the numbers and gave him the results. The AUDIT offers the following treatment recommendations based on the person's score:

1. Alcohol Education
2. Simple Advice
3. Simple Advice plus Brief Counseling and Continued Monitoring
4. Referral to Specialist for Diagnostic Evaluation and Treatment

Robert's score on the AUDIT landed him in the middle of the last category; he had similar results on the MAST. "Congratulations, Robert, clearly you were not hiding anything," I said, attempting to ease the blow. "The instrument suggests that you be referred to a specialist for diagnostic evaluation and treatment." I let that settle in and asked him if he had any questions. He did, and asked, "What do you mean, by 'referral to treatment?'"

"Well," I responded, "since I'm an addiction specialist, you don't need to see someone else. So, let me tell you what I recommend. First, do not stop drinking. Let's simply keep an eye on things and keep talking about it. This is simply a test, and while it shows problematic use, I think it's best for you to absorb the information at a pace that makes sense to you, and for us to keep meeting and discussing what comes up.

"I'm a therapist practicing Family Recovery Therapy," I explained. "I work with families who are seeking help to heal from the harm associated with substance use and the impact of substance use on their loved ones and their family members. Would you be willing to continue to meet with me, and your daughters, and see what we can do to make things better?" I asked.

"Well, yes, but I'm a little confused right now. The results of the test are disturbing, and I'm not sure what I'm to do with my daughters."

"No worries," I replied, "this work is pretty simple and can be a lot of fun. For now, know that you are fine, and we will take this one step at a time. We will continue our weekly family sessions. And, a moment ago I said for you to not stop drinking, to continue as usual, to enjoy yourself. But I'm wondering if you would be willing to notice the urges to drink, the thinking or feelings that inform your decision to have another drink, and maybe how you feel the next day about your drinking?" We were wrapping up the session, confirming the next family meeting, and just before we rose to leave, I said, "Oh, one more thing, maybe best to not drive if you have been drinking." He laughed, "OK Doc, I get the picture." We shook hands, smiled, and I closed the door.

I felt proud. It had taken many weeks to get from that first phone call to this session. Like putting together a jigsaw puzzle, we were slowly doing the work to bring healing to each of the family members, and to the family as a whole. I was also mindful that I was clueless about the future. I was simply working with what was in front of me, one session at a time, using the FRT Principles and my counseling skills to move forward, knowing that both addiction and codependency are thorny problems and that, at any time, the family might resist treatment and terminate.

The following week, I was excited when I saw the family on my calendar for the day. I had received a call from Sue a few days earlier saying that all three sisters would attend the session with their father. And when the four family members had arrived and settled in, I asked the question I often begin sessions with: "What would you like to work on?" I looked around the room at each of them. "Who wants to start?" It was Angie who asked the question that I imagined was on all their minds. "I'm curious how the session with Dad went last week," she said.

Looking at Robert, I asked, "Robert, would you like to talk about that?" "Yes, well," he said quietly, "I took some verbal tests and they showed that I might have an issue that I need to think about. Larry told me not to stop drinking but to take a look at my thinking, what goes on in my mind before I take a drink. And it was a 'no big deal' week. Oh, and I didn't drive when I'd had more than one drink."

I wanted, for the moment, to take the focus off Robert, but before I did, I asked him if it would be okay for me to let his daughters know what we found out. He agreed.

I explained, "Problematic drinking can be difficult to define, so it is helpful to look at it from different angles. We are of course looking at the frequency and amount, but also asking questions about whether or not there is craving or obsessional thinking about drinking. We are also looking for examples of someone losing control or having adverse consequences as a result of drinking. We use a couple of testing instruments that touch on all of those, and end up with a score that indicates where the individual is with their drinking. Robert ended up in a category that was defined as problematic. Robert," I said, looking at my file, "the category you fit in suggests that you be 'referred to an Addiction Specialist for Diagnostic Evaluation and Treatment.'"

I paused for a moment and then said, "I think I have talked about this process before, but let me review. As an FRT therapist, I meet with families who are concerned about the possibility of addiction or alcoholism." I continued, "My method is simply to gather information, educate, and make recommendations that point everyone towards health. Is Robert an alcoholic? The truth is that I don't know. The results certainly suggest that he might be, but I think Robert, if he is honest, will be able to tell us eventually. We have to remember that addiction, and alcoholism is an addiction, has the following hallmarks: inability to control use of the substance, a brain that will crave the substance, adverse consequences caused by using the substance, and chronicity—that the problem has been going on for some time. We already know that there have been some adverse consequences, like the DUI, and possibly the broken arm."

I sensed the sisters' energy rise and was concerned that they would want to focus on the tests and their father's drinking. But it was important to me to stay centered and focused on the whole system, so I shifted to the sisters and asked them, one by one, what they were learning in their support groups and how they were doing with the core message of the support groups: to keep the focus on themselves and not get involved with obsessive thinking or trying to change another person. This led to a discussion that took most of the rest of the hour, as I had intended. Nearing the end, I turned to Robert. "Robert, I have a similar suggestion to the one I gave you last week. Here is what I'd like you to do. I'd like you, when you drink, to notice your desire to drink, sometimes called craving. Notice if you look forward to drinking, notice what happens after you have finished a drink, and if you are able, do this for every drink, even if you have many drinks. Play with this; try to look inward at what is pulling you towards the next drink, and perhaps the next one. Simply notice where that desire comes from, and what might be causing it. Don't necessarily change the amount, just notice it. And," I continued, "would you be willing to report the results next week?"

"Sure," he said. "Great!" I replied. I added, "and also notice if there is a part of you that would, well, I don't want to call it lying, but notice if you might possibly find yourself wanting to minimize what really happens. Problematic drinkers' egos tend to exhibit a form of denial and rationalization and might want to shade the truth." He nodded, letting me know he understood the question, and we ended the session.

In the family sessions over the next month, I continued to gently re-focus the daughters' attention away from their father's behavior and onto their own differentiation process, helping them develop an awareness of their fear and obsessive thinking about their father's drinking. And, of course, Robert's drinking was also central to the discussion in the sessions. He was beginning to discover that voice inside him that craved alcohol.

"Yes," he said, "I do notice something that is weird. It's almost like I realize that I'm missing something, almost like being hungry after missing a meal, an urge that makes drinking seem like something I need, but after a few drinks, I seem to sort of forget I've had one and automatically get another."

"And, do you ever decide to put off a drink for a bit?" I asked. "Sometimes," he said.

"And what happens then, do you notice anything unusual?" I continued. "Yes, I seem to get a little upset and notice that another drink makes that go away."

"Let me check out something," I began, as I got up and walked over to my computer. "I'd like to look up the definition of the word 'craving.'" Looking at my monitor, I read: "Craving, a powerful desire for something, like 'a craving for chocolate.' Synonyms: longing, yearning, hankering, hunger, hungering, thirst, pining, want, wish, fancy, urge, need, appetite, greed, lust, ache, burning, addiction, aspiration; the goal: more."

"Robert, that little voice in your head that is asking for another drink, do you think you could say that it is craving?" "Yes, I suppose so," he replied.

"OK," I said, "I'd like to step back and talk about what might be causing that craving. Certain individuals, perhaps about ten percent of the population, have a brain that is wired a little differently from other people's brains. The brain in these individuals has circuitry and neuronal wiring and pathways that predispose that individual to crave something. It could be alcohol, drugs, gambling, sex, shopping, gaming, or eating in ways that are self-harming and not fully under control. Science and medicine have been delving deeper into the process and we are now fairly certain about how this all fits together. Simply put, the midbrain, a part of the brain that is out of our awareness, sends us a message to seek the addictive substance or behavior, and this individual's mind, their ego, or their thinking, executive function, in their prefrontal cortex, simply goes along with this craving. What the addict avoids noticing is that they can't control this response. Those midbrain instructions override the thinking mind's ability to control their behavior, and, ultimately when we lose control, bad things can happen."

Robert was listening intently as I spoke. I continued, "The medical profession now defines addiction as a chronic disease, not unlike diabetes, asthma, or hypertension. It is progressive—it almost always gets worse without treatment. And," I said slowly, "the fix is relatively simple: acknowledge the problem and get external support to regain control. Here is what I'd like you to do," I looked at him. "I'd like you to continue drinking, but I want you to try to control it. Maybe you decide, ahead of time, how many drinks you will have, even if it's a lot, and then stick to that, or maybe decide to not have any, and see what happens."

Robert had been fairly compliant with the process to this point, but I wondered how he would handle this request. He had been showing up, but was that because of pressure from his daughters—or was he really curious? I wasn't sure. And, I knew that addicts' egos will powerfully defend against accepting loss of control and will act out, even to the point of terminating counseling. Perhaps he would not come back, and his drinking would get worse. I was comfortable, at least, that I had been respectful of his situation, and that the education he had received from our sessions went a long way towards "planting a seed" that, in the future, could lead to him seeking help. I was also well aware of my ego, of my wish for him to "get it." I needed to respect the process that could provoke him to walk out, to know that I had done the best I could, to trust what I had done, and to realize that, if he left, the stage had been set if he chose to get help later.

And his daughters, having by now attended many Al-Anon meetings, were well aware that their father was most likely an alcoholic, and were realizing that they could not, by any means, get him to stop. And they were also realizing how much of their lives, their childhood development, and their own families, had been impacted by his alcoholism. My mind considered the options. Would Robert return and admit his loss of control? Would he drink himself to death? Would the daughters' codependency re-engage into a renewed addictive/codependent downward spiral? Would they distance from him if he backed out of treatment and continued drinking? Or would the work lead all of them to continue to follow the recovery path we were on? I didn't know.

As the family entered the room for our next session, I noticed that Robert was a little withdrawn, and I started with him. "Hey Robert, how are you doing?" He seemed somewhat at a loss for words and I asked him, "I'm wondering how your experiment around controlling your intake of alcohol went?" "Oh, well," he said, "I think I have a problem. I suddenly was aware of that voice calling for a drink, and then another. One night I said that I'd only have two drinks, but by the time my second one was done, I seemed to forget all about the exercise or my agreement with you, and kept drinking. I have to admit that I'm a little scared that I can't control my drinking."

I'd like to pause here, for perspective. In the current paradigm of addiction treatment, providers have a predictable and unified response when an addict says they need help: referral to another resource, either to an intensive outpatient program or a residential treatment center. In the model these programs follow, they treat the client for one to three months and then discharge them, referring them on to someone else, or perhaps giving them suggestions to "continue recovery work," but without specific resources. This assembly-line model results in over half of addicts who receive often-expensive treatment failing to achieve remission—nearly half will relapse before a year is up.

In Family Recovery Therapy, we are not engaged in an assembly-line approach, endlessly sending the mentally ill addict from one place to another. We treat them as clients in a therapist's office, and we do what psychotherapists do. We assess the problem, create a treatment plan, and then stick with the client through at least the first year of continuous sobriety. Even if the addict does a stint in a detox facility or a residential program, we are always in close contact with him, and we coordinate our treatment with the work of any other program involved. Additionally, we deal not only with the addiction, but also with any accompanying mental disorders, and with the myriad problems that addicts typically experience.

Back to the session with Robert and his daughters. I got the sense from all of them that this was an important moment, and it was. Robert was facing his situation, but unsure what to do about it. "So, Robert," I said, "it seems like you are acknowledging that a part of you, a part outside your conscious control, directs you to do something that you don't want to do. Did I hear that right?" He nodded. I suggested that I review the hallmarks of addiction, and they all agreed. "Craving, Robert, which you are now aware of, is one of them." I went on, "And loss of control, the brain's inability to make decisions and then stick with them. From what you said, Robert, I think you would agree that you were unable to control your drinking, that there was loss of control. Yes?" He again nodded. "And, the third hallmark of addiction is adverse consequences. You have mentioned that you had a 'few too many' the night you fell down and broke your arm. And there was a DUI, and also that your daughters have, for a long time, been concerned about your drinking, and have kept you away from some family functions. Is that also a fair statement?" Again, he agreed. "And the last one, chronicity, the fact that this has been going on for some time."

I opened the session to questions. Robert was mostly quiet, but Angie asked, "What does treatment look like?" I couldn't help but laugh, "The reality is that it looks like this; you have all been in treatment since our first meeting. "Look," I continued, "in fact, treatment is pretty simple—get the support to stop enabling," I said, looking at the daughters. "And," I went on, looking at Robert, "to stop doing your addictive behavior for this one day, and then repeat the same thing tomorrow. Along the way we attend to other stuff, but the goal is to stop for one day, and then do it again the next day. We use social support and mutual aid groups, not unlike Al-Anon, to help us, and, of course, we keep meeting and we keep supporting the family and its members' recovery—one day at a time."

As we approached the end of the session, I asked Robert if he had any questions. "No," he said quietly. I reminded him that he could always give me a call if he did have questions, and confirmed our next appointment. I prompted the sisters to go to their meetings, and advised them to speak, if not at group level, at least to other people in their meetings about what they were dealing with, and to get support for themselves.

I anticipated that this would be a difficult time for Robert, and I was not surprised when he called me a few days later. "I'm realizing that I can't stop drinking. I guess I should go to some sort of rehab program." I wanted to laugh, thinking, "What do you think we have been doing?" Instead, I said, "Let's see if we all can schedule a meeting as soon as we can, today if possible, and talk about what your options are. Would that be OK?" He agreed, and I said that I would call Sue and have her contact her sisters.

The role of an FRT therapist, I believe, at times, is not unlike that of any first responder. We drop everything to attend to the client at these critical points, which sometimes means arranging evening and weekend sessions. With Robert and his daughters, I was able to schedule a session that afternoon. I had already contacted a few of my friends who go to AA meetings and asked them to stand by in case I would be sending a newcomer to a meeting that evening. When I met with the family, the air seemed filled with tension—everyone was wondering what was going to happen next. I asked Robert if he would be willing to tell his daughters what he had told me on the phone. Robert repeated that he'd accepted his inability to stop drinking, and that he was ready for help. I mentioned, "And, didn't you mention something about being willing to go to a rehab, if necessary?" He nodded solemnly in agreement.

"A residential treatment program might be necessary, but, in your case, I'm thinking that it might not be the way to go, at least for now, and that we can do the treatment here at home." I went on, "Sometimes a person is so impaired that a residential treatment center is indicated, but I'm sensing that you are well enough, and informed enough, to try outpatient treatment. Would you be willing to try that?"

"Sure, but what does that mean?" "Let me tell you … but first, have you had anything to drink yet today?"

"No," he replied. "Great," I continued. "I have a thought. Your daughters have been going to support meetings and I'd like you to go to one this evening. I've found one that I think would work for you." I turned to his daughters and said, "I'm wondering if one of you would be willing to go with your dad to a meeting?" Sue agreed to go with him.

"OK Robert, I want you to go to a place where other clean and sober alcoholics just like you have found a way to stay sober. I actually have a couple of friends at that meeting who, with your permission, can meet you and help you get settled in. You won't have to do a thing, just show up. And, if they ask at the meeting if anyone is new and you are comfortable doing it, you might introduce yourself. Would you be willing to do this?" I asked. He was naturally anxious, but agreed to go. "Great," I said, "and, would the two of you mind giving me a call after the meeting? I'd like to hear how it was for each of you. And I'm thinking that I'd like to have another session tomorrow. Let's see if we can find a time that works."

Sue called later and reported that she and her father had gone to the meeting. Then Robert called. "Wow, that was odd," he said. "The people were really nice to me and most of them seemed to be pretty happy, considering that they are alcoholics. In fact, they seem to almost brag about it, saying it after they say their name and then everyone welcomes them. I'm not sure about the God angle, but it was OK."

"Great!" I said. "I'm glad you went. And, I have a question, Robert. Do you think you can get to bed tonight without drinking?" "Yes," he replied. We confirmed our meeting for the next day and said goodnight.

I smiled to myself, thinking of my first support group meeting. I had half expected hobos in dirty smelly trench coats. Instead, I walked into a room of laughing, well-dressed people who seemed to be quite happy to be there—it was almost like a cocktail party without the alcohol.

When I met with the family the next day, I asked Robert and Sue to describe their experience of attending their first AA meeting. After they related their impressions, I turned to Robert and said, "When we spoke yesterday, you mentioned that perhaps you needed to go to a rehab. Could you imagine that you are already in one, that this counseling, and that meeting you went to, and a treatment plan that I put together for you—that these could be the rehab that is recommended for you?" I explained, "Addiction is a complex disorder and it has a lot of consequences for us as well as for those close to us. We need to see treatment as a steady, but slow, daily progression from drinking to full remission. I'd like to let you know a little more about my treatment program. It consists of regular involvement in the support groups and counseling. We will look at biological, psychological, social, and spiritual aspects, both for you and your family. We also do random drug tests to help you stay focused on recovery and to let us know if you have relapsed. And, if you are unable to stay sober, then there will be a brief period in a detox facility or perhaps referral to a residential program. But, for now, I'm optimistic. You have shown up for our meetings and become more educated, and you have successfully made it through one day sober. That's how this works: we simply get the support needed from the meetings and counseling to stay sober just for this day, and then repeat it the next day."

Robert and his daughters listened intently to my description of treatment, a process that, in fact, they had already begun. I concluded, "For now, I want you to continue going to meetings and coming in for sessions."

A short digression, to talk about cost. Effectively treating chronic medical disorders can be expensive. And, it is estimated that it is 10 to 12 times more expensive to *not* treat addiction. The earlier it is treated, the less expensive it is. Treating addiction early—as a teen, for instance—could avoid the later expenses of a host of medical treatments, legal fees and court costs (divorces, DUIs, etc.), and more and more residential programs. And ultimately, we can't put a cost on a life that is lost to addiction.

Currently, we see "Call 1-800-GET HELP" ads on TV that claim to offer the caller resources for addiction treatment. Some of these are shady and deceptive, and frankly are fronts for exploitative businesses. Please see John Oliver's YouTube video, *Rehab*, for an eye opening, fun, 19-minute exposition of this industry (Oliver, 2018). In my county, we have a number of residential treatment programs. One costs $16,000 for 30 days, another is $55,000 for 35 days, and the others are priced somewhere between the two ends of that spectrum. In other parts of the country, there are some programs that cost over $100,000, for one month. And all of them will recommend an Intensive Outpatient Program (IOP) like the FRT model, upon discharge. There is a 50 percent chance that the patients treated using the current treatment model will relapse within a year, requiring a return to rehab—sometimes relapsing over and over. I once met an addict who had been to rehab 22 times.

Regarding costs, I do not work with insurance companies. I am a "fee for service" provider and am paid directly by my clients. At my current hourly rate, the initial month of Family Recovery Therapy costs about $400 to $800 per week, and $400 to $600 per week for months two and three—or about $5,000 to $6,000 for the first three months, then $15,000 total for the remaining nine months. That's $20,000 to $25,000 for a year of treatment that is far more effective (close to 100 percent when the protocols are followed) and less expensive when paid out of pocket than the current treatment model—of residential treatment followed by treatment at an IOP—that fails half of their clients, and typically does not include family members.

I do not work directly with insurance companies, but will provide a superbill for a client to submit to their insurance company for whatever reimbursement their insurance plan allows. Many therapists are contracted to work with insurance companies, and insurance quite possibly will cover the majority of the costs of FRT addiction treatment. Regardless, the FRT model is less costly than the dominant paradigm—and has a better success rate at obtaining remission from this disease.

It is important to name this aspect of treatment, because it is a vital consideration to those involved. Yet, when a family is facing addiction, they will often feel ready to "do anything" and are easily exploited. FRT is a saner, more accessible, less costly, and more effective paradigm. Back to our story.

Robert confirmed that he was going to a meeting that evening, and I again asked if he would be willing to give me a call after the meeting. He agreed. There were two more sessions that first week: one with Robert alone; one with Robert and his daughters. I asked Robert to call me to check in on the days we didn't meet. Robert was beginning to see how this "rehab" worked—meet with me and go to meetings and make it to bed each day without relapsing—one day at a time. A week into his sobriety, it was apparent to me that everyone was in much better shape than when I had first met with them. Robert seemed livelier, and his daughters were much less serious. But I cautioned, "Addiction is a very pernicious disorder, and we need to respect its power and stay close to the meetings, and get guidance to stay on track with recovery." This set the stage for me to bring up the Treatment Agreement.

"I have mentioned that there is a treatment plan and that I want to go over it, line by line, and answer any questions." Holding the contract, I started to read, "This is the 'Addiction/Codependency Family Treatment Program' and the following are stipulations of the treatment agreement." I stopped and looked up at them and said, "As an FRT therapist, I'm treating all of the individuals in the family impacted by addiction, but I'm also treating the family system that has been affected by this disease. I break the treatment into three components: the addict, the codependents, and the family system, each of which has specific requirements." I started to read:

Treatment for the Addict:

1. Addict agrees to stop all substance use, detox, and if appropriate, move into a sober living environment.

"Robert, you have already stopped drinking and, at this point you have detoxed. If you are unable to stay sober, I will recommend that you move into a sober living home or possibly go to a residential program, but for now, let's see how it goes. Any questions about this item?"

"No," he replied, and I looked at his daughters to confirm that they understood this as well.

2. Individual and Family Therapy.

"We are already doing that," I said. Looking at Robert, I continued, "I'd like to see you a few times a week for the next week or so, and all of you weekly for the first three months, and then we will reevaluate as you become stabilized and get further involved in your support groups."

3. Addict agrees to attend 12-Step meetings, get a sponsor, work the Steps, go to 90 meetings in 90 days, and then continue to go to regular meetings until graduation from program.

"You are already hearing about sponsors in the meetings. A 'sponsor' is like your personal coach or mentor, someone who will help you work through the 12 Steps."

4. Addict agrees to frequent, random drug testing.

"Drug testing is a part of all addiction treatment programs. It not only lets us know if you have relapsed, but it is also one more tool to help you stay committed to your sobriety, knowing that any drinking will be discovered."

I looked at Robert, and he nodded that he understood.

   5. *Addict agrees to get a developmentally appropriate, honorable, entry-level, full-time job.*
   I laughed and said he could skip this one since he was retired.

   6. *Addict agrees to stay away from "using friends" for 90 days.*
   I looked at Robert and asked, "Do you have any drinking buddies who might not understand what you are doing?" Robert reassured me that he was pretty much a solitary drinker. "OK, just in case, I'd avoid situations, for now, where your socializing included drinking. Perhaps when you are golfing?" I asked, looking at him. "Actually, I have gone to the clubhouse for a few drinks, but it was never a problem," Robert answered. I doubted him, knowing that denial and minimization are common in addiction.
   "OK, I'm wondering if you would be willing, for now, to skip that. Let your buddies know you have other plans and avoid that temptation." "I can do that," he said.

   7. *Addict agrees to go to a detox facility if they relapse.*
   "Addiction treatment needs to escalate if there are relapses. There is a local detox facility where you would spend 72 hours. It is sort of a 'time-out' that can be very helpful to re-focus on the fact that sobriety is hard for some people. Having this consequence, I find, often gives us a deeper understanding of the need to stay close to treatment." Robert nodded in agreement.

   8. *Failure to succeed in this Intensive Outpatient Program (IOP) will result in a referral to a Residential Treatment Program.*
   "Some people are so impaired that they really do need to get away, and get a lot of support to stop drinking, before they can return home and do what we are currently doing in an outpatient setting," I explained. Robert also agreed to comply with this.

   9. *Referral to other 12-Step programs may be made if the need arises.*
   "We know," I said, looking at all of them, "that the addict's brain experiences craving, and its need to get a 'hit' can sometimes draw the person to gambling, sex, spending, food and other forms of compulsive behavior. If I see a need to address anything else that arises as we move forward, I may make a referral for that as well."

   Turning to the three sisters, I said, "And here is the treatment for you guys."

Treatment for the Codependents:

   1. *Individual and Family Therapy.*
   "This is just as we have been doing."

   2. *Codependent agrees to attend a minimum of two Al-Anon meetings each week, get a sponsor, and work the 12 Steps.*
   "Your program will be very much like Robert's—get a sponsor and work the 12

Steps. And, I'm going to recommend that one of the meetings you go to, be a women's meeting," I said, and they all nodded.

    3. Codependent agrees to remain abstinent from substances during the initial two months of treatment.

"I recommend this as a way not only to support Robert, but to deepen your understanding of the ways that our culture often depends on alcohol to socialize, both at family get-togethers and at other social gatherings." I checked in with each of them to get their agreement.

    4. Referral to other 12-Step programs will be made if the need arises.

I had already mentioned this a few minutes earlier in talking about the stipulations of the Treatment Agreement for the addict, and I said, "Codependents, too, can be drawn to cope by turning to unhealthy behaviors that can become problematic." The three sisters nodded their agreement. "And the following is for all of you."

Treatment for the Family System:

    1. Family Therapy.

I looked at Robert and at each of his daughters. "We have already begun this process."

    2. Family agrees to attend, together, three Al-Anon meetings in the first 90 days of treatment (meeting to be chosen by the FRT therapist). (Arrive early, stay at least 10 minutes afterward.)

"Robert, these meetings will give you a good idea of what the family members of alcoholics go through, and what their recovery process looks like."

    3. Family agrees to attend, together, three AA meetings in the first 90 days of treatment (meeting to be chosen by the FRT therapist). (Arrive early, stay 10 minutes afterward.)

"And," I looked at the sisters, "this will give you all an opportunity to see AA in action and to understand more about addiction and what Robert is going through."

Graduation:

    The Intensive Phase ends after all adult family members reach these milestones:

    1. Addict: One year of continuous sobriety and completion of the 12 Steps.
    2. Codependent: Completion of the 12 Steps.

"This is what we are aiming for. One year of continuous sobriety for Robert, each of you doing your 12-Step recovery work, and therapy to heal the damage that's been done and to get your relationships back on firmer ground," I said. "It's actually pretty simple. Go to meetings and take on the next thing that comes up. There will be many things that will come up along the way, which we will deal with. Any questions?" I asked, looking around. It was clear that everyone understood the basic premises, and I said I would review these at each of our sessions.

This was the end of the initial phase. From here, the work would unfold naturally as Robert settled into his meetings, found a sponsor, and reported on his progress. The sisters deepened their recovery in Al-Anon—working with sponsors, they became more knowledgeable about their "codependent relapses," and learned to recognize the obsessive thinking that took them away from the present moment. They also began to face and deal with the issues resulting from growing up in an alcoholic family, issues that had deeply impacted their lives and relationships.

In the initial hours, the first days, that critical first month, the first few "relapse-prone" months, the first year—at all phases—the family needs hands-on care. And, in every session, I'm looking for "red flags," areas where there may be some resistance or lack of commitment. I remind clients to use the tools of the social support groups: going to frequent meetings, getting a sponsor and working the 12 Steps, reading literature, volunteering for commitments, sharing at meetings, reaching out to newcomers, making program calls, arriving early and staying afterward to have in-person, one-on-one conversations. I also remind clients of the importance of each of these recovery behaviors. There are always a few red flags, such as failing to get to meetings frequently or procrastinating getting a sponsor, and I address these lapses in each session. Throughout my years as an FRT therapist, I have found that families have successful outcomes when family members work a thorough and consistent program.

To reiterate what the Clinical Director of the Betty Ford Treatment Center replied when I asked him about the treatment center's recovery rates in 2010 (quoted above, in Chapter 1):

> Those who follow our discharge recommendations have a success rate of staying sober through the critical first year that approaches 100%, and those who do not follow our discharge recommendations have a success rate that approaches zero.

And when asked, "What are those discharge recommendations that result in a 'nearly 100% success rate'?" He replied:

> We advise them, upon discharge, to transfer to a family-based intensive outpatient program, go to daily AA meetings—90 meetings in 90 days—and then keep going—and get a sponsor and work the Steps. And that the family members, the codependents, do the same in Al-Anon. And, depending on the circumstances, for the addict to move into a Sober Living Environment.

Over many years of working with dozens of families, I have found that this treatment model has always yielded successful outcomes, when everyone does their personal work. In the cases that did not succeed, it was because the clients did not follow through. For example, in one situation, the codependent wife refused to do her part. She resisted going to Al-Anon meetings, continued to monitor her husband's behavior, and perpetuated the drama at home. Her husband stayed sober, but after nearly two years of doing his own recovery work, he decided to leave the marriage.

In this vignette of Robert and his daughters, I have combined aspects of a number of cases, but one particular family I worked with was uppermost in my mind. I ran into a member of that family recently, and was delighted to hear that "Robert" was three years' sober, and that everyone in the family was doing well.

Chapter 10

Case Study—Adolescent

"Good luck with this one," a colleague declared on the phone, "I've worked with this 16-year-old girl for a few months, and she has a drug problem that's beyond my scope. I haven't been able to make a dent."

I gathered a little more information from my colleague and asked her to have the parents call me. My default position regarding teens in trouble is to meet with the parents first, and assess *the parents*. They are the ones who will be doing the work, day-to-day. In addition, I've found little success meeting alone with a substance-using teen. Typically, the teen will tell me what they think I want to hear, then continue doing exactly what they have been doing. Only when I can get the teen's parents involved (which may include having them drug test their teen), and help them improve their parenting, can I make any headway with their substance-using child.

The mother of the girl that my colleague had mentioned called me, and I spoke with her for a few minutes. Almost immediately, she launched into a list of her daughter's transgressions. I listened attentively, acknowledged the challenges she was dealing with, then quickly turned the conversation to taking the next step. I suggested that she and her husband come in and talk about what was going on.

Sandra and Gary, the parents of the acting-out girl, arrived for our session. They were both concerned about their 16-year-old daughter, Mary, who had started using drugs. Sandra was a schoolteacher and Gary worked for the county parking enforcement department. They had three children: a daughter, two years older than Mary, and a son, four years older, who were both away at college. I started the session by telling Sandra and Gary a little about me. "I'm a licensed marriage and family therapist, and I specialize in working with families that are dealing with substance abuse and codependency. I've been doing this work for many years. Now," I paused momentarily, "tell me how I can help you. Perhaps talk about the history of the problem and what is happening now."

Sandra began talking. Their daughter, Mary, had been an "OK" student, and she had been experimenting with drugs since her freshman year of high school. But about a year ago, when Mary was a sophomore, she had radically changed her behavior and lifestyle. Her grades in school had dropped precipitously, she had new friends whom the parents had never met, and she had disregarded her parents' expectations about school performance. Most weekend nights, Mary came home intoxicated or high on something. In addition, she seemed unusually tired or irritated during the week, often going to bed and sleeping as soon as she got home from school. Sandra concluded, "We're exhausted and don't know what to do to rein in our daughter."

I listened empathically and asked some clarifying questions. Gary filled in a little more about the situation. He described an incident from the previous Saturday night. "Mary came home at 3 a.m., obviously drunk. When I got out of bed to talk with her, she screamed at me and slammed her bedroom door in my face." Then he added, sounding exasperated, "This isn't the only time something like this has happened." I suggested that they bring Mary with them to the next session. I added, "If she refuses to come in, let her know that the two of you will be coming in, that some decisions will be made that involve her, and that she will probably want to be here. If she doesn't come in, then the two of you keep the appointment, and in the session we will discuss what needs to happen next."

I start to assess the family from their first call to me, putting together a picture of the family dynamics. In the first session, as per my model, I always meet with the "sane ones"—those who witness a problem in someone else. Are they enablers? I have to wait until I know more before I can answer that. Usually, in the second or third session, I have them bring in the "problem person."

At the outset of the second session, I met alone with Gary and Sandra's adolescent daughter, Mary. I wanted to let her know that I'm a family therapist, that I'm here to see how I can bring order and serenity to her family and to the individuals in her family; that I'm not simply an advocate for her parents. I joined with Mary by making a silly joke or two to put her at ease. And then I began, "I met with your parents a few days ago and heard a little about what is going on, as they see it, but I'd like to hear from you. How can I maybe get you guys back to having fun and getting on with your lives? How can I help you?"

"I dunno," she said. "They are always up in my shit and making my life miserable." She was clearly irritated at having been dragged into my office. She would rather not be here, and certainly wasn't excited about opening up to a stranger.

I continued, "Your parents said that you have been behaving differently over the last year, that your grades have dropped. They also said that you might be drinking and using drugs. Any truth to that?" Mary retorted, "So what? All my friends are doing it, I don't see the big deal."

"Do you think you have a problem with drugs?" "No!" she replied.

"Great," I responded. "A lot of people are unable to control their drug use and have a problem like addiction. Sounds like you don't think you have that kind of problem." Again, she responded with a resounding, "No!"

"That's good news," I said, "we don't need to think about drug rehabs or anything like that, right?" She said, emphatically, "No!"

I expected her to say that, but I had purposely planted a seed. I had used the words "addiction" and "rehab" in the context of her drug use, letting her know that I am familiar with those terms. Based on what the referring therapist and her parents had said, I knew these might apply to her in the future, and I wanted to bring them into the conversation from the beginning. I brought Mary's parents back into the room and, with Mary's permission, briefly reviewed what Mary and I had talked about.

Adult addiction almost always starts in the teen years. Looking back on my own life, I recall the events that led me on a path towards addiction. I started "getting high" from sipping vanilla extract (35 percent alcohol, 70-proof) as a ten year old, drank my first beer in eighth grade, got tipsy on my friend's father's homemade wine shortly after that, and was getting drunk whenever I could by the tenth grade.

As clinicians, how do we think about addiction and addiction treatment when the parents are still legally responsible and have the right to place their child into treatment? A little history may be useful here.

During my last internship before I became licensed, I worked for four years in an outpatient, adolescent drug treatment program. It was the mid–'90s, and marijuana and alcohol were the only widely available drugs of abuse. At that time in our upscale community, any teen using or possessing drugs or alcohol, who came in contact with the police, was cited and required to meet with the Juvenile Probation Department, which would refer the teen and his parents to our drug treatment program. The program included three months of individual therapy, family therapy, teen group therapy, multi-family group therapy, and drug testing. The program employed half a dozen counselors—interns like me. We were supervised by licensed practitioners.

Many of the families we worked with had successful outcomes—their kids stopped using drugs, and the parents learned better parenting skills. Twenty-five years later, I still run into folks who were in that program. The program served as a great intervention for substance-using teens and their families.

A few of the teens back then identified themselves as "addict/alcoholics" and entered 12-Step recovery. The majority of the teens got some education, the parents became wiser and better informed, and the families left the program. Adolescence is almost always a chaotic time for both teens and parents, and is especially so if drugs are involved.

When I work with substance-using teens, age 17 and younger, I proceed differently than I do with adults. I work closely with the teen's parents and help them learn to set appropriate boundaries, levy consequences, and monitor their kid's substance-related behaviors. If this isn't sufficient to stop substance use, I sometimes refer the family to juvenile services where the police and courts can provide more support to the parents and additional consequences for the teen. If this doesn't achieve remission, I may refer the family to a family-based, clinical wilderness program or a therapeutic boarding school—both of which provide more structure—in which the teen's sober brain can continue to develop, away from a drug-using peer culture, and the teen's substance use can be addressed. Some teens will grow out of problematic drug use. The longer we can protect a drug-using teen from being seriously impacted by substances, and allow their brain to continue maturing unimpeded, the better chances are that the teen will develop normally. And if the teen grows up and develops a substance-abuse problem later in life, hopefully they will have the maturity, as well as the education about substance use, to acknowledge they have a problem, reach out for help, and benefit from treatment.

Back to Mary's family. When I met again with Sandra and Gary and their daughter, Mary, I recommended that we implement my "Prevention Program," which includes education and counseling in weekly individual therapy and weekly family therapy sessions, plus drug testing for Mary. I proposed a six-month program, and the six months would begin again if Mary relapsed. It was "full-court press" for every family member, and it engaged the parents actively in treatment. I still use this model today when I work with young teens. Basically, there are two possible outcomes using this approach: either the teen stops using drugs, stays sober, and moves on with their life, or, alternatively, if the teen can't stop drug use, we escalate treatment.

I worked with Mary's parents to establish boundaries to contain their daughter's behavior: more study time, a curfew on weekend evenings, no alcohol or drug use, and attending weekly counseling sessions. I explained to the parents, "Kids, including teenagers, need to feel safe and secure. They need boundaries—even though they often squawk about having them—not only to help them learn right from wrong, but to feel cared about and to know that someone has got their back. We don't know yet whether Mary can control her drug use, but we start with giving her some room to make healthy decisions—to improve her school performance, to respect her curfew, to go out and not use drugs—and see how she does." I told them that this was a health and safety issue and that they needed to reassert their authority as parents, so Mary would feel contained and have limits to bump up against.

Over the next several weeks, it became clear that Mary was unable—or unwilling—to stop using substances. While she showed up for therapy and agreed to the program's stipulations, she was unable to regularly produce clean urine samples. And she had acquired a strange habit of going to parties where she would steal other people's money—Mary herself acknowledged this, but didn't think there was anything really wrong with it. "These people have a lot of money, lots more than I do," she rationalized. Mary developed a taste for cocaine, a drug that was not in common use among teens at that time. But she found it and the money to buy it.

After a few more months, it became obvious that the Prevention Program was not keeping Mary sober and we needed to escalate treatment. We placed Mary in a nearby adolescent residential program for acting out kids. Since she was locked down, so to speak, she became clean and sober, although she managed to sneak out on two separate occasions and get high. She stayed in the residential program for close to a year. At that point, the insurance money ran out (this was in the mid-1990s, before insurance companies were required to pay for addiction treatment), Mary was then age seventeen-and-a-half. She returned to live with her parents—and resumed her old behavior: stealing her friends' money and getting high on everything, especially cocaine, if she could find it. And, Mary and her family returned to treatment with me. I referred her parents to Al-Anon for additional support.

In some ways, we were back to where we had started—with a drug-using teen refusing or unable to get sober, and parents unable to effectively contain her. But a new reality was dawning. Mary would be eighteen in six months. By now, Mary's parents were going to Al-Anon regularly, and they were learning what the program teaches: "We can't change another person—only ourselves." I focused treatment both on the parents' letting go of their daughter (asking her to leave the house on her eighteenth birthday if she refused to go into a residential addiction treatment program for adults), and on confronting Mary with the reality of her imminent birthday and the choice that she would need to make then. We didn't know if she grasped that her parents were serious about withdrawing all support when she became an adult. After all, in her mind, they had always housed and supported her, and it was only a birthday.

When I met individually with Mary, I helped her understand how she could support herself: get a job, find a room to rent, take buses, get her own cell phone, etc. I was trying to get her to comprehend the significance of the dilemma she faced. And, I was purposefully raising her anxiety, because her parents' withdrawing support and her needing to support herself were becoming very real possibilities. I was also beginning to trust that through my work with the parents, and their participation in Al-Anon, the parents were learning to implement a consistent message of real consequences for Mary, and I hoped that Mary was beginning to believe that the consequences were real.

I wanted Mary to see residential treatment as a viable option for her, one that would allow her to grow and heal and flourish, rather than her having as her only choice needing to suddenly fend for herself. In my individual sessions with Mary, I presented a rosy picture of what the new residential program would look like. I showed her the website for a good rehab in Washington State, a family-based program that I had visited and liked, and thought would be a good fit for Mary. I told Mary about other families who had successfully used this program. I described some details of the program to Mary, including the groups, the recreation and fun activities, and the beautiful surrounding countryside. She did not show any interest, but I kept at it. The weeks went by, the dirty drug tests kept coming in, the parents kept going to Al-Anon, and the family kept showing up for therapy.

As Mary's eighteenth birthday approached, she became more anxious about her future. She still did not show any interest in going away. Her parents, with my guidance, started telling her the plan: On her birthday, she would either agree to get in the car with them and drive to the treatment program I had recommended in Washington, or they would ask her to hand over her cell phone and leave the house. They told her they would change the locks, and if she set foot on their property without their permission, they would call the police and report her for trespassing.

Meanwhile, I met with Mary's parents and suggested they contact the facility in Washington, both to find out if they had open beds and to get answers to any questions they had. I described how treatment at this residential program would unfold and explained what their part in treatment would be. Mary's parents and I were hopeful that Mary would choose to enter treatment on her eighteenth birthday, rather than obstinately maintaining she could manage on her own and ending up crashing with friends when her parents said she could no longer live at home.

On her eighteenth birthday, Mary relented. She got in the car with her parents, rode with them to Washington, and entered the adult treatment program. As soon as it was clear that Mary intended to go to the program, I reached out to the current clinical director, introduced myself, and told her a little about the case I was referring to them, and would be collaborating on with them. They get a lot of calls like this, but I wanted to put my foot in the door and establish a connection with the person I would be referring to, so that later, when I started working with Mary's counselor and with the discharge staff, they would know me. I was laying the foundation for a partnership between the residential program and my "wraparound" program, and establishing that their program served as only a temporary phase in my long-term, comprehensive, family-based, intensive outpatient treatment program.

In Mary's case, because I'd had extensive communication with the clinical director of the program before Mary was admitted, the staff copied me on the emails to the family about treatment. I requested the name of Mary's counselor from the program director, and asked him to have the counselor call me; the counselor called me on Mary's first day in the program. (I had instructed the parents to make sure their daughter signed a release during her intake that allowed me to talk to the program's staff. This is essential!) I introduced myself to Mary's counselor, gave her my client's background, described the family dynamics, and explained my treatment model, including my ongoing work with the parents. I requested and scheduled a weekly conference call that would include the counselor, the parents, and myself. I also asked about their program's process of discharge, transfer, and step-down to a sober living environment. At the end of the call, the counselor said, "Wow, sounds like a great program, we should get you on our referral list."

"Thank you," I said, "but I don't accept referrals from residential treatment programs (RTCs). I have not had much success working that way." I told her that, based on my experience, an RTC typically locks the "IP (Identified Patient) process" firmly in place. I explained, "Generally, an RTC and the enabling codependents have colluded about the addict being the 'problem,' and, working from a family systems perspective, it becomes much more difficult to get the enablers into treatment once that collusion has been established. The way it could work," I continued, "is for *you to refer to me the enabling codependents who call you* seeking treatment for their child. That way, there is a possibility that I could engage them in the FRT model, and then, if appropriate, I could refer the addict to your program, if I think it's a good fit." (I would refer them elsewhere if another program would be a better fit.)

Once Mary had begun treatment in Washington, we were securely ensconced in the "RTC Phase": weekly conference calls that included Mary's therapist, her parents, and myself; the parents attending a minimum of two Al-Anon meetings a week; and my weekly, in-person therapy sessions with the parents. There was a lot to talk about in the weekly sessions with the parents: what it was like for them to have Mary out of the house and how they were managing the "developmental crisis" and accompanying grieving process that every parent goes through as they launch their child out of the nest and into adulthood. In the parents' weekly therapy sessions, we discussed their work in the social support groups. And we also addressed questions about Mary's current treatment, what discharge would look like, and the process of Mary's moving into a local sober living environment upon her return from the program.

After several weeks away, Mary was clean and sober, and her brain was coming back online and getting healthier. Her days in residential treatment were filled, from early in the morning to the end of the day. There were two group meetings a day, writing assignments, group recreation time, individual counseling, psycho-educational talks, drug and alcohol counseling, scheduled exercise time, and free time. Mary was busy and engaged in her life for the first time as a sober adult!

Like most programs, the center in Washington, views the first 30 days as primary care. For the majority of clients, residential treatment ends after 30 days, and they are discharged. However, some programs have the option for care to be extended to 60 or 90 days. Mary and her parents, advised in part by the program's staff and with input from me, agreed to extend Mary's primary care for another 30 days. I was happy to hear this, because I knew Mary's development had been significantly delayed during her years of substance use, when her growth was "off-line." The endless escalator of life's ongoing development was beginning to start moving again for Mary.

In preparation for Mary's return home, I sent a copy of my FRT Treatment Agreement to Mary's counselor. The counselor and I discussed it at length so that she could introduce the agreement to Mary. A few weeks before Mary was scheduled to return, I had a phone session with Mary to go over the Treatment Agreement with her and answer her questions. She agreed to comply with it. I knew the real work would begin when she returned home and embarked on a new life path, which would be very different from the course she'd been on before treatment. Mary still had the emotional development of a person younger than her chronological age, but she would be expected to step into the adult world—with the help of her support team.

The extension of Mary's stay gave her parents and me more time to prepare for the next stage of treatment, the transfer from the residential treatment program to the step-down, intensive outpatient program. I presented a general overview of the Treatment Agreement to the parents, and they agreed to it in principle—we would go over the agreement line by line in a session that included Mary, when she returned. I had contacted staff at two of my trusted sober living environments (SLEs) and inquired about available space for Mary. The parents picked the SLE that they preferred, and the house manager called Mary to initiate the placement.

Moving from a residential placement to an SLE is a critical process. Many clients are lost to treatment during this transfer—a break in treatment can allow the client an opportunity to return to old familiar places and drug-using friends without support or structured time, which sets up a scenario with a high potential for relapse. Mary had been in a "treatment bubble," and the last thing we wanted was for her to drift back into her "substance-using, peer culture bubble." Fortunately, the Family Weekend at the treatment center occurred near the end of Mary's residential stay, and Mary's parents drove her back from the ranch. I had arranged for Mary's family to come directly to my office on their way back, in order to sign the Treatment Agreement (the same agreement that Mary's counselor had shown her, that Mary and I had talked about on the phone, and that I had discussed with her parents). Signing the Treatment Agreement immediately upon Mary's return was essential to provide continuity and a seamless transition to the ongoing work with Mary and her family. After the session, Mary's parents would drive her directly to the SLE. Mary would go to an AA meeting that night with her housemates, and meet with me the next morning.

One of the stipulations of the agreement was that Mary needed to get a full-time job. Mary had never had a job, and was clearly anxious at the prospect of getting one. Early in her first week back, during an individual session, I drove her around the local community, and we visited the trio of my favorite places: Starbucks, Peet's, and Whole Foods. They all offer "developmentally appropriate, honorable, entry level jobs." I have guided many young adults to their first job in one of these businesses, with nearly universal success. These companies always seem to be hiring, they welcome the applicant who has no prior work experience, and will train them. These types of jobs engage the newly-working addict with other young adults, and with the public. Plus, this kind of job provides a good foundation for their future jobs. Within a week, Mary was hired by Peet's Coffee, and started training.

In her first week back, I met three times with Mary individually and once with her and her parents. I started the family session by asking Mary, as I usually do with someone new to treatment, "Are you still sober?" I wanted to keep the focus on Mary's sobriety. We also discussed the 12-Step meetings Mary was attending, and talked about her challenges living in the SLE.

I also asked Mary and her parents to agree not to have any contact outside of our weekly family sessions "for the next few weeks." I explained that the family members were learning new ways of relating. The parents were no longer responsible for guiding Mary's life—that job had been taken over by the recovery process, the meetings, her sober home roommates, and my work with her. And Mary was coming to understand that she was responsible for her own life, and learning to reach out to people other than her parents for guidance. I explained to the family, "You will have plenty of time later on to have happy times together, but these initial months are a time to learn new, recovery-based ways of relating. In a few weeks, I'd like you to plan 'shoulder-to-shoulder' time together—activities like hiking and movies, where there will be little likelihood of re-engaging in codependent relapses by bringing up some painful, unfinished issue from the past, or having a 'codependent relapse' by offering advice to your now-adult daughter."

The FRT approach was successful in working with Mary's family. Everyone in the family complied with the Treatment Agreement. Mary did not relapse, and she made it, without incident, to the one-year anniversary of her sobriety. Mary's parents and I showed up at the AA meeting where Mary received her one-year chip. Mary and her family continued to meet with me for therapy for four months after Mary's first AA birthday, with weekly family and individual meetings and regular drug testing. At that point, Mary's father completed the 12 Steps with his sponsor; her mother had completed the Steps two months earlier. They had achieved the goals stated in the Treatment Agreement—one year of continuous sobriety for the addict, and completion of the 12 Steps by all family members.

Mary's family left treatment in 1997. As of this writing, Mary has over 25 years of sobriety. She has been active in the AA program this entire time, and she is one of my "go to" people when I have a new woman client who is about to attend her first AA meeting. After getting my client's written permission, I connect my new client with Mary via text message, then have Mary meet the newcomer before the meeting starts and introduce her to other AA members. Mary has sponsored a number of folks as well (see Appendix J for a diagram showing the development of the addict into a healthy self). And her parents are still active in Al-Anon. Whenever I think of Mary, I remember the scrawny, lost kid who could not stop doing drugs, and her parents, terrified that they would lose their child.

Addiction is a terrible disorder, but this traumatic disease can often be used as a catalyst to bring a family together in a transformational process. Recovery can make a family stronger and healthier than it might have been had addiction never entered the picture. And FRT establishes a solid foundation for the next generation to experience healthy, fulfilling lives.

Chapter 11

Stephanie Brown's Developmental Model of Family Recovery and FRT

Now that we have seen the FRT recovery model at work, we can review the case studies from another perspective and place them against the backdrop of Stephanie Brown's Developmental Model of Addiction and Recovery (Brown & Lewis, 1999). Brown and Lewis describe the stages of recovery for a family moving from the throes of active addiction to a time some years after sobriety has been achieved, when the formerly enmeshed alcoholic and codependent family members have re-constellated as a group of autonomous individuals, interconnected in healthy relationships. Brown's stages provide a useful frame of reference for understanding the FRT model.

Stephanie Brown's work has been pivotal for me in understanding how addicted families change and grow. I first met Dr. Brown in 1997, and then met her again when I attended the Harvard Symposium on the Addictive Disorders in 1999. She was the keynote speaker at the symposium and was presenting her then-recent book, co-written with Virginia Lewis, *The Alcoholic Family in Recovery: A Developmental Model* (1999). I have periodically consulted with Dr. Brown since 1997, and have integrated her wisdom and perspective in conceptualizing my own model.

For their book, Brown and Lewis interviewed a large number of subjects who had been in various therapeutic and addiction treatment modalities. Their subjects comprised 52 couples and families whose length of abstinence ranged from 79 days to 18 years. Some of their subjects were currently seeing therapists and some had worked with therapists in the past. Some of the subjects relapsed during the course of the research. The authors also observed three couples with longtime sobriety that they worked with in a monthly couples' group over the course of five years. Brown and Lewis drew upon their extensive interviews and observations in comprising a cohesive model that describes the stages an alcoholic family system and the individuals in an alcoholic family traverse in the process of recovery. Their book is a valuable resource for clinicians who are working with alcoholic families.

The Developmental Model created by Brown and Lewis looks at three domains of experience, or aspects of the family, that are affected by addiction and that change in the process of recovery. These three domains are Environment, Family System, and Individual Development. "Environment" is the context of daily life and includes the "feel" of the home, the degree to which there is consistency and predictability, and the sense of safety and security in the home. The "Family System" embraces both the family structure—the rules, roles, rituals, hierarchies, and boundaries—and the family's process, the communication and interactional patterns in the family. "Individual Development" encompasses biological, emotional, cognitive, and intellectual development of the individual family members, as well as development of the individual in relationship to others. Brown follows these three domains through four "Developmental Stages of Recovery." These four stages are: the "Drinking Stage"; the "Transition Stage" (which is the end of drinking, and consists of two sub-stages, "Drinking," that includes the point at which the addict or family hits bottom, and "Abstinence," the beginning of sobriety); "Early Recovery" (which lasts for several years after abstinence has been achieved); and "Ongoing Recovery," (which generally begins after five years of recovery, and continues, going forward).

Family Recovery Therapy encompasses the first three stages of Stephanie Brown's model: Drinking, Transition, and the beginning of Early Recovery. A family system and its members who are engaged in the intense treatment approach of FRT typically traverse the first two or three stages (and sometimes enter the fourth stage) in the first year of FRT treatment. The families in Brown's study progressed through these stages over a longer period of time because most of them were not engaged in frequent or consistent therapy and group work. It is important to note that Brown's stages are not time-dependent or linear, but are based on an assessment of the family's recovery as seen through the lens of the Environment, Family System and Individual Development.

As someone with long-term personal recovery from addiction, I can look back and see my progression from the Drinking stage, through the slow rewiring of my neuronal networks during the Transition and Early Recovery stages, and eventually arriving at the Ongoing Recovery stage. In Ongoing Recovery, like many others in recovery, as well as normal healthy people, I continue to grow, change, and develop. My recovery process has benefited from many years of personal therapy, group therapy, social support groups, numerous workshops and retreats, as well as extensive education. As clinicians, we support, encourage, and hold hope for the person who seeks recovery to achieve normal development and a healthy life, despite the impact of their growing up in an alcoholic home, or the consequences of an adulthood devastated by addiction, mental illness, or other stressors.

Family Recovery Therapy, like Stephanie Brown's model, views recovery, not only of the individual, but of the family as a whole, as a complex and involved, multi-step process. A particularly bumpy stage occurs, as noted in Brown's model, in the transition between Drinking and Abstinence, when the addict must abstain from drinking while the codependent family members need to focus on their own recovery and refrain from enabling the addict. FRT is particularly useful in helping family members persevere and stabilize during this rocky time.

The challenge of this transition period is apparent in the addicted spouse case study. During the period when Bill is drinking, there is discord in the family. Bill and his wife Jennifer argue, and their 15-year-old son, Vincent, fights with his father. However, there is stability in spite of the chaotic environment—when Bill drinks, each family member engages in behaviors that are familiar and predictable. Everyone in the family knows how events will play out: Bill gets angry, Bill and Jennifer argue, and father and son fight. And the next day, everyone in the family behaves as if nothing happened the night before. When Jennifer starts going to therapy, and then begins to attend Al-Anon meetings, it creates more tension in the household. Bill gets annoyed when Jennifer upsets the household routines by going to meetings. Jennifer refrains from engaging with Bill when he complains. Bill recognizes that Jennifer is stepping back from him, which makes him angry. Then Bill begins to experiment with "controlled drinking," which makes the home environment less chaotic, but also less stable. When Bill actually stops drinking and goes to an AA meeting, it is challenging both for him and for Jennifer; Bill has to squarely face his issue of loss of control—to drink or not to drink—and Jennifer must rely heavily on her support system to keep her focused on her own recovery. Her challenge is to stay with her own process and not to distract Bill from his personal quest for his own truth.

As in Brown's model, FRT holds that, optimally, the old structure of the family—the former homeostasis—must be dismantled completely in order to allow the family members to construct a vastly different entity, a family in which each and every family member can develop an individual self. How long it takes a family to collapse its former dysfunctional structure and then to consolidate the revolutionary individual and interpersonal recovery changes, and to establish a stable, consistent, and secure state, varies with each family, the situation, the obstacles, the kind and frequency of treatment the family is receiving, and the family members' level of motivation. A premise of FRT is that when all the family members—each of whom grows and changes independently, at his or her own rate—participate in an integrated and intensive recovery program as described in this book, the process steadily moves forward.

Families engaged in FRT can move through the stages of Drinking (or substance-using), Transition, and Early Recovery at a faster rate than the subjects in Brown's research who did not have the advantage of treatment in a family-based, comprehensive, and intensive program. In the FRT model, at the end of the first full year of continuous sobriety for the addict, and with completion of the 12 Steps by each family member, the family will be well on their way towards establishing a solid recovery base. This unified, cohesive, integrated approach, with participation of all family members, moves the process of early recovery forward swiftly in the first year of treatment. One year of continuous sobriety for the addict, along with completion of the 12 Steps by each family member, is but one milestone on the path of recovery, but it is an achievable and significant marker for a family moving toward stability and ongoing health, and creates a solid platform for further growth in Ongoing Recovery.

Below, I include an outline of Stephanie Brown's four stages of family addiction recovery, as well as the three domains she describes where change occurs in the process of recovery. To recap, the stages of recovery include: Drinking, Transition (with two substages, Drinking and Early Abstinence), Early Recovery, and Ongoing Recovery. The three domains of change are the Environment (the home environment, or context for the family), the Family System, and Individual Development. I describe each stage of Brown's model and integrate into her model excerpts from the case studies presented in this book.

Stephanie Brown's Developmental Process of Recovery:

Four Stages of Recovery
1. Drinking
2. Transition
   Drinking
   Abstinence
3. Early Recovery
4. Ongoing Recovery

Three Domains of Change
1. Environment
2. Family System
3. Individual Development

1—Drinking Stage

As Brown describes, in the active Drinking stage, drinking is the central organizing principle of the family. The family is trying to deny active alcoholism while also justifying the alcoholic's loss of control, and rationalizing to themselves how it all makes sense—which is crazy-making. It is essential to include this stage in depicting the recovery process, because the reality of addiction is foundational to the family's history and to the growth and change that follow.

Domain: Environment

In this stage, the home environment is characterized by anxiety, tension, and chaos. There is an ongoing attempt to control an out-of-control and unpredictable system. Family members exhibit hostility, anger, shame, and guilt. And the home is unsafe, with possible trauma. In the case study of an addicted spouse, Jennifer reported in our early sessions that she was frightened, even terrified, that Bill would actually assault her, and that he had been physically abusive with their son Vincent, to the point where she had considered calling the police. She never knew when Bill would cross a line, his personality would change, and he would start raging at both Vincent and her. In those early therapy sessions, Jennifer seemed anxious and desperate, and talked about terrifying moments where she actually considered taking her son and "running away from it all."

In the case study that features Peter, a substance-abusing young adult, Peter created chaos in his home environment, even though he was unaware of it. His divorced parents were chronically upset. When Peter went out at night, each parent waited anxiously at their own home to see if or when Peter would return. His parents fought with each other about how best to handle him; they were always on edge, fearing one more call from the school or from a parent reporting yet another example of Peter's crazy behavior—or worse, a call from the police. The chaos and unpredictability continued, no matter which parent's home Peter lived in. He was often intoxicated, belligerent, or hung over. He actively opposed any attempts by either of his parents to integrate him into the normal flow of family dinners, chores, and family outings. Any family activities Peter did participate in typically ended in fights and hostility.

Similarly, in the case study of the adolescent, 16-year-old Mary's drug abuse upset her household. As Mary's grades slipped and she missed her weekend curfews, her parents were at their wits' end. They sought help from therapy and started to go to Al-Anon, but Mary continued to use drugs.

In a situation with an alcoholic parent who is not living in the household, there are repercussions in the homes of the concerned others. In the case study about an addicted parent, three adult daughters living in separate households were concerned about their father, Robert. Sue, the eldest of the three, was particularly upset when her father fell one evening and broke his arm as he walked from a restaurant to his car after they'd had dinner, during which he'd had several drinks. Sometimes when Sue called her father in the evening, he slurred his words as he spoke with her. At daytime family events, Robert appeared present, sober, and engaged, but in the evening, if he'd been drinking, he was very different. Sue and her sisters were worried because they did not know the extent of their father's drinking, and were fearful that he would hurt himself again as he had when he'd fallen. The adult daughters had grown up with their father's drinking, which affected their development. And, as adults, they continued to focus on their father, which distracted them from pursuing their own lives.

Domain: Family System

During the active drinking stage, family members are often in denial that addiction is the real problem. The addict's drinking and its aftermath trigger efforts by codependent family members to rescue the addict and hide their family's reality from outsiders. Family relationships are tense and polarized, with frequent, aborted attempts to create short-term stability—which is always in flux, as family members react over and over again to the "elephant in the room." Drinking becomes the central emotional concern for every family member, derailing the family as a whole from developing healthy norms, roles, and rituals.

In the case study about the addicted spouse, Jennifer reported that Bill's drinking and the conflict in the household had grown worse over their 20 years together, and it drove her crazy—she was upset almost every day and rarely had a good night's sleep. Jennifer shared that their son, Vincent, retreated to his room and became absorbed in computer games to hide from the endless conflict, or sometimes provoked fights with his father to prevent the parents from clashing. Vincent took on the role of a "Spousified Child" and became his mother's confidant, which further interfered with his individual development and movement towards "leaving the nest."

In our addicted parent case study, Sue reported that being with her father at daytime family gatherings when he was sober and engaged was very different from trying to connect with him in the evenings. Her father's drinking impacted the composition and the tenor of family gatherings.

In the case of the 16-year-old addict, Mary, the family was in turmoil, and Mary's behavior became the central organizing principle in the family. Mary had been acting out for some time at the point that her parents sought help. Mary's drug use and consequent erratic behavior derailed the parents' efforts to support and launch a healthy daughter.

Domain: Individual Development

In this arena, the normal, expected, age-appropriate development of individual family members has slowed down or stopped and been replaced by attempts to make sense of the craziness. Individual family members have each developed a "false self," and their behavior is geared towards helping to reduce stress in an out-of-control family—unlike a healthy family where healthy individuals support age-appropriate development for everyone, and quickly resolve conflicts and regain stability. In the case study of the addicted spouse, Bill and Jennifer's son, Vincent, put aside his normal, 15-year-old life to protect his mother. Instead of being interested in friends and sports and girls, like a normal teen, Vincent had turned into a kind of security guard who spent his evenings at home, on alert in case he needed to step in and protect his mother from his raging, intoxicated, alcoholic father. His mother similarly had shifted her focus away from pursuing her own career or other interests in order to contend with the chaos at home and the discord in her marriage.

In the case study of the addicted parent, although Robert's daughters had developed functional, adult lives, their father's drinking was a source of ongoing concern to them. The daughters were upset that they could not include their father in family functions that took place in the evening. Worry about their father became a central focus in the life of each adult daughter, diverting attention from their own lives.

In the case study of the adolescent, Mary's parents were frustrated and at their wits' end trying to manage their daughter's substance abuse, and her resultant poor school performance and disruptive behavior. Mary's development as a healthy young woman, preparing to graduate from high school and leave home for college or a job, was thrown off course when Mary began to abuse substances. Mary's parents were overwhelmed by their daughter's behavior, dismayed at her developmental trajectory, and sidetracked from their own lives and goals.

2—Transition Stage

(The Transition Stage includes both the end of drinking—"hitting bottom"—and the beginning of abstinence.)

Substage: Drinking

At this stage, the family is beginning to acknowledge the presence and severity of alcoholism in the family. The alcoholic realizes he or she can no longer control his or her drinking, and the codependent family members realize they cannot control the alcoholic. This stage is stressful—the old system begins to crumble, old behaviors are no longer effective, and old beliefs cannot be sustained—what was familiar is giving way to questions about the future.

Domain: Environment

The Transition Stage occurs when someone in the family hits a bottom—either the addict or the codependent, or sometimes both. The family is at a turning point. Prior to hitting bottom, problems at home increase, out-of-control behavior escalates, and the rationalizations supporting denial deepen. In the story of the addicted spouse, Jennifer reported that Bill had actually put his hands on Vincent, who got physical in return. Their home was chaotic and unsafe. In the case of the adolescent, Mary's acting-out behavior escalated, causing her parents to hit a bottom and seek help. And in the situation with the young adult, Peter was causing more and more disruption in the homes of both of his divorced parents. The "hitting bottom" moment for the parents—the point at which they sought help to deal with Peter's drug use—was the father's discovery of drugs in Peter's car. In a chaotic home environment, with someone close to hitting a bottom, there can be significant drama—loud arguments, guns fired, TVs thrown through windows, physical fights, injuries, people arrested, and worse.

Domain: Family System

The family is hitting bottom. Reactivity and confusion reign, and things seem to be falling apart. The family systems theorist, Dr. Murray Bowen, described the trajectory of a family in acute distress. He is reputed to have said that the family disease will continue until the repercussions stemming from taking the easy way out on tough issues—the old dynamics—exceed the pain associated with acting on a long-term solution. When family members realize the emotional cost of continuing to try to "fix" an unfixable situation, they give up and seek outside help to find a better solution.

The end of drinking in the Transition Stage is a critical period—the homeostasis that existed for a long time is now in a state of collapse. Things are falling apart. This is the point when a suffering family member may call a "treatment program" or a "rehab" whose ads they've seen on TV or on Google, or search for an "Interventionist," or possibly ask someone for a referral. It is at this juncture when a codependent or concerned family member is likely to contact an FRT therapist. An FRT therapist will join with the anguished family member and guide the caller—who may well be an enabling codependent—to shift their focus away from the addict toward external resources, including therapy and social support groups. At this pivotal point, the addict may vacillate frantically between using and stopping use, while the codependent anxiously bounces between enacting codependency and suspending it. The codependent can benefit from the guidance they've received from the FRT therapist and their support group. When Bill and Jennifer were at this point, Jennifer had to work hard to detach from Bill's ups and downs. She settled into therapy and attended support groups to help her manage the instability of this period.

The family engages in a merry-go-round of grappling with the new and the old—first turning one way, then the other. The family may take positive steps, and then revert to old habits, which may be followed by another round of positive change. Eventually, either the family stabilizes, as family members begin recovery, or continues on its downward spiral.

The cycle of surrendering to outside help and then returning to prior behavior, and then surrendering once more, can play out over days, months, or even years. Each family member must come to terms with the idea of letting go of the old, and accepting guidance with the new, which leads to a path of recovery. The FRT therapist needs to let a family go through its own process—to allow them to become ready to accept help. Some families, even with the best intentions, need a long time before they are ready to make the decision to enter recovery, and the therapist, when working with addiction, needs to remember it's their path, and that recovery has to happen in their time. However, the clinician needs to know when it is appropriate to intervene, to question, to educate, and to offer direction to the family that is struggling with addiction. It is crucial that the therapist both remain involved, and yet maintain sufficient detachment from the family system to not risk pushing a family faster than it can go. Trying to force a family to move to a stage it has not yet organically reached can cause the family to balk and resist treatment.

At this stage, the FRT therapist helps family members understand their predicament, and nudges them to move through their denial, gently challenging their core beliefs. The therapist encourages them to accept the limits of their control—the addict cannot control their substance use, the codependent cannot control the addict. In the spouse and parent case studies, it is at this stage that Bill and Robert each discovered they could not, in fact, control their drinking. This is when, as a therapist, it is crucial not to push the client forward; by allowing them to find that they want and need to make a change, the family system is guided toward a new stability. When Mary, the teen in the adolescent case study, was continuing to come home late and use drugs, it was important for her parents, Sandra and Gary, to learn from their support groups how other parents had dealt with these situations. Sandra and Gary had to come to terms with what they could and could not do to corral their daughter. Sometimes they were successful in holding to their boundaries, and sometimes they slipped back into old patterns. Family members are counseled to use several recovery resources: the therapist, social support groups, contact with others in recovery, and literature about addiction and codependency. When there are children in the household, we work with the parents to stabilize the home environment and provide whatever resources we can to help and support the children, which may include involving the police and Child Protective Services.

Domain: Individual Development

It is hard to imagine any family member at this unstable transitional stage engaging in normal, healthy development—just trying to survive is often the challenge. Each individual is stressed, and struggling to contend with others' increasingly out-of-control behavior. Jennifer, as noted, was very anxious and did not know what to do. She talked about leaving her husband. This is the crisis point, when enabling codependents, more and more stressed and "down to their last nerve," become desperate for a way out of the chaos and despair. Peter's parents, after finding narcotics in their son's car, finally decided to get professional help. Mary's parents felt helpless to control their daughter's acting-out behavior, her bouts of drunkenness, and her dropping grades, and they, too, sought help. And, in the case of the addicted parent, the crisis point occurred when Robert, who had been drinking, fell and broke his arm; his eldest daughter became alarmed and reached out for help.

Substage: Abstinence

The beginning of abstinence is an unstable time for both the addict and the codependents. Each family member struggles to adopt new behaviors to replace the coping mechanisms of the past. Abstinence is fragile, not just for the addict, but also for family members. Family members may see-saw between abstinence and relapse, sometimes refraining from past behaviors, and sometimes reverting to their old, codependent ways to try to manage the alcoholic.

Domain: Environment

As Brown describes, the family at this stage is engaged in the "trauma of recovery." The formerly predictable homeostasis has changed. The chaos characteristic of the home during addiction is replaced by a new and different kind of unpredictability. Confusion reigns as family members try out new behaviors, and cope with the consequences, interpersonal and emotional. While there may be hope for positive change, there is also fear of relapse. And conflicts may persist as a way to maintain emotional connection. In the spouse case study, Jennifer was distraught when she called me, desperately seeking help. She was distressed by her husband's drinking, the chaos at home, and the impact of the situation on their son. Jennifer wanted things to get better, but when Bill stopped drinking, Jennifer vacillated between the recovery path—keeping therapy appointments and attending support groups—and sinking into her prior denial, cancelling sessions, and fighting with her husband.

The old family homeostasis needs to be completely dismantled in order to make room for a new structure and a new reality. As Stephanie Brown points out:

> This finding—the need for family systems collapse—is central to our whole theory of recovery. It is the collapse of the family structures and defense mechanisms that protected and maintained the drinking that clears the ground for the transformative process of recovery. As one family said, "You're not just putting your life back together; it's a new life." [Brown & Lewis, 1999, p.19]

Understandably, when a family makes fundamental changes, there is tremendous emotional and psychological upheaval. The FRT therapist needs to be the solid, compassionate guide who shepherds family members through this period of instability, encouraging them to heed the wisdom of their support system as they begin to construct lives grounded in sobriety, serenity, and recovery. In the case of the addicted spouse, Jennifer needed to rely both on guidance from her therapist and on encouragement from members of her support group, whose experience and understanding could help her weather the tumultuous situation at home. In the case of the addicted parent, the adult daughters were encouraged to attend community support groups well before their father, Robert, became part of the treatment process. And when Robert entered therapy with his daughters, as his FRT therapist, I encouraged him to use AA for support. Mary's parents received assistance from their community support group as well as from therapy. Eventually, we coordinated treatment for Mary, first at an adolescent inpatient program, and later, at an adult residential program. And in the case of Peter, the young adult addict, his parents benefited immeasurably from hearing the experiences of others in their community support group. The stories they heard were vital in helping them learn not to enable their son's addiction and to support his recovery. All of these were examples of reconfiguring the environment in which these families found themselves.

Domain: Family System

Nearly everyone in the family struggles at this stage with the collapse of the prior homeostasis and the fear of the unknown. The old roles, rules, and rituals no longer apply—but nothing has been built yet to replace them. Children complain that they "don't know what is happening," as their parents exhibit new and different behaviors. Meanwhile, parents themselves are trying to incorporate new information and shift the family towards a new, healthier, but not yet established, homeostasis. In this stage, the family is undefined, suspended between the old and the new. In each of our case studies, this is the time when the codependents—Jennifer (married to an active drinker); the parents of the adolescent Mary; young adult Peter's parents; and Robert's daughters—are beginning to get outside support. As they hear others' experiences with similar family systems, they learn new ways to see, name, and approach their own situation.

Domain: Individual Development

This is the time that each family member grapples with developing a new sense of identity as someone who has "let go," but who, at the same time, is not sure what that means. For the codependent family members, prior identities—as helpers, enablers, rescuers, fight-interveners—no longer are appropriate. It is common for individuals to feel depressed and afraid as they struggle to shift their behaviors and their priorities. In the case of the addicted spouse, Jennifer, some weeks into Al-Anon, still resisted "jumping in" and sharing at meetings—she was mostly a bystander, quickly slipping out of the room when the meeting ended. And her husband, Bill, was opposed to the idea of talking in public about his problem, a problem he was struggling to accept. In the case study of the addicted parent, Robert's daughters found it challenging to involve themselves in support group meetings and to shift their focus from their father to themselves.

3—Early Recovery Stage

In Brown's model, this stage begins after abstinence has been achieved and maintained for several years. It is important to reiterate that Brown's model is based on research collected from families that typically have not had the advantage of consistent mental health support or immersion in a 12-Step recovery process. Early Recovery occurs sooner in Family Recovery Therapy, because family members in this model engage in intense and consistent therapy and outside support. In FRT, Early Recovery begins during the first year of sobriety, after which a family transitions into Ongoing Recovery.

The family in Early Recovery is still unstable, as it continues to grapple with the disintegration of the old system. Each family member is focused on his or her independent process of growth and relies on external support for guidance. Recovery is still new enough that codependent family members sometimes lapse into old ways, although they can steady themselves more quickly than during the Abstinence phase. In FRT, with the advantage of weekly individual and family therapy, as well as engagement in group work, significant stability is typically achieved within the early months of treatment.

Domain: Environment

New behaviors, new identities, and changing relationships take shape in Early Recovery. A new stability at home begins to settle in. Routines change and new ones get established as treatment intensifies and involvement in social support groups continues. Homeostasis based on addiction and codependency has mostly crumbled, the former chaos has subsided, and the home environment feels more secure.

In this stage in the addicted spouse scenario, Bill occasionally instigated conflict with his son and wife, even though I, their FRT therapist, suggested that they avoid touchy topics outside of therapy. Bill, Jennifer, and Vincent are resilient enough that, when issues come up, they can be addressed relatively quickly and resolved, particularly with input from the FRT therapist and from Bill and Jennifer's 12-Step sponsors.

In the case of the addicted parent, in early recovery, Sue and her sisters acknowledged they sometimes worried about their father when they heard he was going to an event where alcohol was being served. They also admitted that they were tempted to "check in with him" after he'd been to dinner with friends. However, they knew that their father's drug tests were consistently clean, and that he was immersed in his own recovery work. Their therapist and sponsors reminded them that each family member was solely responsible for their own sobriety and serenity, and that they needed to focus on themselves.

In the case study of the young adult, Peter, his parents needed to shift their relationship with their then-19-year-old son to create an adult-adult relationship to replace the parent-child dynamic of their prior interactions (which had been appropriate when Peter was a minor). Peter was employed, sober, and solidly working on his recovery, but his parents occasionally slipped into "codependent relapses" and offered Peter advice he hadn't requested, as if he were a child. Peter, however, was quick to point out these "slips" to his parents. Peter's parents needed to continue their recovery work and allow Peter to grow into an autonomous young man. In general, his parents seemed to trust that Peter was moving forward in a good direction.

Domain: Family System

In the family, at this stage, a new, healthier, homeostasis is beginning to develop. Family members demonstrate more respect and appreciation for each other's autonomy. Conflict arises less frequently than in the drinking and early abstinence phases; any conflict that occurs is brought into individual and family therapy, and is quickly resolved. New rules, roles, and rituals are gradually taking hold based on the 12-Step principles and the guidance from the FRT therapist. There is a sense that the family is beginning to establish a new foundation, albeit shaky, which can support continuing growth and individuation of the family members. In the spouse case study, it was during this stage that I would hear from Vincent that he was having fewer fights with his dad. Jennifer and Bill at this stage were generally able to engage in conversations that were calm and respectful.

Domain: Individual Development

While family members suffer bouts of fear, confusion, anxiety, depression, and sadness as they move forward in this intense period of change, they also experience intervals of calmness and serenity. Family members begin to shift their orientation from others to themselves, and to concentrate on the new things they are learning. This is a period of intense self-focus as each family member gradually begins to absorb the wisdom of recovery and to build a new identity as a recovering person. The once-foreign idea of turning their lives over to a power other than themselves had seemed impossible to embrace when they were in the throes of maintaining the illusion of control, but they have begun to grasp this concept, and consequently to experience serenity and a growing sense of optimism. The FRT therapist gently acknowledges their uncertainty, encourages them to let go, and offers perspective and hope as they gradually shift and grow, one day at a time.

Individuals in the family case studies exhibited personal progress in early recovery. Six months after Bill stopped drinking, Jennifer began to settle down. She reported that she was sleeping through the night for the first time in years. She relied on recovery friends for support, and enjoyed some social engagements with them as well. Peter, the young adult, was solidly on a recovery path several months after his relapse, active in his support groups, and working full time. His parents had each settled into their own recovery groups, and both of them appreciated having more serenity in their respective households. In family sessions, Peter and each of his parents were more articulate about their needs and feelings, and able to be respectful of each other, even in the face of disagreement. Eighteen-year-old Mary was well-established in her sober home, participating in support groups, and working full-time. With the ongoing guidance of weekly family therapy, Mary and her parents were building solid, adult-adult relationships. They often enjoyed Sunday evening dinners together. And in the case of the addicted parent, once Robert was firmly ensconced in treatment and doing his own recovery work, his adult daughters were able to focus on their own recovery and begin to address the repercussions on them of growing up in an alcoholic family. Robert was welcomed back into their homes for evening events, to celebrate birthdays and holidays, and to spend time with his grandchildren.

4—Ongoing Recovery Stage

Ongoing Recovery, in Brown's model, occurs after five years of recovery. It takes a long time to let the prior homeostasis completely collapse and to construct a new foundation. Individuals by this time have established solid recovery identities, consistent abstinent behaviors and independent goals. The strong individual recovery of family members provides a foundation for building healthy family interactions and new, recovery-based norms, roles, and rituals.

Families engaged in comprehensive FRT treatment may begin to build this foundation by the end of the first year of the addict's sobriety, and continue to enrich and expand their lives in the process of ongoing recovery. When I encounter members of families I have worked with in the past, it is always a joy to witness their engagement in life—to see Ongoing Recovery in action.

Many years ago, when I interned as a therapist at a treatment center for families of teens, I worked with a 16-year-old boy and his mother. The mother stopped enabling her son's drug use, her son stopped using drugs, and the mother and son developed a healthier relationship. The boy grew up and became a healthy, sober, adult man. He developed a career as a CPA, married and had a child, and the mom became a happy grandmother who regularly babysits her granddaughter. Another time, I worked with a 22-year-old opiate addict and his parents. I guided the family through treatment as the young man attended a Residential Treatment Center (RTC) and then continued outpatient work near the RTC. That was 12 years ago. Today, he is a licensed mental health professional and works at a wilderness program for young adults. What a pleasure it is to witness this young man's transformation, and his trajectory from young addict to therapist working with young addicts.

Domain: Environment

During Ongoing Recovery, the home environment comes to resemble the environment of a home that has not been impacted by addiction and codependency. The specter of relapse has receded. The home feels safe, secure, and stable, and supports the absence of addiction and codependency. Conflicts are fewer and are quickly resolved as family members keep the focus on themselves and actively engage in their recovery behaviors, which are now the new normal. Differences are no longer volatile, and there is an atmosphere of accountability and mutual respect.

In the spouse case study, Jennifer, Bill, and their son, Vincent, enjoyed happy family vacations—these were a welcome change from the tense and miserable trips during the years when Bill was drinking. And in the case study of the young adult, Peter, both of his parents enjoyed Peter's visits to their respective homes. The parents and Peter were able to discuss and quickly resolve differences.

Domain: Family System

In Ongoing Recovery, the family has become stable and predictable in healthy ways and can handle crises, tension, and illness as they arise, metabolizing them and returning relatively quickly to a state of stability and serenity. The family is firmly grounded in reality. Each family member brings more of themselves and their personal strengths to the family, which allows the family to grow and establish developmentally appropriate relationships. In the case study of the addicted parent, the father, Robert, became a trusted listening ear for his daughters when they wanted to talk about their families.

Individual Development

The movement towards differentiation has become the norm—each individual has developed a stable sense of personal identity, as well as the capacity for healthy interpersonal connections. Each family member has a strong sense of self and is capable of self-examination and insight, and can recognize his or her shortcomings and defenses, as well as strengths. Individuals may pursue new interests, or may resume old ones with a new perspective on their significance. Family members continue to utilize social support groups, and perhaps therapy and other resources, to further their personal growth. In the case study of Peter, the young adult, Peter chose a new and unexpected career direction as a registered nurse. His parents kept up their participation in social support groups. In the case study of the adolescent, the formerly drug-using and acting-out teen, Mary, became a longtime AA member and sponsored other young women with histories of alcohol or drug use.

Conclusion

Stephanie Brown illuminates the long view of family recovery from addiction, which unfolds, stage by stage, over a span of many years. FRT facilitates a concentrated and focused recovery process that can move a committed family through several phases of change within a year, and lay the groundwork for recovery to continue along the path that Brown describes. Families that engage in Family Recovery Therapy exhibit strength and solidity.

For the FRT therapist, it is a joy to observe family members make fundamental changes through each stage in succession. Each therapy session provides snapshots of positive change at home, in all three Domains—the Environment, the Family System, and Individual Development—as individual family members choose to behave in new and healthier ways in the minute-to-minute unfolding process of their lives.

Family members who do the work of Family Recovery Therapy, and who continue to pursue ongoing recovery, can build satisfying and fulfilling lives and manage life's ups and downs with greater awareness and emotional skill than was the case prior to treatment. Therapists who know Brown's work will find FRT to be a deeply satisfying and highly effective approach to addiction treatment.

PART THREE

Using Adjunctive Resources

Chapter 12

Working with Other Treatment Providers

Central to this book is the theme of systems coordinating with systems. In the FRT treatment model, the FRT therapist facilitates work with the family system, and interfaces with the addiction treatment system—other providers involved in a family's treatment to achieve a cohesive recovery process. The FRT approach is grounded in science and in evidence-based research that point to the benefits of an integrated system of professionals who come together to treat the family system, which is comprised of all those impacted by, and impacting, an individual's addiction.

As defined by the American Society of Addiction Medicine (ASAM) (see Chapter 3), addiction is a medical disease that has biological, psychological, social, and spiritual implications. Recovery from this disease requires input, coordination, and treatment by a team of providers who contribute to the common goal of helping the addict, the family, and all those impacted by one family's addiction—which can include the extended family, friends, employers, and others. The FRT model seeks to change the current addiction treatment protocol to a new paradigm, a systems-based approach. FRT Principle 5 speaks to the FRT therapist's collaborative work with other adjunctive services involved in a family's recovery process:

FRT Principle 5
As the treatment team leader, the FRT therapist guides the family throughout the continuum of care and collaborates with all supportive therapeutic services, which may include other treatment providers, interventionists, treatment programs, physicians, and any other adjunctive services.

Asking practitioners to adapt to this paradigm shift is challenging. But I believe we must implement this perspective—to fail to do so is an abdication of what evidence-based research and science have proven about effective addiction treatment (see Chapter 4 regarding the parallels between FRT's principles and the guidelines of the National Institute on Drug Abuse).

Today, the "recovery process" is informing and changing America's collective awareness of our number one mental health problem in a way that perhaps religion has done in the past. The explosion of 12-Step programs is a symptom of our collective need for connection, community, and inspiration. For many people, "drug treatment" is an entry point into major lifestyle change. This has profound implications for a future where disparate medical, psychological, and spiritual disciplines collaborate to treat people holistically, using the recovery process as a template for partnering with and integrating various disciplines.

I would like to use myself as an example of someone who, not unlike millions of other addicts, has recovered by utilizing appropriate professional and paraprofessional resources. As mentioned earlier, my life's journey began in an abusive, loveless alcoholic family. I attended 13 schools in six states before graduating from high school. I progressed through 25 years of active addiction, hit a "bottom," began early recovery in my late 30s, and finally evolved into my current life of long-term recovery.

During my recovery process, I have been privileged to hear thousands of loving, wise words from men and women in thousands of social support groups, and from a handful of mentors—with whom I have spent hundreds of hours, in coffee shops, their offices, and their homes—who have provided guidance and taught me how working the recovery principles could alter my core emotional, psychological, social, and spiritual condition. I have received additional assistance from many mental health professionals who have helped me understand how my childhood shaped me, and who slowly have helped me rewire my brain, which has allowed me to "wake up" and "grow up." With this assistance, I have been able to reach a point in my development close to where I believe I would have been, had I received appropriate caregiving early in my life and not succumbed to addiction. With a lot of support, I have finally been able to become a functional, healthy person, capable of functional, loving relationships, as well as to become a contributing member of society.

I recovered what had been lost, I healed what had been broken, and I learned what I had never been taught. And, it took "a village."

What does it take to heal? Everyone's path is different, but, for illustration, I'll continue to describe my individual journey as one example, one story, of how an addict pursued recovery with the help of a team of providers.

A few years after I detoxed and stabilized, medically and physically, I sought out the services of licensed psychotherapists. Some innate wisdom told me that I was "broken," "not yet well," and that I needed outside help from various professionals to guide me back to wellness. I experienced a profound awakening when I was able to connect authentically with a wise mental health professional in a way I had never been able to do with anyone before. The magic and mystery of psychotherapy allowed me to connect with a trusted other, to see parts of myself that had been hidden, and to strengthen my capacity to live life in "recovery mode." Over the years, I have worked with therapists using a variety of approaches, including cognitive behavioral, humanistic, existentialist, psychodynamic, psychedelic, and somatic. Also, I spent eleven years in a professionally facilitated men's group, and I have attended countless hours of couples' and family therapy. And occasionally, I have turned to psychiatrists who have recommended a brief course of medication to help stabilize me during a crisis.

While I never received treatment at a residential addiction program, I have attended dozens of three- to ten-day intensive residential retreats for codependents and adult children of alcoholics, Gestalt therapy groups, meditation retreats, and men's retreats. These retreats have expanded my awareness and contributed to my recovery. I still enroll in residential retreats on a regular basis to further my growth, deepen my ability to play and have fun, and to make loving connections with others. These experiences have contributed to my ongoing development, which was impeded by growing up in a loveless and emotionally barren alcoholic home.

In addition to the experiences I have gained from social support groups, therapy, and education—which have helped me deepen my relationships and enrich my life—my capacity to be mindful and peacefully present has been furthered by attending three, ten-day silent Buddhist meditation retreats and several shorter retreats.

I have turned to medical doctors, on many occasions, to treat and correct a variety of, sometimes serious, afflictions I have suffered from. Today, as I practice good self-care, eat healthy food, and exercise, I am grateful for a healthy body that is vital and free of chronic diseases—in my seventies.

I attribute my growth to the help I have received from many healers, whose skill and love have facilitated my progress as I have worked to become a healthier person. In this process, I have discovered a deep desire to continue to grow, to optimize my biological, psychological, social, and spiritual potentials. I attend social support groups twice each week where, without fail, I get love, hugs, and connection with my fellows, some of whom have, like me, been attending meetings for decades. And I have the opportunity, just about every week, to reach out to and connect with someone new, someone just like I was, 40 years ago—sick, lost, confused—and maybe to say something helpful, or to spend some time, and perhaps to save a life, as someone saved mine. I have discovered a quiet place within myself, from which I continue to seek more of the inspiration, wisdom, and guidance that each of these connections has provided. I still meet weekly with a wise psychotherapist who continues to help me unravel and reveal the unconscious drives from my childhood that continue to impact me. His support gives me the courage to face—head on—and celebrate, the existential realities of my brief moment on this planet.

I am very grateful to have made it from that alcoholic family of my childhood to the life I currently live. While I thank my good fortune (and hard work), I'm aware of the addicts and codependents still suffering today, and of the opportunity for all of us professionals to do better—to become better informed, to integrate our treatment with that of other professionals, and to further our understanding of addiction and of this family-systems treatment approach. When it comes to the malady of addiction, my hope is to inspire treatment providers to become, or to coordinate their work with, an FRT therapist—this new-paradigm professional who will case manage a team of providers and treat the addict, the codependents, and their family system.

In my 25 years working as an addiction therapist, drug counselor, and treatment program director, I have coordinated with numerous professionals and paraprofessionals, including medical doctors, psychiatrists, psychologists, therapists, social workers, lawyers, police departments, probation officers, the courts, educational consultants, interventionists, treatment program clinical directors, and sober home managers. Below, I address those working in several of these professions and make recommendations for an FRT therapist to better coordinate treatment with members of these disciplines. Using this new model that provides a continuum of care can improve outcomes for our clients (or patients) and their families.

Medical Doctors

Physicians are highly trained, skilled, and experienced professionals. However, as mentioned earlier, they typically have little training in addiction and little knowledge about the addicted family system. And yet, they are the "go-to" professional when it comes to medicine and are highly likely to come into contact with addicts, including those in the earliest stages of their disease, as well as with those who have an addicted family member. Because they have been poorly educated about addiction—either about its symptoms, or about the denial that obscures it—they are unlikely to assess for addiction in the short time they typically have available to address and treat the many symptoms their patients present. There are probably 30 million addicts in this country who will interact with a medical doctor at some point. I believe it is vital that physicians come to understand that roughly ten percent of their patients are likely to be in the early stages of addiction, or are active addicts, and that physicians begin to use their access and authority to assess for addiction, to educate, and to refer for further evaluation, when in doubt. During the years I was a practicing addict, I probably saw a dozen medical doctors who failed to assess me for possible symptoms of addiction—and one who did. That doctor helped save my life.

As an addiction treatment provider, I have, on occasion, contacted medical doctors to discuss an addict we were both treating—typically an individual in crisis. My calls with them have usually been brief. I have yet to have a medical doctor refer a family to me for addiction-related treatment. Nor have I collaborated with a doctor who then consulted with me, long-term, on a case. Communication with a physician regarding a client has always been initiated by me. This may be, in part, due to the way medicine is practiced today: The old-fashioned "Family Doctor" has been replaced by insurance-driven, keep-it-brief, medical care. As I've mentioned, when I first met my current, long-term personal doctor, I described to him my brain disease of addiction, its chronicity and potential for relapse, and the kind of support I needed from him. Now he asks me each time I see him, "Have you been going to your meetings? Still talking to your mentor?" He understands, or at least pretends to understand, that the patient in his consulting room has a medical disorder, a potentially fatal brain disease that can kill the patient, if he stops taking his "medicine"—attending the social support groups that remind him that he has a disease—and that tell him not to drink or use drugs, or to engage in addictive behaviors, just for today.

I would love to coordinate treatment with a client's doctor and have their authoritative voice and support in encouraging the family's acceptance of a long-term, integrated addiction treatment approach. The addict's family members would benefit from their doctor's prescription to follow the FRT therapist's recommendations, and it would be one more voice backing the family's recovery, even while the addicted family system's resistance and prior homeostasis tug them the other way. This is what I believe the FRT paradigm makes possible.

I was a fortunate addict. A doctor-created chain of events led to my recovery. At the age of 38, I went into a seven-day, residential, stop-smoking program. I knew I was addicted to nicotine, and I was highly motivated to stop smoking, but I was still in denial about my alcoholism. During the intake appointment, I met with a doctor who asked me about my alcohol and drug use. (At various points in my adult life, I had consulted with other doctors who asked me about my substance use, but did not thoroughly assess the patient sitting in front of them—me, an alcoholic in total denial—who exhibited numerous issues that could be caused by substance abuse.) I wanted my nicotine addiction treatment to succeed, so I was honest with this doctor about my history with drugs and alcohol. My response to his questions led him to refer me for an assessment with an addiction specialist in their program. The addiction specialist asked me a series of questions and administered a simple test. Based on my answers, he told me that I was at "high risk" for alcoholism and recommended that I seek treatment. I was aghast! I immediately blocked out his words and worked frantically to reconstruct my denial.

But prompted by one doctor's referral, followed by a single interview with an addiction counselor, I was motivated—eight months later—to attend a social support group and begin my recovery. (And I have remained sober since that day.) Prior to attending that first meeting, I had been in active addiction, I had been depressed and increasingly suicidal—but one medical doctor was thorough and persistent. I owe my life to that doctor's thorough assessment and referral.

Residential treatment programs that include appropriate medical treatment are typically focused on the addict, and rarely include regular involvement of the codependents in the long-term clinical treatment. In these facilities, doctors may prescribe suboxone for opiate addicts, and release them with a suboxone prescription—then cross their fingers as they discharge these clients, often witnessing them relapse because the doctors failed to solidly ensconce the clients in a family systems-based step-down aftercare program. If these centers were working with an FRT therapist, who was involved in an addict's treatment from day one, there would be a structured continuation of care upon discharge from the residential program, into an IOP. An FRT therapist would oversee treatment from the outset, make the referral to the residential program, work with family members during the addict's residential treatment stay, as well as be involved with inpatient treatment planning for the addict, and manage ongoing treatment of the family and the addict during and after the critically important transition from residential care.

While medical doctors have some familiarity with addiction, unless they have received special training, they may not recognize possible symptoms. For example, meth addicts notoriously have poor teeth, those who snort cocaine and other substances are subject to sinus inflammation and infection, and heavy alcohol users can exhibit elevated liver enzymes. Furthermore, doctors may not be aware that addiction creates unusual stress for loved ones of addicts.

When I refer an addict or a family member to a medical doctor in the course of Family Recovery Therapy, I inform the doctor about my treatment process and my need for their collaboration. I explain that my work with families is evidence-based, and I describe the treatment for the family as well as for the addict. I explain that addiction is a family disease, and discuss the benefits of family-based treatment. I also explain that it is my job, as an FRT therapist, to oversee and manage treatment, and to coordinate care with other professionals treating family members. I clarify that the doctor plays a vital role in monitoring and treating the patient medically, and also in collaborating with me about the patient's treatment. I will often send the physician a generic copy of the Treatment Agreement so that they can understand the process and support all aspects of it.

I want doctors both to know the signs of addiction, and to understand what constitutes effective addiction treatment. Also, doctors typically do not understand the systemic nature of the disease. A doctor may not consider that someone who presents with stress-related physical problems, and who complains about their young-adult addict child or their spouse who drinks too much, could in fact be helped by Al-Anon or another similar support or mutual aid group for family members of addicts. I want to educate doctors about addiction, codependency, and the addictive family system, because this is information they are unlikely to have acquired in their training. Doctors armed with this knowledge will be better prepared to collaborate with an FRT therapist, and can work cooperatively to best serve their patients struggling with these afflictions.

Psychiatrists

Psychiatrists are medical doctors who are the mental health professionals authorized both *to assess* psychological problems and *to prescribe* medication to help relieve symptoms. It is imperative that the FRT therapist work collaboratively with the prescribing psychiatrist when a client is taking psychotropic medication, and that an FRT therapist have a psychiatrist to whom they can refer a client who might benefit from medication. It is important that the psychiatrist understands the nature and complications of the mental health issues of addicts and codependents. Psychiatrists that specialize in addiction possess this expertise, but only a fraction of psychiatrists get this training.

Psychiatrists, as well as other mental health professionals, refer to the *Diagnostic and Statistical Manual of Mental Disorders* (*DSM*) for assessment purposes. The

DSM-5 (American Psychiatric Association, 2013) lists a number of symptoms that can result from substance abuse. These include depression, anxiety, problems with sleep, eating, or sexual function, and psychotic symptoms. Ideally, a psychiatrist assesses every mental disorder symptom as a sign of a possible substance-related or addictive disorder—and refers the patient to addiction treatment if needed.

Because psychiatrists address the psychiatric needs of our clients, coordination of treatment between the FRT therapist and the psychiatrist is essential. I have found that many of my clients are taking psychotropic medication when they enter addiction treatment. However, the "symptoms" for which they are taking medication often turn out to be caused by their substance use, and not due to a pre-existing mental disorder. Their mood disturbances, sleep problems, obsessive patterns, impulse control issues, and other psychiatric symptoms often abate when the addiction has been put into remission, and the client's medical needs change. Sometimes, the client no longer needs any medication. This is true for codependent family members as well, who find that treatment and support—learning to set boundaries, determining when to engage and when not to, establishing new behaviors and ways of coping—relieve some of their stress and allow them to navigate life without reliance on medication.

If there is a psychiatrist involved in some aspect of my client's treatment, I describe my treatment process and goals, and explain how the psychiatrist and I can work together. Psychiatrists, more than members of most other helping professions, seem to understand and welcome our approach, because often they have witnessed failures resulting from ineffective addiction treatment. Many psychiatrists understand the chronic nature of addiction and readily support addiction treatment. It's important that any involved psychiatrist understand and fully support the details of the treatment plan. I let psychiatrists know that a patient's need for psychotropic drugs may shift in the process of recovery. As addicts and codependent family members change their behavior and learn new ways to manage their thoughts and feelings, they may experience fewer, or less intense, symptoms—symptoms which they formerly managed with the help of medication. When I collaborate with a psychiatrist, I stress both the significance of their role in understanding and treating psychiatric symptoms, and the need for close coordination with me as I oversee the treatment progress of all members of the addict's family.

Psychologists and Psychotherapists

Education in addiction and codependency is underemphasized in graduate work for psychologists and other mental health professionals (Marriage and Family Therapists, Clinical Social Workers, and Licensed Professional Counselors). From my personal experience, mental health practitioners have a blind spot when it comes to addiction treatment. These professionals are trained to help their clients get control over their problem. They fail to understand that a client with an addictive disorder, by definition, is someone who will never be able to *control* their hijacked prefrontal cortex. An addict suffers from a medical disorder, and their disordered brain renders them unable to resist their "medicine," which is their substance or addictive behavior. Addicts are already trying to "control" their dysphoric feelings, by using drugs and other addictive behaviors. The addict needs specific addiction treatment and is unable to use the advice of these well-meaning practitioners. I once heard someone say, "An addict needs to have eight years of sobriety before they can benefit from depth therapy." While perhaps an exaggeration, there is some truth to the statement that an addict needs to embrace recovery and achieve a basic level of emotional, physical, and psychological stability before they can receive significant benefit from depth psychotherapy. Digging up old, long-buried wounds too early in the recovery process will add to the client's anxiety at the very time the goal is to reduce their anxiety and stabilize them.

"Harm reduction" is the clinical approach used by most clinicians when they address substance use problems. Andrew Tatarsky, one of the leading proponents of harm reduction, has described his experience of integrating psychotherapy with outside social support group participation for his substance-abusing clients (2002). This cognitive behavioral approach is appropriate for the majority of clients grappling with substance issues. However, I believe that clinicians who adopt this approach, as mentioned above, sometimes fail to recognize, or to refer for appropriate assessment and treatment, those clients who suffer from the brain disease of addiction. That some clinicians fail to grasp the possible presence of addiction contributes to the tragic failure of the current addiction treatment paradigm to provide adequate treatment.

Many mental health professionals have misconceptions about addiction treatment and recovery, and fail to address treatment for the impacted family members. One local psychotherapist sent me a number of families struggling with addiction, families that I treated successfully using my family-based treatment approach. I was taken aback when she told me, "Larry, you should play down the 12-Step recommendations. 12-Step programs are cultish, and it is affecting your reputation," even though utilizing social support groups, including 12-Step, is a widely accepted protocol for addiction treatment. This kind of statement indicates a "blind spot," or simply a lack of education among mental health practitioners about the value and efficacy of community-based social support groups.

The FRT therapist is the addiction-trained, family systems provider who case manages addiction treatment. Sometimes treatment entails coordinating with another therapist. Typically, when a therapist views addiction as a primary problem, the non-addiction-specializing therapist terminates with the client and transfers their client to this addiction specialist. But sometimes a client may have a long-term relationship with another psychotherapist, and I will, of course, need to coordinate treatment with them. On occasion, the referring therapist does not understand addiction treatment and has countered my recommendations, which has undermined the addiction treatment.

Chapter 12. Working with Other Treatment Providers

The code of ethics for Licensed Marriage and Family Therapists requires that therapists coordinate treatment with other professionals involved in a client's care. When addiction is the primary issue and a client is working with another therapist, if the other therapist is unwilling to coordinate care and support addiction treatment, I suggest that the client terminate treatment with the other therapist and focus on their addiction treatment with me. I do this *only* when I have clarity that *addiction is the primary issue* and needs to be the focus of their therapy. Unfortunately, there are therapists who view a client's psychological problems as the root of their issues with addiction or codependency, and oppose the client leaving therapy. If the client is unwilling to follow my recommendations, I must let go, and accept the client's choice and the reality that I cannot provide the kind of treatment for the client that I believe would be most useful. Sometimes in these situations, I can provide limited consultation to the therapist or client, make treatment recommendations, and hope for a good outcome.

On occasion, a client needs to establish a relationship with another therapist to work on a specific ancillary issue. In these cases, I get written permission from my client to consult with the other therapist. I inform the other therapist about my treatment process, and ask that we consult with each other in order to support each other's work.

Mental health professionals need to understand that social support groups are a vital part of addiction and codependency treatment. As an FRT therapist, I educate psychologists and psychotherapists who are not well-versed in addiction about the fact that addiction is a *family disease*. Recovery, I clarify, is not simply about recovery of the individual addict, but recovery of the family system. I let them know that social support groups are a critical component of treatment *both* for addicts and for family members—that in their respective support groups, addicts and codependents develop a community of others in situations similar to theirs. Though these groups are not clinical in nature, there is extensive evidence that social support groups can be a valuable adjunct to psychotherapy, and play a role which psychotherapy cannot fill. These groups provide a place for addicts or codependents to learn from others who have had experiences similar to theirs and who have found ways to manage and even thrive, despite their situation. This peer support empowers clients in ways their individual therapy sessions cannot. Those in recovery receive invaluable gifts from social support groups: reassurance that they are not alone, empathy from others who understand and have been there, inspiration from those who have made peace with their circumstances, and encouragement to stay the course. In time, they find that they are able to join with others, to laugh, and even hug others—something that is often lacking in their addiction-focused lives.

Mental health professionals who are working with individual family members need to understand that the FRT therapist will coordinate and oversee treatment of the family. If the adjunctive therapists are not trained or educated about addiction, the FRT therapist needs to educate them about addiction and the attendant codependency. Any mental health professionals involved in a family's treatment must support both the FRT model and the treatment plan. The FRT therapist will collaborate with the mental health professional, who is a part of the family's treatment team, both to support the other therapist in working with their client, and to ensure that the family as a whole is moving forward in the recovery process.

Once again, as noted in Chapter 2, the words of addiction psychiatrist Timmen Cermak, address the need for coordination in the treatment process: "No one deserves to be a part of this (treatment) continuum unless they do it in a way that's integrated with what came before them and what comes after them. Their services need to be constructed in that way" (personal communication, 2018).

Lawyers, Probation Officers, and the Courts

Evidenced-based laws, attitudes, and approaches are slowly replacing the practice of criminalizing addiction. My local community has moved steadily in this direction. Twenty-five years ago, I interned at a program working with substance-using teens and their families. At that time, whenever the police found a juvenile in possession of drugs or alcohol, the teen was cited and referred to juvenile probation for consultation. I regularly talked to probation officers and visited my clients in Juvenile Hall. Several years later, I played a small role in developing a local teen Drug Court. Those of us working with this population learned to bring families, treatment, courts, and the law more on track with the guidelines of evidence-based addiction treatment.

My experience is that those who work in the courts and probation departments understand the significance of addiction treatment. They welcome collaboration with addiction treatment professionals, because they understand the benefits of treatment over incarceration. It is very helpful for addiction treatment providers to coordinate with lawyers, judges, probation officers, and parole departments. Involvement of the legal system can support addiction treatment, particularly when legal consequences for non-compliance can be integrated into the treatment plan. The simple message, "comply with the treatment recommendation or go to jail," often keeps an addict in treatment long enough to "wake up" from their addiction sufficiently to comprehend the benefits of ongoing recovery. Probation officers typically welcome collaboration from addiction treatment providers in developing the stipulations of a probation agreement. However, in some circumstances, I have found that being proactive and initiating contact with the probation officers is necessary. They are often overworked and focused on urgent cases, and occasionally fail to follow up on cases they imagine are going well. We can help keep an addicted client in treatment, and aware of the consequences for non-compliance, by reminding them of our ongoing communication with their probation officer.

Some lawyers are very savvy when it comes to handling clients who have addiction problems. They will work collaboratively with their clients, the courts, and addiction treatment providers to structure a legal outcome that both protects their clients from adverse legal consequences and ensures that an addict receives appropriate treatment. For example, instead of pushing to have the case dropped, a lawyer can work with the courts to mandate treatment, and agree to drop the case only upon successful completion of treatment.

However, some lawyers do not understand addiction and will advocate for their client's release or for dropping charges, even when it means that an addict, who is in dire need of addiction treatment, escapes consequences. The client continues his addictive behavior, which can lead to even more serious consequences—for the addict, and for others. When I talk with a lawyer about a client, I educate them about how addiction works and why it is necessary for addicts to experience the natural consequences of their disease—which can include mandatory addiction treatment.

Educational Consultants (ECs)

Educational Consultants (ECs) are certified practitioners who are the "go to" experts for placing at-risk students into specialized settings, including residential placements. While education is their primary concern, placement can be complicated when substance abuse treatment is needed. The certification process for ECs requires them to visit many specialized schools and residential programs every year so they can identify the right program for a particular client. They work closely with a family and with other providers to assess a family's specific needs, and then coordinate the transfer of the young person to a residential placement. The EC continues to be actively involved with the family and the young person during the initial stages of treatment, and then, I find, often slowly disengages as the residential program takes charge of the case. The residential program may make further recommendations for treatment, with or without ongoing collaboration with the EC.

This differs from the FRT model in which the FRT therapist coordinates a client's placement in residential treatment and continues to oversee the case, including the client's transition to aftercare, and treatment for them and their family going forward.

Sadly, I have been involved in a number of "who is in charge?" conflicts with ECs. We are members of two different professions, with two different treatment approaches. Educational Consultants are the liaison between families and alternative schools or placement options, and are skilled at making referrals to appropriate institutions. Since ECs visit and evaluate a large variety of schools and alternative facilities for children, teens, and young adults, their familiarity with these resources can outweigh the knowledge of an FRT therapist regarding placement options. Family Recovery Therapy encompasses a broad range of concerns that extends beyond the choice of a residential placement for the child. FRT therapists are focused on recovery for the family as a whole. Whether, when, and sometimes, where it is appropriate to send an adolescent or young adult child needs to be evaluated in the context of the family recovery trajectory. In the FRT model, treatment of the family continues, both while an adolescent or young adult child is attending a residential center, and after the child returns home. Reintegration of the child who has been away, and returns to the continuing-to-heal family at home, is an important phase of treatment, and this process sets the stage for ongoing individual and family recovery. Educational Consultants are typically focused only on their young client and do not address family issues.

On occasion, ECs and I have stepped on each other's toes and failed to offer the concerned parents a single, coordinated set of recommendations. I have had families that I was effectively treating terminate treatment with me and choose to work with an EC. And I have had cases where the parents were working with me and with an EC at the same time, and the parents dropped the EC, much to the chagrin of the EC and against my recommendation. In some cases, the parents were resistant, and chose a path that required less parental involvement rather than a more rigorous approach. Family Recovery Therapy, of course, requires parental participation, and, optimally, the FRT therapist and the EC coordinate to offer the family a unified treatment recommendation.

Collaboration between the EC and the FRT therapist best serves the needs of the family seeking assistance. It is important to inform Education Consultants about our model and how it works, and to coordinate closely with them. This is helpful, both so the family can understand our unique roles, and so the EC and the FRT therapist can be on the same page regarding treatment recommendations, particularly at the critically important "returning home" phase. In complex cases, where an addicted young person has co-occurring issues (another psychological problem, in addition to addiction), it would be appropriate for the EC to help coordinate placement and treatment with the FRT therapist, and have the FRT therapist (with the EC's involvement, as appropriate) coordinate the transfer home and continue to direct the intensive outpatient aftercare treatment. This collaboration offers the family the best possible chance of a successful outcome.

Interventionists

I am a long-time member of the Association of Intervention Specialists (AIS) and a Certified Intervention Professional (CIP). Most AIS members are also certified as Certified Intervention Professionals by the Pennsylvania Certification Board. AIS members are bound by a code of ethics which stipulates, among other requirements, that they neither be affiliated with nor be employed by any residential treatment program. There are no legal or licensure requirement for interventionists, and many non–AIS interventionists have financial relationships with particular treatment programs. When an interventionist's potential financial gain plays a role in the referral process, there is a risk that the client may not be referred to the most appropriate treatment program.

"Intervention," as it is applied to addiction, is a wildly misunderstood process. In the 1960s, an Episcopal priest by the name of Vernon Johnson developed the concept of intervening on an addict. He proposed that an interventionist—usually a recovering addict with some training in drug counseling—convene a group of caring family members who could persuade the addict to go to treatment. These "surprise" or "Johnson" model interventions sometimes succeeded in getting the addict into treatment, but not in keeping him there. The addict, realizing that he'd only agreed to enter treatment because he had been pressured by his family, often changed his mind and discharged himself. He frequently relapsed and returned to his dysfunctional family. His resentment at being scapegoated as "the problem" often led to more discord in the family.

As those in the field of addiction treatment began to better understand the role of family dynamics in addiction, and witnessed the ineffectiveness of pushing an addict—who was unprepared to receive help—into treatment, the "systemic intervention" was developed to replace the surprise model. Since enabling, codependent family members may unwittingly support the addiction, it became clear that an effective intervention must include those family members. But, almost by definition, an intervention, as practiced by interventionists, is a time-limited process: get the addict, and perhaps the codependents, into treatment, turn the case over to the treatment program, and then, in most cases, have little or no contact with the family.

It is important to understand that FRT does not view "intervention" as a stand-alone event, but as the *process* that engages the family in treatment. In the FRT model, the intervention begins when the FRT therapist receives the first phone call from a concerned family member, and continues through the early work with the family, and lays the groundwork to treat the family system through the first year of continuous sobriety.

Residential Treatment Center (RTC) Clinical Directors

As noted earlier, in the FRT Model, a Residential Treatment Center (RTC) may be a valuable resource during one stage in the overall treatment process. RTCs help stabilize an addict and ground them in early recovery. However, the crucial work follows the inpatient stay, when the addict returns home and he and his family continue on the recovery path throughout the critical first year of continuous sobriety. While RTCs may initially resist this concept, it is essential that they grasp this key element of Family Recovery Therapy, which is central to the paradigm shift in FRT's treatment approach: the work with the family and the addict *following* an addict's treatment in an RTC is critical to recovery; the RTC serves as but one phase in the overall treatment process.

To reiterate what the clinical director of the Betty Ford Treatment Program once said:

Those who follow our discharge recommendations have a success rate of staying sober through the critical first year that approaches 100%, and those who do not follow our discharge recommendations have a success rate that approaches zero.

We advise them, upon discharge, to transfer to a family-based intensive outpatient program, go to daily AA meetings—90 meetings in 90 days—and then keep going—and get a sponsor and work the steps. And that the family members, the codependents, do the same in Al-Anon. And, depending on the circumstances, for the addict to move into a Sober Living Environment.

As an FRT therapist who has referred many clients to RTCs, I have witnessed the nearly universal success of sustained recovery among those individuals and their families who have followed this advice—which is basically the same protocol as the FRT model. But it has required, in nearly every case, that I educate the staff at these residential programs about my model. As mentioned earlier, it is vital to communicate to a residential treatment program that they are a partner for only one phase of our extended treatment program. Given the prevalence of the current treatment paradigm, this can be challenging for staff at RTCs to grasp, because RTCs have always seen themselves as the "Top Dog," in that paradigm—the ultimate and most complete level of care. Staff members at RTCs often do not understand that we are offering a far more comprehensive treatment plan than simply residential placement for an addict. This is understandable, because the FRT model has yet to be widely disseminated or accepted.

When I consider making a referral to an RTC, I tell the RTC staff that they need to coordinate care with me regarding the family's involvement in their program, and they must discharge the client into our intensive aftercare program. Should an unusual circumstance arise, the RTC staff and I together determine if the client would be better served with a different treatment plan. (I've never had that happen with an adult client.) We need to expect them *not* to understand this, initially, since they routinely operate much like a factory, and simply refer their discharged clients to the same places they have in the past—which makes sense, since previously they did not have other options. In my experience, the RTC staff are generally aligned in following their usual procedures, and this model may at first be hard for them to get their heads around. But explaining the protocol of Family Recovery Therapy, and engaging them in following it, will produce good results. They are typically delighted once they understand the model and grasp that I will work with the RTC *and* the family, from day one, and that I will coordinate the addict's discharge and aftercare with them. My participation relieves them of the responsibility of planning the next step for the client, clarifies that their role is limited to the period during the addict's stay at the RTC, and reassures them that treatment will continue after the client leaves the RTC. This is—once they understand it—exactly what they *want* for their client: comprehensive, wraparound, family-based treatment for the addict and the addict's family for an extended period of time.

I am always skeptical when a potential client comes to me and says he has already chosen to attend a specific RTC. I wonder what led him to his choice. And I suspect this individual either does not understand my approach, or does not want to enroll in comprehensive treatment. There are good, well-established programs, and there are many programs that are sub-par, or dreadful. Again, John Oliver's *Rehab* (Oliver, 2018) is worth watching. Even a good program can go "bad" if, for instance, it was bought out by another program and the former director and staff left. I consult with my peers before recommending *any* program, even if I have had good experiences with it in the past. And, if I have not used a particular program, I will speak to the clinical director to confirm his acceptance of the FRT model and establish at the outset that I can readily coordinate with the addiction counselor who will be treating my client.

There has been a recent increase in the number of residential treatment programs that offer "extended care" at their local sober living homes. From my experience, this is contraindicated in almost every case, because nearly every addict eventually returns home, and must, adapt to living in his home environment. Again the phrase, "You have to stand up where you fell down," is apropos. When an addict returns home to the same family, the same drinking or drug-using peer culture, and the same community where they were enabled and became addicted, relapse is common unless a tightly structured, comprehensive, family-based, wraparound program is in place. I'm in favor of treating the family system *in the community where they live and where the addiction thrived*. A trip to a spa-like retreat is of little help for the addict who then returns to the prior challenges of an enabling family and drug-using friends.

The programs that understand my approach—involve the family in treatment and return the client to me for aftercare—have been a joy to work with. Collaboration with like-minded residential program staff has significantly furthered treatment and recovery for the families in my care. The excellent results of such collaborations provide real evidence for the efficacy of the FRT model at work.

A note to staff members working at Residential Treatment Centers who would like your center to update its treatment approach to employ the model laid out in this book. First, know this: the approach currently used—treat the addict short term but do not treat those who enable the addict's addiction—is entrenched, and with few changes, has been the dominant paradigm since AA was founded in the 1930s. Unfortunately, the current approach will fail half your center's clients. The directors who run the center where you work quite possibly went through treatment themselves at a similar program—and replicated what they knew, and created a new program based on their experience—or learned from other treatment programs using the same model. The model is well established in our nation. Change will have to come from the top down. Show your colleagues this book. Bring up this approach in staff meetings. Talk to the directors of the program. And, if that fails, start your own program based on the FRT model.

Sober Living Environments (SLEs)

Nearly one hundred percent of my young adult, and some of my adult, addicted clients, will return from residential treatment and move temporarily into a "step-down" facility, often called a sober home, a sober living environment (SLE), or a halfway house. These facilities are typically sobriety-focused and recovery-oriented residences where individuals eat and sleep, and from which, each day, they go to work and to 12-Step meetings. Generally, all the residents are in recovery and attend daily social support groups. Young adults who had been living at home with parents before treatment typically live in an SLE until they can get their feet on the ground and establish their own independent living arrangements. Not uncommonly, young adults spend six to twelve months at an SLE. Older adults may stay in an SLE for a shorter period—perhaps three months—before moving back in with their families or moving into independent living. Of course, some adults may benefit from either a shorter or longer stay at an SLE; the optimal length of stay will vary, case by case.

There are a wide range of SLE housing options. There are inexpensive, two-people-to-a-room accommodations in a modest home, located in an unassuming neighborhood, where six to twelve residents live, and where each individual typically is responsible for their own food. There are more expensive facilities, with one person to a room, in a well-appointed house that is located in an upscale neighborhood, and that perhaps provides chef-prepared meals.

Sometimes the line between an SLE and an RTC can get blurred when an SLE provides counseling. Some SLEs market themselves as having "supervisory staff" on location that "treat" the clients in residence—for an extra fee. This latter model, from my perspective, can complicate aftercare, and may leave the client wondering who is in charge of treatment, unless the SLE counselor and the FRT therapist clearly define and tightly coordinate their roles.

It is vital for the FRT therapist to coordinate with the manager of an SLE where a client will reside. The FRT therapist needs to make sure the SLE manager is on the same page regarding treatment. I have seen SLEs that are simply poorly run boarding houses inhabited by relapsing addicts with little recovery, and who perhaps are just out of jail. I have seen homes that accommodated six men on cots lined up in a row in a dirty basement. At one point, I had a client working as a "house manager" at the same time he was dealing drugs! These are unsuitable placements that I would never use, but these facilities are in business to house those who lack the money to pay for better places. I use a few highly reliable SLEs—I know the owners, and I know they have trusted staff members who keep a close eye on the sobriety of their clients. However, even some seemingly solid SLEs have had rough patches, with some residents engaging in drug use and relapsing.

Even in the best scenarios, some clients relapse, because addiction is a relapsing disease. This raises the question, "Why use SLEs?" The simple answer is that a good placement provides housing during the critical transition period for the addict after leaving residential care and before either moving back home or into an independent living situation. Moving too soon into the prior, unrecovered enabling home environment and peer culture is typically contraindicated for an optimal treatment outcome. Our overarching treatment goal is to help restore family members to healthy development. With a young adult addict who had been living with his parents before treatment, our goal is to launch the individual out of the nest, into an independent and sober adulthood. A good SLE is an invaluable stepping stone to true independence, and we encourage the addict's progress towards stable and sober independent living.

Here is what I have learned over the years about the SLEs that, as an FRT therapist, I recommend:

- Know the owner of the SLE. Meet with them. Ask about their approach. Visit their SLE. Are the clients drug tested? How often? What happens when someone relapses? (Typically, a client who relapses is discharged and required to go to a detox facility, and is not allowed to return to the house for at least 72 hours, then drug tested before returning, to confirm they are clean. The resident may be kicked out permanently after the second relapse.)
- Get a release from the client to talk to the house manager. See if the client's "story of the house condition" matches the owner's "story." A house can "go bad" when a resident brings drugs into a home undetected which can set off a cascade of relapses.
- Ask other SLE owners about the SLE's reputation. They know who are reputable SLE owners and who are not.
- Let the "sobriety" of the SLE be part of the counseling session dialogue. Transition to living in a sober home is a critical adjustment during a precarious point in treatment. It is not unusual for a client, after a few months, to move to another sober home that may be a better fit.

I usually tell an SLE owner something like this: "It sounds like X House is fairly stable, and I'm going to recommend it to my family. I will be getting a release from my client to speak to your house manager so I can check in and see how my client is doing, how the house is doing, and I will also ask the house manager to contact me if anything gets sideways."

The FRT therapist coordinates treatment with all of the involved providers. It is easy to see how any single provider, acting independently, can make the addict's recovery problematic. Having the team work together, as the FRT therapist guides the treatment process, optimizes the chances of the addict successfully getting through the critical first year of sobriety.

County or Government Agencies

Family Recovery Therapy is an evidence-based model that can be applied in city, county, or government agencies and nonprofits—as well as when the FRT therapist is self-employed and working in an individual or group private practice. However, agencies need to recognize the enormity of the shift in treatment approach that employing the FRT model entails. Government agencies are notoriously burdened with entrenched bureaucracies and fiefdoms resistant to change. They are hardly in a place to start from scratch and overhaul their operation in the way that will be required for them to implement the FRT model, this new paradigm. An individual practitioner within an agency must monitor and guide the treatment process for an addict and their family—the addicted family system—from the beginning of treatment until the addict has achieved one year of continuous sobriety and the family has established a stable foundation of recovery. It is this protocol that can prevent the fragmentation and poor results characteristic of the current fragmented treatment paradigm.

This is what I might say to an employee working in addiction treatment at a county, state, or other government agency who wants to introduce this approach into their treatment planning. "First, thank you for the work you do. You are doing some very hard, yet rewarding work—saving the lives of addicts. Second, this approach will take some effort to implement. You are up against the homeostasis of an organization embedded in a system that is wedded to the status quo—the old paradigm: treat the addict briefly, refer them on, give little attention to those who enable their addiction, and accept that this treatment will have limited success. Many of your clients will fail to establish long-term sobriety and, in the majority of the cases, will relapse. Possibly they will become homeless, be incarcerated, or worse."

And I would also say, "Changing bureaucracies is almost impossible unless there is a compelling reason. My hope is that this book will be the spark that sets off a cascade of changes leading to a paradigm shift in addiction treatment. Show this book to your colleagues, bring up the subject in meetings, talk to the Big Dogs, rattle some cages. Treatment programs, like addicts, want to get better. This book describes a better way. It can be done."

I believe that, if properly presented, agencies will understand the efficacy and rationale of this approach. And I hope that gradually, agencies and other governmental addiction treatment providers will integrate this model into their work, and eventually will use it to replace the current, outdated paradigm of addiction treatment.

Chapter 13

Social Support and Mutual Aid Groups

We are an affiliative species. Our earliest ancestors survived and thrived because they lived in tribes. As infants, we depend on our caretakers for sustenance and survival. If we are fortunate, we are loved, nurtured, and protected for many years. But many of those who later are prone to addiction didn't have this early loving connection with dependable caretakers. As the physician and addiction specialist, Gabor Maté, describes in his book, *In the Realm of Hungry Ghosts: Close Encounters with Addiction* (2010), the down and out, the homeless—the street people—disproportionately come from broken homes. For these individuals, the most reliable source of comfort and escape from pain is often their addictive substance or behavior. The addict becomes dependent on a substance or behavior to reduce pain. The addict typically affiliates with other addicts. They have often been fired from jobs, kicked out of families and marriages, and estranged from those with whom they were previously close. The addict is often bereft of potential closeness to another person, to family members or to peers.

Recovery for the addict entails giving up the very thing that has been their most consistent and trusted companion. Healthy, stable, reliable connection with other people, albeit often daunting, is foundational to recovery. This is why "social support groups," or "mutual aid groups," are a vital resource for addicts in their transition away from dependence on addictive behaviors or substances. Residential treatment programs virtually always include group therapy as well as attendance at social support groups in their treatment protocol. It is in these groups that addicts find the supportive and loving connection that has been absent from their lives.

Codependents are also "addicts." Codependents become addicted to the compulsive and controlling behaviors they hope will save their loved one from the harmful consequences of substance abuse and addiction. And codependents—ever hopeful they can change their loved one—repeat these behaviors over and over again, despite experiencing pain and suffering as a result (Cermak, 1986). Let's take another look at the current definition of addiction adopted by the American Society of Addiction Medicine (ASAM) in September 2019:

> Addiction is a treatable, chronic medical disease involving complex interactions among brain circuits, genetics, the environment, and an individual's life experiences. People with

addiction use substances or engage in behaviors that become compulsive and often continue despite harmful consequences.

Prevention efforts and treatment approaches for addiction are generally as successful as those for other chronic diseases.

Codependents, like addicts, often come from families lacking differentiation and close, loving, and dependable connection. They have often grown up without the benefit of secure attachment to reliable caretakers. Recovery for codependents entails learning to refocus their attention on themselves and to rewire their neuronal networks. Codependents benefit from connection with others who understand their plight and can be supportive, which social support groups can provide.

In these groups, those new to recovery can connect with others who have had experiences similar to theirs. The people comprising social support groups are peers—individuals who themselves have suffered from the disorders of addiction or codependency, and who therefore can understand and be empathic with the addict or codependent who is new to recovery.

Addicts who enter a residential treatment program are often introduced to the concept of social support groups early in their recovery process. Detox facilities and residential programs may host a couple of different kinds of social support group meetings for their clients, in order to expose them to various options that are available.

Addicts will find in these groups others who suffer from the same medical and mental disease they are afflicted with. Remember, addiction is a disease of the brain. It is chronic—it never goes away—and addicts, like those suffering from other chronic diseases such as diabetes, are prone to relapse and will benefit from ongoing support for the rest of their lives. The stories, the literature, the lore, and the friendship that addicts experience in these social support groups remind them that they have an unremitting, pernicious disorder. They embrace the concept of "recovery" (not "recovered") which normalizes the process of healing from addiction, and acknowledges the chronicity of the disease. These groups supply the "medicine"— the healing environment—that is fundamental to treatment (Erikson, M., 2020; Chappel & Dupont, 1999). Diabetics rely on insulin, heart patients on statins, and addicts on their support groups.

There are a number of social support, or mutual aid, groups for recovering addicts. Among the most common of these are 12-Step (Alcoholics Anonymous), SMART Recovery®, LifeRing Secular Support, and Secular Organizations for Sobriety, although there are others as well (see Appendix K). 12-Step programs are by far the most available and best known of these groups, but an addict can find help through any group of peers who meet regularly, share their experience, and support each other in maintaining sobriety.

Availability of a group is an important consideration for the addict. Initially, and throughout the first year of sobriety, it is recommended that the recovering addict who used substances on a daily basis take their medicine every day, which means go to a meeting every day. Craving and recent memory of past drug-related experiences make the newly recovering addict vulnerable to "forgetting" that they have a diseased brain—a brain that tells them many times each day that their former "medicine," be it drugs or alcohol or other self-harming substances or behaviors (including codependency), can instantly ease their discomfort and distract them from their problems. If someone has diabetes, he regularly checks his blood sugar level and takes measures to stabilize it. If someone has heart disease, he takes his heart medicine daily. Social support and mutual aid groups are the "medicine" for the addict's diseased brain. In Marin County, California, where I live, which has a population of 250,000 people, there are over 300 12-Step meetings a week for alcoholics and addicts. The foreword to the fourth and most recent edition of *Alcoholics Anonymous* (2001) reported that there were over 108,000 AA groups in 150 countries, and that the worldwide membership of AA was estimated at 2 million or more. LifeRing Secular Recovery, Secular Organization for Sobriety, and SMART Recovery®, in total, have fewer than 10 groups per week in the county, other than those that are under the auspices of a treatment program or part of a doctor's private practice.

Though non–12-Step programs provide infrequent, and often not readily available, support to addicts, for some people, these groups are invaluable. Non–12-Step groups offer tools to help individuals make and sustain behavioral change. They also provide a community of peers, of recovering addicts, that can relate to each other's stories and support each other's recovery. However, it is challenging to get to daily meetings, "a meeting a day, 90 meetings in 90 days," when there are only a few meetings each week.

Unfortunately, "non–12-Step treatment programs" for addicts are often marketed not by addiction specialists or addiction doctors, but by unscrupulous businesses endeavoring to attract those looking for a "softer, easier way." Perhaps these programs appeal to those who do not grasp the nature of addiction, or who fear that, with the 12-Step approach, they may be getting involved in a "cult" or a "religion" (12-Step programs are neither a cult nor a religion). Ads for these programs might say, "Non–12-Step," "Not for life," "No need to admit powerlessness," "Not a religion," "Not abstinence only." Unfortunately, many such programs are sub-par, money-driven businesses that fail to effectively treat the addict. The majority of addiction treatment programs clearly favor the 12-Step model for social support groups, because these groups have demonstrated their efficacy and value for over 80 years, and their prevalence makes them accessible to a large number of people.

Some of the advertising slogans used by non–12-Step programs are clearly anti–12-Step, such as, "Not for life." This advertisement suggests that 12-Step programs *require* that a person continue going to meetings "for life," meaning "forever." There is no such requirement. It is up to the individual to decide if they want to continue attending meetings. In AA, it is clear that recovery is "one day at a time." This message is ubiquitous and is alluded to regularly in AA parlance: "Can you stay sober today?" "Can you make it to bed tonight without relapsing?" "How can I help you stay sober just for today?" Although many 12-Step participants find ongoing attendance at meetings helpful to staying sober ("for life"), the program focuses only on *this* day, one day at a time.

The claim, "Not a religion," is simply misleading. The book *Alcoholics Anonymous* (2001) makes quite clear that AA is *not* a religion, and that each member gets to choose their own guidance, their own "Higher Power"—some source of wisdom beyond their own ego. AA, not unlike transpersonal psychology, invites the individual to acknowledge that he is more than his ego, certainly more than the ego that first arrived at the door of an AA meeting and desperately needed some "higher" or "other" source of guidance which could override his disordered thinking. AA is *spiritual* when it recommends that the addict believe in some kind of wisdom or resource other than his own willpower. The Steps do mention "God." Step Three states, "Made a decision to turn our will and our lives over to God as we understood Him." AA's deity-based language stems from its beginnings. Bill Wilson, co-founder of AA, and primary author of the book, *Alcoholics Anonymous* (1939), achieved his early sobriety as a member of the Christian-based Oxford Group, an organization which helped some alcoholics become sober in the 1930s. Wikipedia, in its entry, "Alcoholics Anonymous," describes the origins of AA as follows:

> AA sprang from The Oxford Group, a non-denominational altruistic movement modeled after first-century Christianity. Some members founded the Group to help in maintaining sobriety. "Grouper" Ebby Thacher was Wilson's former drinking buddy who approached Wilson saying that he had "got religion," was sober, and that Wilson could do the same if he set aside objections to religion and instead formed a personal idea of God, "another power" or "higher power" [Alcoholics Anonymous, n.d.].

It is important for the clinician to educate the addict or the codependent about the *clinical* wisdom of working the 12 Steps, and to differentiate AA's wisdom and foundational principles from its historical origins. Clinically speaking, ideas that reflect aspects of several approaches to psychotherapy—cognitive, behavioral, existential, humanistic, psychodynamic, relational, and transpersonal—can be found in the 12 Steps.

"No need to admit powerlessness" is another line used by some non–12-Step programs in their marketing. As we have seen, an addict's midbrain hijacks the executive function of his prefrontal cortex. This is the medical basis of the brain disease of addiction. The addict's admission of powerlessness is, in fact, necessary for them to accept the reality of their medical condition. The addict—no matter what program or group or resource they turn to—reaches out precisely because they know they cannot stop their addiction by themselves, and they need help to achieve remission. "Powerless" does not mean "helpless" or "irresponsible." It means acknowledging that their prefrontal cortex has lost control over volition in regard to drug use and that they need the help of others to stop using.

It is worth noting that 12-Step programs do *not* advertise. In fact, it is specifically stated that the program relies on "attraction, rather than promotion"—people come, one day at a time, because it works. No 12-Step program profits from having members in attendance; they exist solely to support the recovery of their members.

The first three Steps of the 12-Step programs emphasize the concepts of "powerlessness" and the need for "a power greater than ourselves," a power wiser than the thinking that prolonged an addict's addiction. Any addict who has accepted that they have a medical disease, and chosen to pursue recovery, can attest to their lack of control over their disease and their need for outside guidance.

I expand on the 12 Steps later, but briefly, the first three Steps in AA are:

> STEP ONE: We admitted we were powerless over alcohol—that our lives had become unmanageable.

Admitting loss of control and powerlessness are central to an addict's understanding of their condition (Twerski, 1997). For the addict, coming out of denial, and realizing that they have a potentially fatal medical disease that requires treatment, is fundamental to their recovery and sets the stage for the next Step.

> STEP TWO: Came to believe that a Power greater than ourselves could restore us to sanity.

For the newly recovering addict, a room full of sober addicts, many with long-term sobriety who are solidly on their feet, have happy lives, and have resumed normal development, is surely an example of "a power greater" than themselves—a power, an inspiration, that perhaps can help them stay sober, one day at a time. Addicts new to recovery are encouraged to rely on this group—this source of wisdom beyond themselves that can restore them to sanity.

> STEP THREE: Made a decision to turn our will and our lives over to the care of God as we understood Him.

We all turn our will and our lives over to the care of "powers greater than ourselves" on a daily basis. As mentioned earlier, if we get a flat tire, we turn our will and our lives over to the care of our car mechanic. If we need medical help, we turn our will and our lives over to our doctor's care. If we have a toothache, we turn our will and our lives over to the care of our dentist. The addict is wise to turn his or her will and life over to the care of a power greater than themselves—often simply a bunch of recovering people who have figured out how to stay sober and to put this medical disease into remission.

Newcomers who express some resistance to "The God Thing" are often asked if they can turn their alcoholism over to G.O.D., a Group Of Drunks. This often makes complete sense to them.

The ubiquity of 12-Step groups in part explains why, in my estimation—based on visiting numerous treatment centers—over 95 percent of treatment programs refer their clients to 12-Step programs for social support and mutual aid. In addition, 12-Step groups have significant longevity. It is not unusual to find 12-Step groups that have been meeting at the same time and in the same place for 50 years or more, and to find members with many decades of recovery who are still active in these meetings, still sponsoring newcomers, and still supporting the recovery of their peers. An AA tradition states that the primary purpose of AA is to "help the alcoholic who still suffers." AA members offer the newcomer support, and when the newcomer is on solid ground, he in turn reaches out to the next newcomer and offers support, just as others reached out to him. The practice of providing support for newly sober addicts, as well as for long-term recovering peers, is at the core of AA and its philosophy—and supplies the addict with something that is often lacking in their lives—a loving and supportive sober community.

Worldwide, and in nearly all countries, Alcoholics Anonymous has developed thousands of meetings that serve over two million addicts, including meetings that support various subgroups of the population. For example, there are AA groups that have been formed to support women, men, gay men, lesbians, transgender people, lawyers, nurses, Spanish-speaking individuals, and those who speak other languages. There are also meetings that take place over the telephone or online, for those who may need to attend remotely. During the COVID-19 pandemic which began in 2020, many meetings transitioned seamlessly from an in-person to an online, live video format.

Social support and mutual aid groups for codependent family members provide an important foundation for recovery from codependency, just as the social support groups for addicts are an invaluable resource for recovery from substance-based addiction. Family members are often lost and confused when their addict enters recovery. Their lives have been focused on the addict—the addict's behavior, the consequences of that behavior, and their response to the addict's behavior. For the family members and the addict to heal, differentiate their thinking from their feelings, and develop very different relationships with each other, they need to make fundamental and dramatic changes in their own lives. As Virginia Lewis, Ph.D., and Stephanie Brown, Ph.D., say: "This finding—the need for family systems collapse—is central to our theory of recovery. It is the collapse of the family structures and defense mechanisms that protected and maintained the drinking that clears the ground for the transformative process of recovery" (1999, p. 19). The most available recovery resource for codependents is Al-Anon, the 12-Step program which has been helping family members of alcoholics and addicts since it was founded in 1951. While some residential treatment programs for addiction offer a family weekend, or a series of family weekends, codependent family members will need ongoing support and guidance to change long-standing behavior patterns, which will help the family system to "collapse" in order for family members to resume normal development and build functional relationships.

Codependents in recovery need to learn to focus on themselves and allow the addict to take responsibility for his own addiction and his sobriety. By the time they seek help, codependents are often emotionally distraught, worn out, and physically depleted. They have lived from crisis to crisis for a long time, and have attempted to accomplish an heroic but impossible task: to get their loved one to change, to stop his or her addiction. Codependent family members may have struggled for years and sacrificed their own wellbeing and personal goals trying to save their addicted loved one. Addiction and codependency have resulted in dysfunctional family patterns. Each codependent family member needs to focus on his or her own development and recovery—only in that way can the family system heal.

FRT Principle 2 states that "Codependents may need lifelong recovery support." Addicts have a chronic brain disorder and almost certainly need ongoing support to counteract their midbrain's "memory" of the rewards of drinking or using. Codependents similarly benefit from ongoing support because they need to significantly alter their focus, thinking, and behaviors. Their lives have become entrenched in dysfunction over time—perhaps years—of interacting with an addicted loved one. For codependents, shifting their focus can be like turning an ocean liner. Their challenge, as stated so aptly in the "we version" of the *Serenity Prayer*, is to "change the things we can," which is only themselves, and to "accept the things we cannot change," which includes the addict. It can take a long time to resume or grow a healthy life when everything has been turned upside down by addiction in the family.

When do we stop developing? We don't. (See Appendix A.) And this is one of the hallmarks of 12-Step programs: members often speak of the never-ending process of recovering, learning, developing, and growing. The recovery process encourages both the addict and the codependent to adopt lifestyles that support the family system's ongoing development. As clinicians, we need to recognize the momentum of the recovery process and support it. We need to respect and encourage a lifestyle based on the premise that individual development—psychological, social, emotional, and spiritual—is ongoing. For every individual in the family, differentiation is the goal: the ability *both* to develop a healthy self *and* to develop close intimate emotional connections with others. There is no end to the process of self-individuation, and there is no limit to the extent of emotional availability and connection we can develop with another person. Social support groups, and 12-Step groups perhaps most effectively, are a pillar of this process. They are a powerful resource for the codependent and the addict; whenever they are needed they are available, whether that is early in recovery or many years later.

The remainder of this chapter will explain how the 14 Principles of Family Recovery Therapy, with the guidance of the FRT therapist, work together with 12-Step recovery principles, both for addicts and for codependents. Let's first review the FRT Principles that specifically refer to recovery support or to social support and mutual aid groups:

FRT Principle 1

Addiction is a chronic, relapsing, treatable medical disease with profound mental and physical consequences. Addicts will need long-term, possibly lifelong recovery support, which can take many forms.

FRT Principle 2
Effective treatment of addiction usually involves treatment of codependents, because codependents enable addiction. Codependency is a chronic relationship pattern that has profound mental and physical consequences and is characterized by an obsessive focus on other people. Codependents may need lifelong recovery support which can take many forms.

FRT Principle 6
The FRT therapist must be well-versed in the 12 Steps and have a thorough understanding and appreciation for the fundamental role that mutual aid programs play in recovery from codependency and addiction.

FRT Principle 7
The FRT therapist, who is a state-licensed medical or mental health professional, must be knowledgeable and experienced in many paths to growth and recovery. Ideally, the therapist is engaged in a personal recovery practice, whether 12-Step or other, in which capacity, the therapist stands shoulder-to-shoulder with the family members.

FRT Principle 8
Since addiction and the codependency that enables it are chronic conditions, it is recommended that the addict and codependents develop ongoing support beyond the first year of continuous sobriety.

Healthy individuals, couples, and families depend on a number of communities for support, including their extended families, friends, neighbors, religious groups, co-workers, government entities, social organizations, and recreational groups or clubs. Addicts and their families, even if they are members of various community groups and organizations, benefit from social support and mutual aid groups specifically focused on recovery from addiction and codependency.

Below, I discuss non–12-Step support groups briefly, and then focus on the social support provided by the 12-Step programs of Alcoholics Anonymous and Al-Anon. I call the non–12-Step groups "secular groups," to differentiate them from the spiritually-based 12-Step groups. To reiterate, neither the non–12-Step groups I mention, nor 12-Step groups, are religious, although various religious organizations do have support groups for addicts. I elaborate on 12-Step groups because they are widely available and therefore have helped many more recovering people than have secular groups. As noted in the FRT Principles above, addicts and codependents may need lifelong recovery support, which 12-Step social support groups can provide. Since FRT Principle 6 states that an FRT therapist must be familiar with the 12 Steps, I discuss the 12 Steps here in detail.

Secular Recovery

Secular recovery groups provide peer support for the recovering addict based on the premise that the recovering person needs self-empowerment to heal. Rather than turning to an external source of strength, as is the case in 12-Step philosophy, in secular approaches, the addict focuses on his own courage and capacity to shape his life. Secular mutual aid groups support recovering individuals to build motivation, control craving, resolve underlying problems, improve relationships, and build meaningful lives.

The most widely available secular group is SMART Recovery®, an acronym that stands for Self-Management And Recovery Training. Its meetings are available in a number of countries, and the organization offers online resources. There are over 1,500 meetings worldwide. SMART Recovery® does not use the terms "addict" or "alcoholic," does not endorse the belief that addiction is a disease, and suggests that the individual participate in the program for only as long as it seems useful.

SMART Recovery® offers the individual evidence-based, cognitive therapy tools. One example is the "ABC Problem Solving Worksheet," which addresses Activating events, Beliefs, and Consequences. On the worksheet, the participant writes about the Activating event, its Consequences, his (dysfunctional) Beliefs about the event, and how he can dispute the Beliefs. He specifies both the effective, new Beliefs he can use, and what anticipated, improved, emotional Consequences those new Beliefs will produce. The participant is also encouraged to do an inquiry about his addiction, how it serves him and what he will and won't like about giving it up. SMART Recovery® provides skill building and rational coping tools to help the participant manage anxiety, increase frustration tolerance, prevent relapse, and build confidence. The coping strategies taught by SMART Recovery® are solid, practical, and useful. For those who do not need more available or ongoing support, or a perspective that incorporates the concept of powerlessness to control addiction, SMART Recovery® provides a solid foundation for the recovering person to lead a healthy life, unencumbered by substance abuse (Horvath, 2000).

Other secular programs, listed earlier, including LifeRing and Secular Organizations for Sobriety, similarly offer a harm reduction, cognitive behavioral-based approach to recovery. There are over 200 weekly LifeRing social support meetings in the United States and Europe.

For those who need more available support, or for whom cognitive behavioral tools are insufficient to maintain sobriety, AA may be a better fit.

12-Step Programs

As mentioned earlier, Alcoholics Anonymous is the recovery program for addicts, and Al-Anon is the recovery program for family members. Both AA and Al-Anon use the 12 Steps as their foundation. The Steps for the two programs are identical, except for one word in Step Twelve: AA encourages its members to carry the message of recovery to "alcoholics," while Al-Anon's Step Twelve encourages its members to carry its message to "others." The Steps spell out the philosophy and the principles of the programs.

Let's review the 12 Steps of AA, one at a time. It is vital for the FRT therapist to fully understand the Steps, as well as to have some knowledge of the Traditions, which are described in AA literature, and to become familiar with the language and customs common to 12-Step programs. Comprehending the essence and value of 12-Step programs will enable the FRT therapist "to stand shoulder-to-shoulder" with their clients. In reality, much of the "clinical" work of recovery transpires outside of our consulting rooms: in the meetings, with sponsors, and with members of the program, all of which provide a 24/7/365 container for recovery, not only during the course of treatment, but after clinical treatment has ended.

The 12 Steps were initially described in the book, *Alcoholics Anonymous* (1939)—also known as the Big Book of AA—which was written in the 1930s by several early members of AA. Although several editions of the book have been printed since then, the language of the book's first 164 pages dates from the era of its first publication. As noted earlier, the religious tone of the book reflects the influence of the Oxford Group on the beginnings of AA as well as the personal histories of Bill Wilson, Dr. Bob, and some other founding members of AA who authored the book. The program and the writings have a spiritual orientation, but do not have any religious affiliation or content. I have noted this earlier, but it bears repeating, because there is a common misunderstanding that the 12 Steps are "religious"; they are not, but they do embrace the *spiritual concept* of a wisdom beyond the thinking ego (see Appendix L). The wording of the 12 Steps sounds a little archaic today because it has not been modified since the 12 Steps were originally composed in the 1930s.

> STEP ONE: We admitted we were powerless over alcohol—that our lives had become unmanageable.

Physiologically, the addict is powerless over their addiction. Another way to say this might be, "We admitted that our midbrain had hijacked our prefrontal cortex, that we were unable to resist craving, that we continued practicing our addiction, and that our lives became unmanageable."

This Step sets the stage for the transpersonal and interpersonal psychology of the later Steps. The addict admits that, in order for him to get stable, his ego needs some sort of "power greater than itself—something outside of himself." The addict has two options, "I'm fine" or "I'm in trouble." We can't do much for the first guy, but the second guy hopefully is now ready to accept the help and guidance which will enable him to achieve remission from his disease, one day at a time. This experience of ego deflation is critical for an addict. As Zen masters say, knowing nothing, having an empty mind, allows us to learn everything.

Some say an addict has to "hit bottom" before his ego is destabilized enough to acknowledge powerlessness over his life and to become willing to follow the guidance of others. While this is certainly true for many addicts, including the author, it is not always the case. As an FRT therapist, I have discovered that it is possible to create a family-based systemic intervention that encourages the addict to slowly accept the reality of his powerlessness. A well-crafted family treatment plan can lead the addict to acknowledge that they have met the criteria for addiction—*loss of control, adverse consequences, craving, and chronicity*—and to accept help to guide them on a path toward remission. One of the 13 "principles of effective treatment" of the National Institute on Drug Abuse (2018) is that treatment does not need to be voluntary. For example, if a judge tells an addict to choose whether to go to AA or to jail, the addict may choose AA. As he attends AA meetings, he may come to understand the nature of his problem. If a spouse tells an addict to get help for his addiction or she will file for divorce, the addict who is motivated to save his marriage may find they actually benefit from getting help. The specter of jail or divorce can create a "bottom" for an addict. Once he has achieved sobriety and his head has cleared, the addict may understand the value of recovery and embrace and comply with treatment. Also, of course, the parents of a non-compliant substance-abusing teen can set limits and require the young person to get treatment. Teens in drug treatment can benefit significantly from learning about substance abuse and addiction. Understanding about potential consequences of drug use may help prevent them from becoming ensnared by the allure of substance use, if they choose to use drugs later in their lives.

Many clinicians do not understand how Family Recovery Therapy works—how a clinically-guided shift in the family's homeostasis over a period of time, which involves individuation of family members, can result in the addict's recognition of his condition. When an FRT therapist guides the codependent family members to stop trying to control the addict, the family dynamics change. Here is an example of how it can work, reported to have been heard in an AA meeting:

> I was doing fine, oh, maybe I drank a little too much now and then, but I didn't see I had a problem—it was my wife's problem. Then my wife started going to those damn Al-Anon meetings. She was going out every night, on the phone all the time, laughing—it was weird. She got off my case, and the next thing I knew, I was going to AA. Somehow, thank God, it rubbed off on me and I started to check it out. That was ten years ago—I owe my recovery to her going to those Al-Anon meetings.

I also use Family Recovery Therapy to change family dynamics with substance-using teens and young adults. The young adult may demonstrate the symptoms of addiction, but his denial prevents him from acknowledging he has a problem. I work with the parents who have been enabling the young adult's substance use, and I suggest they think about establishing consequences for his behavior. I slowly guide them to stop enabling their young adult child. The young adult, in the course of family therapy, gradually grasps that he will not be able to continue living at home if he persists with his drug-related behavior, and chooses to enter treatment. For example, the parents of a young adult addict might get to a point in treatment where they say, "We love you and are concerned about you. We've witnessed your behavior, and we think you need to go to residential addiction treatment. Of course, you are an adult, and you are in control of your life. But if you choose to refuse help, we will ask you to leave the house, and give us your cell phone and car keys." From my experience, the young adult addict, who is accustomed to living comfortably at his parents' home, would rather go to a warm safe place with a bed and food instead of suddenly needing to fend for himself. For instance, Peter, in the young adult case study (Chapter 7), was motivated to attend the wilderness program to avert the prospect of homelessness. In treatment, the young person detoxes and learns about substance abuse and addiction. He describes his crazy, out-of-control behaviors, in front of both treatment center staff and his recovering peers, and comes to understand his susceptibility to drugs, and the possibility he might have the disease of addiction. What he learns in this process about loss of control and craving can help him recognize these symptoms of addiction—the unmanageability of his life—if he relapses in the future. Relapse with this population is common because young people are in a process of individuation: they want to make their own decisions, and they question whether they have a disease.

A stint in detox is usually the wake-up call needed to refocus the young addict. Once detoxed, they review their thinking and behavior, learn more about addiction, and renew their involvement in social support groups, all of which help them grasp the nature of their addiction at a deeper level. They can, perhaps for the first time, comprehend Step One—that they are powerless to control their drug use without asking for help.

Codependents entering Al-Anon may also have a difficult time initially accepting their powerlessness, not so much "over alcohol" as "over the alcoholic." For a long time, their lives have been centered on their addicted loved one, and shifting that focus, as mentioned earlier, can seem like turning an ocean liner. Codependents new to Al-Anon usually have spent a long time attempting to control the alcoholic, her behavior, and the consequences of her actions. Giving up that endeavor may provoke significant anxiety—codependents fear that something terrible will happen to their loved one. And something terrible may happen. But terrible things have already happened, things they have not been able to prevent. Codependents face tremendous loss as they reorient their lives away from their addicted loved one and instead look at their own lives. They become aware of all they have given up in trying to save their addicted loved one.

Like many substance-using addicts, by the time codependents get to Al-Anon, they generally recognize that their lives have become unmanageable. They are aware of their distress and despair, and they can see that their lives have become chaotic, and their personal interests and development have been sidelined. But for codependents, as for addicts, acknowledging that there is a problem is the first step toward recovery.

> STEP TWO: Came to believe that a Power greater than ourselves could restore us to sanity.

Another way to say this might be, "We came to believe that someone or something *other* than our mind or our ego could help prevent our midbrain from hijacking our prefrontal cortex and persuading us to take our drug." For codependents, the wording might be, "We came to believe that someone or something other than ourselves can relieve us of the insanity of our fruitless efforts to control or change the alcoholic. We realized these attempts were not sane."

The wisdom of this Step naturally flows from Step One. If we are powerless over something, if by ourselves we have become stuck and can't fix the problem, we understand that we need help, and that help is available. *We all do this all the time.* If we have an infection, we go to a doctor; if our lights go out, we call an electrician.

The beginning phrase, "Came to believe," indicates that there is a *process* involved in adopting the idea of "a power greater than ourselves." In attending one 12-Step meeting, then another, and then more meetings, over time the addict (or the codependent) learns slowly and incrementally about the program. Grasping the concept of "a power greater than ourselves" initially may be confusing (and may even seem "religious"), but gradually, it begins to make sense (and we see there is no religion involved at all). "Coming to believe" is a journey towards recognizing that the very help we need exists. It's hard to "come to believe," both for the codependent who has felt responsible for solving every problem, and for the addict who is sure they know what "medicine" they need. "Believing" develops over time.

Sometimes an addict has a problem with the idea of "a Power greater than ourselves." If he has had any negative experiences with religion, he may resist the notion that some God-like entity can help. The FRT therapist needs to differentiate "religion" from "spirituality." He needs to explain that religion involves following a specific ideology, and that religions often dictate certain truths about reality and the purpose of life. Spirituality, however, allows the individual to develop a personal sense of what has meaning. Spirituality embraces universal concepts and realms beyond the ego. Religion frequently is imbued with fear and the potential for negative consequences, whereas spirituality is trans-egoic and invites us to expand our awareness. The FRT therapist assures the addict that "a Power" does not mean God or anything god-like, but simply *something* beyond his own distorted thinking—perhaps the collective wisdom of the members of the meeting he attends. As noted earlier, sometimes in AA parlance the suggestion is made to use "G.O.D., Group Of Drunks," as a power greater than oneself. Or the addict can choose something like the calm of nature or a specific place where he feels peaceful. For the addict who acknowledges his loss of control, it is essential that he understand that the solution requires more than his own defective thinking. Perhaps a "Group of Drunks" is just the medicine he needs to stay sober for just today. There is an oft-used 12-Step slogan (from a quote attributed to Albert Einstein) that speaks to this issue: "You can't solve a problem with the same thinking that created it." Usually, the addict can admit that his best thinking has not kept him sober or helped him refrain from drug use.

Frequently, those new to Al-Anon similarly resist the concept of "a Power greater than ourselves." If they have had negative associations with religion, or are atheists, they complain, "religion does not work" for them. As in speaking with the addict, the FRT therapist needs to clarify to the codependent that 12-Step programs are not religious, but they do have a spiritual component; the programs use the concept of "something greater"—or other—than the individual, but each person can conceptualize his own, personal, concept of what works for him. For the codependent, that power can be thought of as "G.O.D., or Good Orderly Direction," which is certainly more rational than their own obsessive thinking. Alternatively, the codependent may choose to use nature, or the universe, or the fellowship of Al-Anon. Some say that they feel a sense of a Higher Power flowing through the meetings. The FRT therapist reminds the codependent that they have already acknowledged that their own attempts to solve the problem have not worked. While their beliefs about a Higher Power may change over time, the concept of "a Power greater than ourselves" is integral to comprehending and implementing the remaining Steps.

> STEP THREE: Made a decision to turn our will and our lives over to the care of God as we understood Him.

As noted earlier, the references to "God" in the book *Alcoholics Anonymous* have their roots in the teachings of the Oxford Group, a Christian organization that worked with alcoholics in the 1930s. Followers of the Oxford Group, some of whom participated in early AA meetings, believed that religion was essential to attaining sobriety. However, many early proponents of AA disagreed. While the first printing of *Alcoholics Anonymous* in 1939 contained frequent references to God, in the Second Edition, published in 1955, the authors added an appendix called "Spiritual Experience" to clarify that AA is *spiritual* and not *religious*. In this appendix, the authors note that the first printing of *Alcoholics Anonymous* had given the erroneous impression that religion or "God-consciousness" was necessary to attain recovery. The authors further explain that the changes that occur in recovery are mostly of the "educational variety" and develop slowly over a period of time—that most AA members gradually come to identify their own concept of a "Power greater than themselves," which they think of as "the essence of spiritual experience." They add that the spirituality of the program need not be a source of difficulty, because "willingness, honesty and open mindedness are the essentials of recovery. But these are indispensable" (p.570) (see Appendix L).

Of course, since this Step explicitly says the word, "God," those who have trouble with the concept of "a Power" in Step Two are likely to be bothered by the word "God" (and perhaps by the use of the pronoun "Him") in Step Three. The FRT therapist needs to emphasize that the wording of the Step is, "God, *as we understood Him.*" This Step does not refer to the God, or gods, of any religion, or to God as defined by anyone else—whether male, female, non-binary, non-anthropomorphic, etc. Instead, "God" in this context is whatever concept or entity the individual chooses to use, to remind them that they cannot *think* their way out of addiction, that they need to rely on something other than their own mind for help—which could be the program, or the fellowship, or a sponsor, or the wisdom of those who have traveled the recovery path before, or the FRT therapist. As one wise person reflected, God can be anything, so long as it is "not me."

Step Three could be rephrased as, "We made a decision to follow the guidance of those who have discovered how addiction recovery works, and who know how to stay sober, just for today."

This Step is challenging. Most addicts have been fighting an epic battle, trying to control their out-of-control brains. The thought of turning over their ineffective efforts at achieving sobriety to a fellowship, or to a concept or an entity they don't even understand, may seem baffling at first.

Spirituality, the belief in something beyond the ego, is fundamental for many people grappling with the human condition. Many of us believe in something—God, Nature, Heavenly Order, Divine Presence, Spirit, Mother Nature, Divine Wisdom, etc. The addict, sadly but not unusually, often has had little experience with love, spirit, or connection. This Step invites the addict to consider the possibility that there can be more to life than what he's known.

The idea of accepting God as part of recovery is sprinkled throughout all editions of the book, *Alcoholics Anonymous,* and many people, including this author, have wanted to rewrite the book in a more secular manner. Even the alcoholics who composed the Big Book understood that the concept of "God" might be difficult for some alcoholics to embrace, which is why they added the critical words at the end of this Step, *"as we understood Him."* These last four words, despite the use of the popular pronoun of the time, leave room for each person to form their own personal view of a concept or power greater than their own ego or thinking mind.

As noted earlier, it is common for those with some recovery in AA to encourage the God-resistant newcomer to substitute his own version of a higher power for God. Those with longer recovery ask the newcomer, "Can you turn your will and your life over to G.O.D., a Group Of Drunks?" Those who have had some time in AA understand that it takes time to build trust in the program and its concepts, and they encourage the newcomer to move forward as slowly as necessary, but to stay with the process—and not drink, one day at a time.

It is also important to point out to the individual embarking on the Third Step that there is a difference between *making a decision* and *following through.* Consider this anecdote, which is said to be repeated often in 12-Step meetings: "Two frogs are sitting on a lily pad. One decides to jump off. How many frogs are left?"

Most people answer this question with "one frog is left." But, no, there are still two frogs sitting on the lily pad: one frog only *decided* to jump, but did not *actually* jump. We invite the addict simply to be willing to consider the possibility that there may be something beyond their, typically impoverished, ego that could help them, and to be open to hearing advice from "a power more informed than their ego/their own thinking mind." This "power," as suggested above, could be the group, a drug counselor, a fellow member of the support group, a sponsor, a mentor, the FRT therapist, or a trusted individual who supports their recovery path. For the recovering addict or codependent, "making a decision" precedes the act of actually *choosing to rely* on that power.

Even choosing to turn one's situation over to a higher power is not a one-time event. Instead of a once-I've-decided-I've-decided-forever scenario, for the addict, making the decision to trust something or someone other than his own thinking mind is something he will need to do over and over again as new situations emerge. And naturally, it is easier to embrace the concept of a higher power guiding the way when things are going well or if there's nothing major at stake. In 12-Step meetings, it is not unusual to hear, even from seasoned program members with a firmly established belief in a higher power, "There was a crisis, and I took back my control—I thought I knew best," or "I just couldn't trust at that moment." Developing willingness to trust external guidance takes repetition, perseverance, and time.

Step Three in Al-Anon is identical to Step Three in AA: "Made a decision to turn our will and our lives over to the care of God, *as we understood Him*." Newcomers to Al-Anon, just like newcomers in AA, can be taken aback at the idea of turning their *lives* "over to the care of God as we understood him." For codependents, experiences with religion at earlier times in their life may color their concept of "God." They may consider themselves atheists or agnostics and want nothing to do with anything that sounds even slightly religious. Seasoned Al-Anon members can help newcomers grasp the idea that they get to create their own higher power or "God of their understanding," a higher power that is quite different from any sense of God they may have had previously. Their "God" or "Higher Power" can be any entity, or concept, or belief that works for them. They may choose the wisdom of the Al-Anon group itself, recognizing how much they benefit from hearing Al-Anon members share at meetings. Many Al-Anon members say they feel better leaving a meeting than when they arrived. Others may choose nature, or the beauty of a flower or a tree, or "G.O.D.—Good Orderly Direction"—as a higher power. It's important they choose something that reminds them that addiction and codependency are problems *they cannot solve alone*. The solution requires embracing a perspective broader than that of a lone individual fending off the chaos of an out-of-control situation.

However, the very idea of relying on anyone or anything other than themselves is daunting for the codependent. Codependents new to Al-Anon recognize they are in trouble, and that what they've been doing hasn't worked, but they are loath to trust anything beyond themselves. Most codependents have learned to be singularly independent and self-reliant, and *not* to trust in anyone or anything except themselves (Beattie, 1986; Cermak, 1986). Experienced Al-Anon members can remind newcomers that learning to trust is a *process*. In the context of FRT, Step Three can be phrased as "made a decision to turn our will and our lives over to the unfolding process of FRT therapy" or "to the guidance of the FRT therapist."

Accepting the first three Steps is the foundation of 12-Step recovery. The Steps help the addict grasp the insanity of trying to control their disease, their need for help, and the reality that help is available. If they understand and follow these three

Steps, addicts can maintain sobriety. And there are addicts who stay sober simply by following these three Steps and going to meetings. At meetings, their brain-diseased peers remind them they have a chronic, relapsing medical disease, and that the solution is to keep going to meetings, and to refrain from drinking, one day at a time. However, sobriety is not the same as recovery, and Steps Four through Twelve help the addict move from sobriety to a place of psychological and emotional wellbeing. In recovery, the addict learns to rewire his brain and rebuild his psyche and his life. In time, he can rejoin society at the developmental level of his peers whose lives and development have not been disrupted by addiction.

Steps Four and Five are about discovering the nature of ourselves and the consequences of addiction and codependency in our lives.

STEP FOUR: Made a searching and fearless moral inventory of ourselves.

The addict's hijacked midbrain has driven him to self-medicate. His single-minded focus on getting drugs has impelled him to go to great lengths in his ceaseless quest for medicine. The addict will often do whatever he needs to in order to satisfy his midbrain's craving for relief from his pain, problem, or dilemma—whatever upsets him—and to acquire his addictive substance. Addicts use drugs or behaviors to manage life:

- Addicts use to numb pain.
- Addicts use to relieve boredom.
- Addicts use to give themselves courage.
- Addicts use to feel calm enough to handle scary situations.
- Addicts use because they are depressed.
- Addicts use to help themselves sleep.
- Addicts use to relieve anxiety.
- Addicts use to find joy and transcendence.

Typically, by the time the addict gets to Step Four, he has been sober for a few months and has "worked" the previous three Steps with his sponsor or mentor. Step Four invites the addict to look inward and to acknowledge all the things he has done, good and bad.

Codependent family members embark on a Fourth Step in Al-Anon just as the addict does in AA. Some of their codependent behavior has had negative consequences, not just for the addict they have been trying to save, but for other relationships, and for their own personal wellbeing. In Al-Anon, you may hear a member say something like, "I never took care of myself. I thought I was supposed to do everything for everyone else. There was never enough time for me."

Most of us harbor memories of things we have done that are embarrassing, shameful, or painful—things we would just as soon keep to ourselves and not think about. For a healthy person, it's not a big deal to let go of past mistakes that don't affect them in the present. However, as Freud and others have pointed out, unconscious drives can run our lives in ways that don't serve us, and we function and feel better when we get help to bring troubling material into awareness, to process it, and to integrate it. We are then better able to manage our painful dilemmas. By reflecting on our past, and by doing the work to mend past errors, we can reduce our shame and begin to heal our wounds.

Addicts may have amassed a lifetime of terrible behavior resulting from their addiction—broken laws, damaged relationships, lost jobs, past betrayals. Facing and taking responsibility for their past is essential to moving forward with their growth and development. There are many approaches to working Step Four, but typically a sponsor or other AA member asks the addict to write down everything they can remember that they did wrong, everything that they feel guilty about, and everything they feel shame or resentment about. This can be a lengthy but vital process. To become conscious of these events, feel the feelings associated with them, and share this material with another person are significant accomplishments. Codependents similarly have accumulated a large repertoire of poor behavior—attempts to rescue, control, or vilify the addict, or to manage other people or situations. They, too, benefit from doing a thorough inventory of their own misdeeds. Over time, this process allows the addict or codependent to let go of shame and guilt about these events and to view their past behavior with self-compassion.

Of course, this is also material that the FRT therapist can integrate into the therapeutic process. Dealing with wreckage from the past is essential to healing. In the course of treatment and recovery, each family member does a Fourth Step with their own sponsor. Later, at Steps Eight and Nine, each individual takes responsibility for their behavior and considers making amends to others they have harmed, including other family members, if appropriate.

> STEP FIVE: Admitted to God, to ourselves, and to another human being the exact nature of our wrongs.

In Step Four, we list our wrongs, and in Step Five, we share these with another person. Both addicts and codependents are often plagued by obsessive and distorted thinking. Their inner thoughts become more tolerable when shared with a compassionate and non-judgmental listener. In Step Five, the addict or codependent chooses a trustworthy individual, one who can listen with compassion, and reads out loud the inventory he compiled in his Fourth Step. This Step is invaluable in helping the addict or codependent free themselves from onerous psychic baggage from their past. They learn that they need not feel shame about their past or hide it, that their past does not define them, and they can begin to let go of the weight and ignominy of their old behavior. The power of deep listening in 12-step programs reminds me of the qualities evoked by Thich Nan Hanh's prayer to the Bodhisattva Avalokiteshvara:

> We invoke your name, Avalokiteshvara. We aspire to learn your way of listening in order to help relieve the suffering in the world. You know how to listen in order to understand. We invoke your name in order to practice listening with all our attention and open-

heartedness. We will sit and listen without any prejudice. We will sit and listen without judging or reacting. We will sit and listen in order to understand. We will sit and listen so attentively that we will be able to hear what the other person is saying and also what is being left unsaid. We know that just by listening deeply we already alleviate a great deal of pain and suffering in the other person [Hanh, 2008, p. 30].

Here is how one recovering person describes his Step Five experience:

My personal experience of doing a Fifth Step went like this: My sponsor scheduled an evening with me at his modest home. He had set out a six-pack of Coke and a can of Planters Peanuts. I sat across from him, got out my Fourth Step list, and started reading. Every now and then he would ask for clarification. I was anxious, because I had so much shame about a few things I had done that I wondered if I would be able to say them out loud. I think my sponsor anticipated this, and told a joke about something that a drunk did while intoxicated that was so gross that I will not repeat it. But the humor gave me courage to feel more comfortable sharing my Step Four writing. When I had finished, he said, "Good job. Let's head to Step Six."

It was remarkable. As I left his home, I felt lighter, freer, that somehow more space had opened up in my psyche. It would take many years of ongoing personal therapy before I could fully understand how my abusive, alcoholic family system and my years of drinking had skewed my character, behavior, worldview, and approach to nearly everything, but I had made a beginning and a major step in the process of trusting another, opening up, unburdening myself, and heading down the path towards wholeness.

Each family member's Fourth and Fifth Steps reveal material that is useful to process in therapy. The FRT therapist guides the addict and the codependents to bring up past events that have been problematic, and to express feelings and attitudes that have negatively impacted other family members. The therapist encourages each individual to be considerate and respectful in broaching topics that may be sensitive or wounding, and guides family members to listen thoughtfully and attentively. Participating in Family Recovery Therapy and working the Steps with a sponsor mutually enhance the recovery process for the family.

STEP SIX: Were entirely ready to have God remove all these defects of character.

Step Six can seem elusive, because it does not spell out exactly what the recovering person is to do. But its meaning becomes clearer to the recovering addict or codependent as they continue to engage in the recovery process.

Prior to working Steps Four and Five, both the codependent and the addict experience disorganized and distorted thinking. But as they work those Steps, certain thinking and behavior patterns begin to emerge. They can begin to observe these patterns, which AA and Al-Anon call "character defects," and they can become willing to have them removed through the ongoing recovery process. Some people shy away from the term, "defects of character," but in essence, these are behaviors which doubtless served as useful survival mechanisms in the past. The attitudes and behaviors the addict or the codependent may formerly have relied on to cope, and to stay sane and safe, are no longer effective. In fact, they get in the way of leading a full and healthy life.

Step Six is the same in Al-Anon as it is in AA. "Defects of character," for codependents, can include the fear that fueled their behavior and the actions they took in their attempts to control, monitor, change, or compensate for their addicted loved one. If the codependent grew up in an alcoholic or dysfunctional family, they may have developed coping mechanisms from childhood such as people-pleasing, perfectionism, over-responsibility, and low self-esteem, which no longer serve them as they move toward developing healthier lives and relationships.

A secularist might re-write this step to say, "Were entirely ready to have others help relieve us of our shortcomings and neuroses."

What does the concept of being "entirely ready" mean? For both the addict and the codependent, this means becoming willing to no longer use the unhealthy attitudes or behaviors which they relied on before recovery. They must continue their recovery work, doing their best, one day at a time, to accept themselves as they are, including their flaws, and do what they can to change, become healthy, and live well. There is ongoing recovery work for the individual to do, but when and how a particular defect of character will be removed is a process. It's not simply a matter of "waiting," but of engaging in the ongoing tasks of treatment and recovery.

In the clinical sessions, the FRT therapist checks in with the family members, encouraging them to keep working the Steps with their sponsors. The process of recovery continues in therapy sessions also, as family members explore behavior that had negative consequences, and learn new ways of thinking and acting.

STEP SEVEN: Humbly asked Him to remove our shortcomings.

The initiative for anyone to change, of course, typically comes from within. And most people are happily or unhappily settled into their homeostasis and may not be motivated to observe their shortcomings and mend their ways. But we are working with a very special situation—a crisis that has affected family members so deeply that they are willing to embark on this "re-boot" of their psychological, emotional, spiritual, and social patterns, and of their family system. This is not an easy "sell," but fortunately, there are many examples of those who have successfully boarded what interventionist Kristina Wandzilak calls the "Recovery Bus" (Wandzilak & Curry, 2006). There are numerous people attending social support groups who have done what is necessary to engage in recovery and to restore personal and systemic development—and the recovering person will hear these inspirational stories at nearly every social support meeting.

The Steps build on each other, and their order is intentional. For addicts and for codependents, these Steps are the same, even though the character traits and problems of the addict are different from those of the codependent. In Step Seven, the addict or codependent specifically requests that their recovery process remove the defects or shortcomings that, in Step Six, they became "entirely ready" to have removed.

The wording of Step Seven suggests the addict or codependent "humbly ask" that their character defects be removed. Some people confuse "being humble" with "humiliation." Being humble, or "having humility," means accepting yourself as you are. This Step speaks of being humble enough to ask for help from the source the individual has chosen to rely on—whether their sponsor, their therapist, the social support fellowship, or their own concept of their higher power. This is an acknowledgment that the problems—the shortcomings that hamper the addict, or codependent—are more burdensome than what the individual alone can tackle. Each addict or codependent has strengths, but additional assistance is necessary to deal with shortcomings. The hijacked midbrain, whether of the addict or the codependent, needs guidance. Remember: we can't solve a problem with the same thinking that caused the problem.

In working Steps Six and Seven, the recovering person may spend several hours with a sponsor discussing recovery tools they can use to increase their awareness, and decrease the enactment, of their shortcomings. In time, more defects of character may come to light as the individual continues to observe his own thoughts and behavior.

The FRT therapist continues to help each family member gain more clarity about their character defects, and more willingness to let them go. The work of Family Recovery Therapy augments and deepens the Step work that each family member pursues in their ongoing growth and development.

> STEP EIGHT: Made a list of all persons we had harmed, and became willing to make amends to them all.

The newcomer to AA or Al-Anon, upon first seeing Step Eight, can become discouraged at the prospect of actually apologizing to people they have hurt. It is important to repeat that *the Steps are taken in order*, slowly and deliberately, one step at a time—at a pace that is generally guided by a sponsor. A phrase often heard in AA meetings is: "Easy does it, but do it." Working the Steps is a process that unfolds, and the recovering person completes the first seven Steps before embarking on Step Eight. The newcomer, once he accepts Step One, is ready to consider Step Two, and so on … one step at a time. In some sponsor/sponsee relationships, the Steps are worked at a pace of one Step each month, but every case is unique. For some individuals, working the Steps can take several years. By the time the addict or codependent reaches Step Eight, he may be eight months, or considerably longer, into recovery. An addict or a codependent who is this far along in recovery has probably already talked with his sponsor about some of the people he will list in his Eighth Step.

Both the addict and the codependent have doubtless harmed others in their misguided attempts to get their needs met. The addict's behavior was driven by his midbrain's craving for relief from pain; the codependent's behavior was driven by a desperate need to control an at-risk loved one or an out-of-control situation. Both the addict and the codependent's behavior profoundly impacted their connections with those close to them.

In Step Eight, the recovering person *makes a list* and *becomes willing*—nothing more.

Making a list is generally the easier part—it's just a list. But willingness can be problematic. Some sponsors recommend dividing the list into three categories: those you *are* willing to make amends to, those you *may be* willing to make amends to, and those you, at this time, are *not* willing to make amends to. With continued recovery and more time in the program, a person may become *more willing*, and be ready to make amends to some people that he was not willing to when he started this Step.

An FRT therapist can work with individual family members to investigate any obstacles or resistance that come up in working this Step. When a person *may be* willing, or definitely is *not* willing, to make amends to someone, there is an opportunity in therapy to explore his resistance and the blocks that contribute to it. Usually, these explorations lead to greater self-compassion as well as a deeper commitment to recovery.

> STEP NINE: Made direct amends to such people wherever possible, except when to do so would injure them or others.

Step Nine, like Step Eight, is an action Step. The directions in Step Nine are simple. The list from Step Eight is the template for Step Nine. The individual has already decided to whom she needs to make amends, and the challenge in Step Nine is to follow through, to "make direct amends wherever possible." An addict or codependent in recovery is expected to take responsibility for her actions and behavior in relationship to other people. The goal is simply *to make amends* for the behavior that caused harm. The reaction of the person she is making amends to is not the concern—this Step simply gives the recovering person the opportunity to acknowledge any wrongdoing and to apologize to the person she has harmed. Sometimes hurt feelings will soften and a healing will occur that both parties welcome. And sometimes the person receiving the amends will not be willing either to accept them or to modify his attitude or behavior toward the one making amends. However, the purpose of this Step is to free the recovering individual from the burden of guilt for her misdoing, not to elicit a particular response from the other person. In both AA and Al-Anon, the goal is to "clean up our side of the street."

Making amends can take many forms. Amends can be made by letter or phone, as well as in person. The recovering addict or codependent discusses with her sponsor the nature of each amends. The circumstances often dictate the method. Some of the people an individual has wronged are no longer living; others may not be geographically near the recovering individual. When the person is no longer living, or it is not appropriate to make amends directly to them, there are other options. The recovering individual may make a "living amends" by changing her present-day behavior—perhaps being kinder, or more compassionate, or more helpful—in situations similar to those in which she harmed the other person. Or, to atone for wrongdoing that can't be addressed directly, the recovering person can make an anonymous gift or donate time toward a cause relevant to the harm he inflicted.

Often, the recovering individual needs to put herself at the top of her amends list. The addict or codependent herself is often the person she has hurt most. Her ways of coping have resulted in significant self-harm. Learning to care for oneself is important in the philosophy of both AA and Al-Anon. For the addict, whose use of alcohol, drugs, addictive substances or enactment of addictive behavior, clearly entailed self-harm, replacing self-destructive behavior with healthy behavior is fundamental to recovery. The codependent, who formerly paid attention primarily to the addict, has ignored her own needs and her own development. Making herself and her own wellbeing a priority is antithetical to her previous self-neglect and self-harm. Learning and implementing habits of self-care are critical to the codependent's recovery.

While accepting an amends is not a part of this Step, a family member that has witnessed the commitment and work of other family members may be happy to receive an apology. This acceptance not only helps mend the relationship of the two family members involved, but also impacts the overall family dynamics. Furthermore, one person's amends can encourage other family members to similarly take responsibility for their own misconduct and to apologize for past wrongs.

There is an important caveat built into this Step: "…except when to do so would injure them or others." Avoiding harm in making amends is essential, and if a "direct amends" cannot be made without hurting another person, the recovering person refrains from making a straightforward apology. As noted, an addict or codependent consults with his sponsor, or others in the program, before making amends. Talking about the situation helps to clarify what constitutes an appropriate amends. For example, a woman might refrain from making amends to an ex-husband for an affair she had during their marriage, because revealing that information would be hurtful to her former spouse and possibly harmful to the other person involved.

For the recovering person, completing the first nine Steps is a significant accomplishment that often improves the individual's self-esteem and sense of wellbeing. This Step exhibits one of the clinical strengths inherent in the 12-Step "treatment" approach—it fosters self-responsibility in relating to others, which builds self-respect and self-worth. Step Nine invites the addict or codependent to take responsibility for his actions and repair the damage he has caused in his relationships. This can create a new foundation for developing functional, healthy relationships, going forward. The concept from the revered Hindu teacher, Nisargadatta Maharaj, is apropos. He describes that the mind creates separation or an abyss and that the heart crosses that abyss (1973). The distorted thinking and behavior of the addict or codependent has hurt prior relationships. Step Nine is an opportunity to heal wounds from the past.

While there is more recovery work to do, by completion of Step Nine, sobriety has become the norm for the addict, and increased serenity for the codependent. The recovering individual establishes a new lifestyle, many prior concerns are no longer problems, and new hope arises as the process of recovery continues to unfold.

>STEP TEN: Continued to take personal inventory and when we were wrong promptly admitted it.

Steps Eight and Nine have enabled the individual to take responsibility for his past actions. But addicts and codependents, like everyone else, make mistakes in their daily lives—it's human nature. Step Ten takes this into account, and guides the addict or codependent to continue to notice his attitudes and behavior and how they affect other people in his daily life. The phrase "when we were wrong, promptly admitted it" encourages the recovering person to make amends, in present time, to any person they have been rude to or hurt, and to not let memories of any mistakes or wrongdoing fester, even for a day. Owning up to and apologizing for mistakes as soon as possible is important to maintain healthy and respectful relationships. Also, some actions cause self-harm, and it's best to acknowledge and remedy these quickly, lest they become patterns that undermine our wellbeing or prevent us from having close and connected relationships.

In 12-Step parlance, the act of promptly admitting wrongdoing is spoken of as "doing a Tenth Step." Some people make an amends immediately upon realizing they have made an error. Others reflect on the day's events in the evening, and do a daily Tenth Step for the day, perhaps noting any amends they need to make. Doing a Tenth Step assures that the recovering individual continues to become more honest, to maintain and grow his self-esteem, and to develop healthier interpersonal relationships. A simple, "I screwed up, I'm sorry," becomes easier for the aware and responsible addict or codependent. Furthermore, making amends may include not just an apology, but a resolve to not repeat the offending behavior.

Step Ten invites the recovering person to notice if he is upset or if his behavior has upset another person, and particularly to note whether he has been dishonest, selfish, or resentful. If he can stay alert, he can get clues to his misdoings, and take responsibility for his behavior. If he is feeling distressed, this Step can be an opportunity to do a written inquiry, perhaps using the following format:

1. Who: The person causing the upset, me or someone else
2. What: Description of the upset or wrongdoing
3. Caused What: My reaction, the negative effect on my _____ (i.e., loss of serenity)
4. My Part: My ego (my self-will, my behavior, my fear, my neurosis)

For example, one client reported that he stopped for coffee, returned to his car and started driving, and then discovered that the cup of coffee he just bought was not hot. He got upset, and could have spent a bunch of time being angry and ruminating about the barista who screwed up. But he said that mentally he did a Tenth Step, and quickly got over it. He thought: "Who": the barista who sold him the coffee; "What": the lukewarm coffee; "Caused What": his anger, his obsessive thinking, his resentment; "His Part": his ego, his expectation that everyone should be responsible—and coffee should be hot!—and his failing to consider that there were a number of legitimate reasons why the mishap could have occurred. With a little distance, he was able to take a breath, laugh at his "self-will" and expectations, and be grateful that he even *had* a cup of coffee; then he could let go, and move on.

This Step provides an important tool for the addict or codependent to use as he continues to grow and to go about the business of living life among his fellow humans. And, as with the material that emerges in previous Step work, Family Recovery Therapy provides a supportive venue for examining and processing current events which may be distressing for the recovering addict or codependent. In therapy, we can effectively help our clients move on from previous events and into the present moment.

> STEP ELEVEN: Sought through prayer and meditation to improve our conscious contact with God as we understood Him, praying only for knowledge of His will for us and the power to carry that out.

The first part of Step Eleven encourages use of prayer and meditation for the purpose of improving "conscious contact with God *as we understood Him*." Both prayer and meditation are tools the recovering person can use to strengthen their spiritual connection with whatever wisdom or power they choose to turn to, the God of their understanding. Prayer and meditation invite the recovering person to thoughtfully reflect on their life, attitudes, and behavior. Sometimes it is said that prayer is asking for help, and meditation is listening for guidance.

Some individuals have a religious background and can easily reach out to God in prayer, perhaps even reciting a prayer they know. For others, prayer may be as simple as acknowledging some small event unfolding favorably, or feeling gratitude for some aspect of their lives. Occasionally when the topic of prayer comes up in 12-Step meetings, someone quotes the thirteenth century German theologian, Meister Eckhart, who said, "If the only prayer you say in your entire life is 'thank you,' that would suffice." (Fox, 1983, p. 109). The practice of expressing gratitude is encouraged in 12-Step programs.

Prayer, for others, is the act of asking for help. It may involve a "Please help me..." followed by a specific request. For those unused to seeking help, the concept of prayer may feel foreign initially. However, as with adopting so much of the 12-Step program, the idea and practice of using prayer becomes more comfortable over time. And it is important to note that expressing gratitude and asking for help are universal concepts, not religious practices.

Meditation has been practiced for thousands of years by people from numerous cultures, and today it is considered beneficial for almost everyone. "Meditation" can take many forms, from observing simple mindfulness in conducting daily affairs, to setting aside a specific time, or choosing a particular way to breathe, or sit, or walk. Meditation practices can include tracking the breath, repeating a mantra, or mindfully focusing on an object. Mindfully paying attention to the present moment is a helpful practice, and is of particular benefit for those who are distracted by worry or ruminate about the past or future. Meditation, like prayer, is personal. Over time, an individual's meditation practice may develop or change. Many 12-Step groups will include a brief period of meditation as part of a meeting's format. A colorful two-minute video entitled, *Meditation 101: A Beginner's Guide* (Harris, 2015), offers a simple and accessible introduction to the practice of meditation.

The second part of Step Eleven, "praying only for knowledge of His will for us and the power to carry that out," specifically instructs recovering addicts and codependents to seek guidance beyond what their ego or thinking mind alone can conjure up. This means that the recovering person must differentiate what her ego thinks is the solution to any particular problem—her self-will—from what is higher guidance or sounder wisdom—and then, consider relying on the latter. This is not an easy task, especially for someone new to the idea of asking for help. But we refer the recovering person to Step Two, "Came to believe that a Power greater than ourselves could restore us to sanity," and remind her that she has already chosen to look beyond herself. The process of seeking wise guidance can become more comfortable with continued practice of prayer and meditation. It is the willingness to search for answers that characterizes the approach of the recovering person on her journey toward wellness.

> STEP TWELVE: Having had a spiritual awakening as the result of these steps, we tried to carry this message to alcoholics, and to practice these principles in all our affairs.

As noted earlier, in the wording of the second clause of Step Twelve, Al-Anon substitutes the word "others" for "alcoholics," but otherwise, this Step is the same in both programs.

Step Twelve has three parts. The first clause, "Having had a spiritual awakening as the result of these steps," can seem very odd to the newcomer, or to someone who has not already worked the previous eleven Steps. However, the majority of people who have completed the first eleven steps will usually say something like, "Some things radically changed for me once I got into recovery. I saw the world differently. Yes, I had a spiritual awakening—I opened up to love and began connecting with others in a new way." Let's remember the desperate addict in his disease, and then consider the process of his getting sober, going to treatment, attending hundreds of social support and mutual aid groups, as well as dozens of therapy sessions, and connecting deeply with many others in recovery. On his journey through the first eleven Steps, the addict's attitude and brain have become fundamentally altered. The phrase "spiritual awakening" can be hard to embrace for some people in recovery, even after months or longer in the program. However, the recovering addict acknowledges that he is profoundly different from his former self, and that he has been transformed by the recovery process. Similarly, the codependent who is immersed in the recovery process and completes the first eleven Steps undergoes equally significant changes in attitude, perspective, and worldview. No longer wracked with worry and false hopes, trying to control what she could never control—another person—the codependent has come to know serenity and tranquility.

Seldom is a spiritual awakening an event; rather, it is a process, much of it unconscious, that happens over time. It unfolds as a result of participating in many aspects of recovery. Both the addict and the codependent have stopped their active, daily struggle to survive. They have acknowledged that there are resources other than themselves that they can turn to for guidance. They have completed a thorough inventory, dredged up past events and the names of those they have harmed, made amends, and possibly introduced prayer and meditation into their lives. They have unearthed and made conscious material that had cost them considerable psychic energy to repress. They are more able to give and receive love, to live a full life, and to seek guidance from sources wiser than their thinking mind. For both the addict and the codependent, these radical shifts comprise the spiritual awakening that evolves from working the first eleven Steps.

The second clause of Step Twelve in AA, "we tried to carry this message to alcoholics," harks back to the origins of Alcoholics Anonymous. AA was founded on the simple concept of one drunk helping another drunk stay sober, just for that one day. Step Twelve reminds the recovering addict to reach out to the new person, just as many others have reached out to him. This foundational principle is hardwired into the culture of 12-Step meetings. Even the nearly-new attendees are encouraged to reach out to the brand-new people, even though the nearly-new folks have only recently joined the program. It is in this process that the new addict gets to experience the program's fundamental premise: "we get to keep what we have only by giving it away." The following was overheard at an AA meeting:

> When I was only a few weeks sober, I was approached by this man. He said, "You're new, yes?" And then he said, "See that guy over there with the red shirt? I think he just started yesterday. Go talk to him. You've been sober for a few weeks, and I've been sober for three years. Who is he going to believe?"

Al-Anon's Step Twelve encourages members to carry the message of recovery to "others," meaning to other individuals struggling with a loved one's alcoholism. Al-Anon's Preamble says that "Al-Anon has but one purpose: to help families of alcoholics … by welcoming and giving comfort to families of alcoholics…" (Al-Anon Family Groups, n.d.-c). Al-Anon members extend the message of recovery to others affected by the disease of alcoholism. Today, the wording has not changed from its 1950s' language, but the fellowship welcomes those with a family member suffering from any emotional problem, including drug abuse, overeating, sex addiction, gambling, other addictions and compulsions, and mental illness.

The final clause of Step Twelve, "to practice these principles in all our affairs," reminds addicts and codependents that the 12 Steps are a *foundation for living*. The recovering person is mindful of the 12-Step principles, and uses them for guidance in his daily life. Doing so encourages continued sobriety for the addict and continued serenity for the codependent.

To manage the complexities of day-to-day life, the person in recovery turns to the process outlined in the 12 Steps. Steps One, Two, and Three remind the addict daily that he is powerless over alcohol, that he has a medical disease, that his life is unmanageable, and that he needs to rely on wisdom beyond his own thinking ego. The first three Steps remind the codependent that they suffer from obsessive thinking and they cannot control others. Many people in recovery repeat the first three Steps to themselves many times each day.

Steps Four and Five provide tools for the individual, to look inward, to uncover and explore unhealthy behaviors or patterns that crop up as his recovery continues to unfold. It is not unusual to hear someone say in a meeting, "I decided to do a Fourth Step about..." (a particular situation). Taking this kind of inventory, and sharing it with a trusted sponsor or other program member, can help the individual better clarify and comprehend his part in a distressful relationship or situation. In Steps Six and Seven, the individual can become more aware of how this issue manifests and less inclined to repeat the unskillful behavior, and become willing to have the attitude or behavior removed.

Steps Eight and Nine provide tools to acknowledge behaviors that have harmed others, or that have been self-injurious. These Steps also guide the recovering person to atone appropriately for any misdeeds or to correct his behavior.

Steps Ten, Eleven, and Twelve are sometimes deemed "maintenance" Steps. They provide a roadmap for the addict or codependent not only to sustain recovery, but to live responsibly as an accountable and respectful adult and a functioning member of society. By implementing Step Ten, the recovering person continues to observe and evaluate his thoughts and behavior, and to make restitution to others immediately. Step Eleven encourages him to pray and meditate in order to strengthen his awareness of a wisdom beyond himself and to rely on that wisdom for guidance. And finally, Step Twelve points out that a spiritual awakening has occurred. This Step reminds the recovering person that he is part of a larger context, that there are others still suffering from the disease of alcoholism and codependency, and that he can reach out a helping hand to them, as others have reached out to him.

The Steps are grounded in values that are basic to many philosophies for living life well and in harmony with others. They include aspects of cognitive behavioral therapy, family systems therapy, existential therapy, psychoanalysis, and transpersonal therapy. The durability of the 12 Steps is an historical fact. Alcoholics Anonymous has grown and flourished in the past 80-plus years, and today there are over two million members of AA and over 118,000 groups in approximately 180 nations (Alcoholics Anonymous, n.d.-a). In addition, as mentioned previously, there are many dozens of offshoots from the original 12-Step program of Alcoholics Anonymous. A few of the better-known 12-Step programs include Smokers Anonymous, Overeaters Anonymous, Gamblers Anonymous, Sex and Love Addicts Anonymous, Cocaine Anonymous, Co-Dependents Anonymous, Narcotics Anonymous, and Internet and Technology Addicts Anonymous. And there are many dozens of less well-known 12-Step programs, each offering its respective members support and guidance for diminishing use of harmful behaviors and living a better life. The spread of 12-Step programs speaks to the efficacy of the Steps, and to the significance of human connection in recovery.

Witnessing the power of a family working together on these Steps, in the process of healing and restoring development, brings tears to my eyes. I know of no other method of psychotherapy that so effectively supports healthy development in a family in such a short time. Below is a brief story of healing in a family I worked with.

> Samantha was an out-of-control 17-year-old with upper middle class, divorced parents. She did not have a driver's license, and had "borrowed" her mother's or father's car on several occasions, had stayed out all night without permission, was doing a lot of drugs, and was failing at school. Her parents contacted me. I met first with the divorced parents together to get a picture of the family and the separate households, and then with them and their daughter. My goals were to stabilize the system and to understand the stressors causing the acting out, as well as to help the parents learn to manage the relationship with their possibly-addicted daughter.
>
> Samantha wanted no part of this attempt to rein her in. On more than one occasion, she stormed out of a session, loudly slamming the door behind her. It was clear, after a half dozen sessions, that outpatient therapy was not going to work in this situation. Samantha needed residential treatment. Samantha's parents and I coordinated "transporting" Samantha to a wilderness program in Colorado. Two experienced transport workers, one a former policeman and the other a social worker, picked up Samantha in the middle of the night, flew with her to Colorado, and drove her to the wilderness program.
>
> Over the next ten weeks, the residential placement staff and I coordinated a family systems treatment plan that comprehensively "re-set" the family system dynamics. The parents met with me individually and together. They joined a weekly conference call with me and the field therapist who was coordinating Samantha's treatment in the field. The staff and I worked with the parents to help them set aside their personal animosities towards each other that led to their divorce, and to focus on coming together as parents for their child. And the wilderness program also helped this now-adult young person (she turned 18 while in the wilderness) to understand her behavior and motives and to focus on what she wanted—as opposed to reacting to her parents.
>
> With input from the residential placement staff, I put together an intensive aftercare treatment plan for Samantha that included her residing in a sober living home, finding and maintaining full-time employment in a suitable entry-level job, and fully immersing herself in social support groups. In addition, she and her parents were going to continue weekly individual and family therapy with me to support Samantha's individuation process, and each parent would also attend Al-Anon meetings.
>
> Samantha and her parents came to the weekly family therapy sessions, Samantha became involved in her social support groups and started waiting tables at a local restaurant, and her parents became active participants in Al-Anon. Each parent chose a sponsor and actively pursued the recovery process in Al-Anon, along with their active participation

in therapy with me. In working Steps 4 and 5, the parents realized how their behavior had harmed not only their relationship with each other, but their relationship with Samantha. In Step Nine, they made amends to each other as well as to Samantha. The parents made amends to one another for vying to be Samantha's "favorite parent," and to Samantha for not listening to their daughter or setting boundaries when she'd most needed them to. Samantha made amends to her parents for her behavior—being disrespectful, using drugs, driving their cars without their permission and before she had a driver's license, flaunting her curfew, and failing at school. The relationships among the three family members improved significantly through the process of making amends.

Samantha successfully completed the aftercare program, including the 12 Steps, and achieved a year of continuous sobriety and nearly a year of employment at her restaurant job. Completing the 12 Steps was a significant milestone for Samantha. It both signified and solidified her dedication to recovery. She came willingly to her individual sessions with me. She no longer slammed the door of my office. A year later, she moved into her own apartment with some of her co-workers. That was five years ago. Today Samantha is about to graduate from a local college. She is still active in social support groups, and she enjoys good relationships with her parents and with peers.

This story may seem simple—almost linear. In fact, if clients follow the Steps of recovery in AA and Al-Anon, it *can* be a truly simple, even if sometimes painful, path to healing and freedom.

At both AA and Al-Anon meetings, participants share many stories of healing the wreckage from their past. Family members—addicts and codependents—speak about the support they received from their respective groups that helped them repair damage from the past, heal and grow, and then build healthier relationships. It is vital that the FRT therapist be well-versed in the 12 Steps, so they know and understand the process their clients are engaged in, and appreciate the skills they are learning—in so doing they will both witness recovery from addiction in action, and partner in their clients' recovery process (see Appendix C).

Social support and mutual aid groups have long been a part of comprehensive addiction treatment. In these groups, addicts and codependents find the help, connection, and community necessary to support their return to normal development and to sustain their ongoing sobriety and serenity.

Chapter 14

Drug Testing

In this chapter, I discuss the necessity for drug testing in treating addiction, describe factors that contribute to getting reliable test results, and provide some information about retention rates for various drugs of abuse. The primary drugs of abuse are alcohol, opiates, benzodiazepines, amphetamines, cocaine, and marijuana. There are many other drugs which are less commonly subject to misuse, such as synthetic cannabinoids, barbiturates, and phencyclidine (Angel Dust).

Drug testing is essential to effective addiction treatment. Addicts are hardwired to use substances—their brain circuitry, which has been altered by substance use, renders them dependent on drugs. Only by testing for the presence of drugs is there certainty whether or not the addict has used. For an addict in recovery, drug testing can be the incentive that deters him from using. The significance of drug testing in Family Recovery Therapy (FRT) is reflected in FRT Principle 11:

FRT Principle 11
   Regular drug testing is a powerful tool and will be used in addiction treatment.

Drug testing can be done by a local reputable service (that works with a licensed, certified toxicology lab) that will report the results directly to you, or you may collect samples and send them to a licensed, certified toxicology lab for screening. If you choose to personally drug test your clients, the process can be straightforward and routine. The effort required to drug test is negligible, particularly when weighed against its significance for a client who is struggling to achieve and maintain sobriety. The procedure can be easy to set up and administer. For your information, if you choose to incorporate drug testing into your practice, the next paragraph includes a brief description of the process.

First, set up an account with a licensed, certified toxicology lab. The lab need not be in your immediate vicinity as samples are delivered by mail to the lab, and labs generally provide results online. The lab will send you collection bottles, labels, and mailers. The process of sample collection is simple: hand the client a labeled container and send the client to the restroom. When the client returns with the capped container, check the temperature gauge on the side of the container (to verify that the sample is fresh), place the container in the mailer provided by the lab, and drop the mailer in a mailbox. The process requires little time or effort, and it is a routine practice in all drug treatment programs.

I didn't learn about drug testing in my graduate school class on addiction. Yet, drug testing is an essential tool in addiction treatment. Addicts in treatment *expect* to be drug tested—all addiction treatment programs include drug testing. Drug testing benefits the addict and helps her stay sober. It is a tool that reinforces the message of recovery for the addict. The specter of drug tests can counter the addict's craving. I hope the information in this chapter will help therapists who have not received education and training in drug testing to understand its necessity and value in addiction treatment.

As I mentioned, early in the course of my training to become a therapist, I interned at an adolescent drug treatment program that treated families of drug-using teens. Drug testing—urine testing—was included in the program's routine protocol. I learned that drug testing is an incentive for adolescents in treatment to remain sober, if they can. Plus, their families were relieved when test results confirmed that their child was drug-free.

During that internship, I became accustomed to performing drug tests on a regular basis. When I started my private practice in 1996, I opened an account with a licensed toxicology laboratory that provides reliable results for drug screens. I learned that drug testing needs to be *verified, frequent, and random*. Verification includes checking the temperature gauge on the outside of the container to determine whether the temperature of the sample is in the appropriate range. A temperature check is essential to ensure that the client isn't substituting someone else's clean urine for his own, when there is a possibility that his urine may be contaminated with drugs.

Verification also includes having samples processed by a licensed, certified toxicology lab. Laboratory-verified test results are necessary, because non-regulated tests (at-home tests) are not always reliable. As mentioned, the FRT therapist can collect samples and mail them to the lab for analysis, or the FRT therapist can refer to a facility that performs *verified collections* and provides *certified results*. With a Google search, you can locate appropriate labs in your area.

A funny story:

> Just before meeting with my weekly peer group of recovering teens, I downloaded their latest toxicology reports. I noticed that Joe's test was positive for methamphetamines. After we got settled into the group, I reviewed the reports with the group members. Looking at one report, I said, "Hey, Joe, you were positive for meth!"
>
> "*You said it would be clean*," Joe screamed at Rob, the teen sitting across the room from him. Clearly, Joe was using drugs and wanted to get away with it by substituting Rob's urine—except that Rob was also using drugs!

Clients will slip clean urine—or urine they think is clean—into the collection bottle if they can. You can Google "faking drug tests" to discover the countless techniques people use to beat drug tests. Drug users will plot beating a test with the intensity that burglars plot robbing a bank! Fake penises filled with urine, and battery-powered, temperature-controlled, hand-held devices that contain clean urine are but two of the clever inventions available. I've heard of individuals who have been catheterized to inject clean urine into their bladder. And rumor has it that a $20 million-a-year professional ball player had his bladder injected with clean urine so he could get away with illicit steroid use.

Frequency of testing is another significant factor in getting useful test results. Drugs are retained in the body and detectable in the urine only for a short period of time (the length of time is specific for each drug, but is usually two to three days). Infrequent testing can create opportunities for drug use to go undetected. And test results both inform the therapist whether or not the client is sober, and motivate the client not to use. For the client, each clean drug test serves as another milestone on his recovery path.

The time between tests needs to be short enough to discourage an addict from using. An addict in early recovery may be subject to intense cravings and may obsess about getting and using substances, especially if they think they can get away with it. When there is a small enough "window" between tests, the addict will be less likely to act on their cravings or to start seeking drugs. It is a service to the addict, and a boost to their recovery, to have frequent negative drug tests.

Initially, testing can take place daily, every other day, or at least several times each week. If the addict thinks there is no way to fit in drug use between tests, he will stop using—if he can. And if he can't stop, we need to know that, and we need to know it as soon as possible—and then rapidly escalate treatment. Also, testing at some frequency must continue throughout the duration of treatment—particularly if there is suspicion that a client's commitment to treatment and recovery has diminished, or if he is vulnerable because of unusual life stressors.

Retention rate is sometimes a consideration in determining frequency of testing. The retention rate—the length of time after use that metabolites of the drug will show up in the urine—varies for each substance. For most substances, the lab results will not quantify the amount of a specific substance present, but simply note whether the substance is present (positive) or not (negative). However, when marijuana is screened, the lab can typically ascertain both the presence and the concentration of THC.

The retention rate for THC varies from one individual to the next, and the level depends in part on body composition. THC is stored in body fat, and an individual with a high percentage of body fat may test positive for THC for a longer period of time than someone with less body fat. THC values also vary depending on the frequency, amount, and duration of use. Someone who has smoked marijuana on a daily basis for a long time may test positive for up to a month after his or her last use. However, someone who smokes pot once a month may test positive for THC for only one to three days after using. Regardless, the amount of detectable THC will trend downwards if the person has stopped using. Most of the other common drugs of abuse will test positive for only two or three days after use. Below is a chart showing the approximate retention rates for common drugs of abuse. The data is based on information from Redwood Toxicology Laboratory, Inc., which is located in Santa Rosa, California.

Drug Retention Times

Drug	Retention Time
Amphetamines	2–4 days
Barbiturates	Short-acting (e.g., secobarbital): 24 hours Long-acting (e.g., phenobarbital): 2–3 weeks
Benzodiazepines	3 days, if therapeutic dose ingested
Cocaine	2–4 days
Methadone	Approximately 3 days
Opiates	3 days
Cannabinoids (Marijuana)	Light smoker (once a week): 1–3 days Moderate smoker (3–5 times a week): 3–10 days Heavy chronic smoker (Daily): 5–30+ days
Phencyclidine (Angel Dust)	Approximately 8 days
EthylGlucuronide (EtG) (Alcohol)	Up to 80 hours

(For more detailed information about specific substances, please refer to the references cited from Redwood Toxicology Laboratory, Inc., n.d.-a–j.)

A licensed, certified toxicology lab can test for hundreds of drugs and can create a panel that fits your specific needs. Currently, I use a panel that screens urine samples for 13 of the most commonly abused drugs: alcohol (ethanol), amphetamines, fentanyl, benzodiazepines, buprenorphine, cocaine, Ethyl Glucuronide (EtG) (the metabolites created by alcohol usage, which stay in a person's system for up to 80 hours after use), Methadone, Tramadol, opiates, Oxycodone/Noroxycodone, and THC (marijuana). For a supplementary fee, a lab will screen for numerous other substances, including nicotine, synthetic cannabinoids, and designer drugs.

The lab also measures a sample's creatinine level, which is an indicator of the sample's concentration. Creatinine is a metabolite that is normally present in urine. If the creatinine level registers under 20 mg/dl, the lab deems the sample "dilute": The sample is insufficiently concentrated for the lab to reliably detect the presence or absence of drugs.

A normal, healthy, naturally hydrated person will typically produce a sufficiently concentrated sample. A motivated addict may try to mask drug use by overloading on water before the collection, and then produce a sample that is too dilute for screening. Dilute samples are considered invalid, and may signal the possibility of drug use. When an individual produces a dilute result, it is important to collect a new sample as soon as possible.

Samples sent to a certified toxicology lab are analyzed by sophisticated immunoassay and chromatography methods. A board-certified medical toxicologist oversees the process. Results from a certified lab are considered the "gold standard" of drug screening, and are sufficiently accurate to be admissible in court for parole or probation violations, or in divorce and child-custody cases.

Special containers are available that will provide instant results, including instant tests for EtG. Instant tests can be helpful when rapid results are an asset—in early recovery, when sobriety may not yet be established, or at any point in treatment when there is suspicion of drug use. The collection jars that are used for instant tests have been fitted with chemically sensitive strips embedded on the sides of the containers. When the jars are filled with urine, the strips change color to indicate the presence of specific drugs.

However, instant test results are considered presumptive, and confirmation of results by a lab is always advised, because the instant tests are less accurate than the sophisticated screening performed by a lab.

Effective drug testing also needs to be *random*. The unpredictability provided by random testing means that the client cannot plan drug use to coincide with times he will not be tested, because he does not know when he will be called in for a test. Often, when frequency of testing is reduced, random testing is implemented. For example, when a client has established a solid and consistent recovery program, and has produced clean tests for many consecutive months, the testing protocol may be reduced in frequency and shifted to random testing. In this situation, drug tests may be performed only once or twice a month, and then, gradually, the frequency could be reduced further. However, these drug tests are scheduled at *random* times. The client is told that, at any time, he may be given twenty-four hours' notice to come in for a drug test.

Testing at any point, even infrequent and random, supports recovery. The addict typically welcomes testing to confirm what they already know, that they are clean! But the fact that testing is random, and that they may be tested 24/7 with 24 hours' notice to come in, supports their continuing sobriety and acts as a deterrent to offset drug using.

A random drug test can catch drug use if there has been a relapse, and, if the sample tests positive, it indicates the need to escalate treatment, step up recovery work, and increase testing frequency. Clients in our program understand that, as per the Treatment Agreement, a relapse may require a 72-hour stint at a detox facility, and will entail a new sobriety date, starting the 12 Steps over again with their sponsor, and escalation of treatment.

I witnessed the consequences of non-random testing several years ago. At that time, in Marin County where I work, local juvenile probation officers visited high schools in the area to drug test teens who were on probation for drug violations. The probation officers used a regular testing schedule: "High School A" on Monday, "High School B" on Tuesday, and so on, week after week. Drug-using kids are generally well informed about a drug's retention rate. In my experience, teens regularly peruse drug information websites (Erowid, n.d.)—and they love to brag about beating the system. They knew, for instance, that if they were going to be tested on Monday, they could smoke pot after the urine collection, and then could use almost *any* drug (except pot, which has a longer and more variable retention rate) for the next four days, and they could even get intoxicated for the next six days and always come out clean! (This was before the EtG test was available, which picks up alcohol metabolites for three days after use.) Eventually, the probation department caught on and started mixing up the collection days.

Bottom line, the testing needs to be frequent enough and sufficiently unpredictable to minimize the opportunity for the addict to use substances without his use being detected. The FRT therapist needs to establish a balance between what is clinically necessary and what comprises a realistic frequency, so as to avoid unnecessary expense. For instance, with someone who has completed many months of treatment, and who has a solid commitment to recovery work, it would be appropriate to schedule random tests once or twice a month for the remainder of their initial year in treatment.

On occasion, I may also use Breathalyzers™ to calculate blood alcohol level. When I work with an alcoholic whom I know is struggling to stay sober or who is in early recovery, I may use a Breathalyzer™ to help the client establish sobriety. Breathalyzers™ only measure alcohol use that has occurred within the past few hours, but it is vital to catch alcohol use quickly if it occurs. Once, a client who had been in treatment with me for about three months came in for a session. He seemed "off," and I asked him to blow into the Breathalyzer™. He then admitted that he had been drinking, and acknowledged that he wasn't sure he could stop. He spent the next 72 hours in a residential detox facility, as per the Treatment Agreement. This experience of relapse and detox was pivotal for him—it convinced him that he was *powerless* over alcohol. The client renewed his commitment to treatment and remained sober for the next year. Had I collected urine from him, his urine would have tested positive for alcohol, but we wouldn't have received the results until a few days later, and we would have missed an opportunity to provide an immediate intervention.

Drug testing is not expensive, and its value in establishing or ensuring sobriety is essential. The lab I work with typically charges around $20 to perform a 13-panel screen. I charge the clients an additional fee to cover the cost of supplies and my time to handle the collection and shipping process.

The value of verified, frequent, and random drug tests cannot be overemphasized. When I'm treating substance-using teens and their families, and meeting with the teenager once or twice each week, I will enlist the parents to test on days their teen is not coming in for a session. In situations when I have had clients who have left the area to attend college elsewhere, I have set up testing for them at a facility near their college. Some of these resources have worked out well, but I have also encountered a few that I would not use again. Due diligence is important in choosing a drug-testing service.

Conclusion

Family Recovery Therapy (FRT) suggests a radical shift from the current perspective on treating addiction, and proposes a comprehensive, effective revision of addiction treatment. This new paradigm transforms addiction treatment in three significant areas: involving enablers in a treatment process in which the *family system* is seen as the client; inserting a *licensed professional* as overseer of the recovery process in a treatment industry which has traditionally lacked regulation; and providing a cohesive, integrated, and effective approach to addiction treatment in which the licensed FRT therapist is case manager and primary treatment provider, from the initial phone call through the first year of continuous sobriety.

Nearly all addiction, as we have seen, is enabled to some degree by those close to the addict. The first vital piece of this new paradigm changes the focus of the current model of addiction treatment—which focuses primarily on the addict—to include the family system and the broader social systems in which an addict lives. The addict-centered approach, the current model, has largely disregarded the significance of family and peers in the life of the addict—the very people who often enable the addict's disease, and are in a position to support an addict's recovery, if they embrace the recovery process. The FRT therapist not only treats the addictive/codependent family members, but typically *initiates* treatment with the enabling codependents. In most cases, it is a member of the enabling family who reaches out to an addiction treatment provider for help, and the family members are almost always in as much need of assistance as is the addict. They are doing their best to stay afloat, but they generally lack the tools and skills, much less the perspective, to repair the family system that has allowed addiction and codependency to thrive.

The second way the FRT model departs from current addiction treatment is that it introduces the concept of a *licensed professional* as the overseer of care. The addiction treatment industry has largely lacked regulation. For decades, there was little money available through health insurance to cover the cost of addiction treatment. The Mental Health Parity and Addiction Equity Act, which was passed in the U.S. in 2008, required health insurance companies to reimburse treatment for the medical disease of addiction at the same level they cover treatment for any other medical disease. Businesses discovered that a lot of money could be made by stepping into the addiction treatment industry. Many treatment programs popped up and were massively overbilling for lab tests (urine tests), there were reports that rehabs were trolling the streets looking for homeless addicts with insurance, and "treatment" sometimes meant a bed with a TV and food until the insurance was cut off. Because government or industry regulation of addiction treatment was rudimentary and not well-enforced, there was a lot of leeway for slick rehab centers to charge large amounts of money but provide little effective care.

Many of the "old paradigm" rehabs do good work, but many well-known national programs quickly degraded when they were bought out and the core staff left. Having a licensed professional, the FRT therapist, oversee the treatment process, including choosing and coordinating treatment with a reputable rehab center when that kind of treatment is warranted, assures consistency and professionalism throughout the course of treatment.

The third essential element of the new FRT paradigm is consistent, interconnected, and coordinated treatment, led by the FRT therapist. The addiction treatment model which has prevailed in the United States for many decades lacks the cohesion and consistency that can provide a solid therapeutic foundation for addiction recovery. The current model is much like a factory assembly line. The addict is passed from interventionist to rehab to outpatient treatment. Each step along the way is typically overseen by a different, *nonprofessional* provider—all the while ignoring the addict's partners-in-addiction, the enabling codependents. These treatment providers vary widely in their training—some are highly experienced, and some are barely sober. In many rehabs, the addict may only briefly encounter a licensed professional during treatment. The provider in the FRT model is a single, licensed professional who is in intimate contact with the family, the addict, and the enabling codependents, from the first phone call through the initial year of continuous sobriety. Furthermore, the FRT therapist coordinates the care of the family with other providers and ancillary services throughout the recovery process. This ensures continuity of care for the family and for the addict. As noted by the addiction psychiatrist Timmen L. Cermak, M.D. (personal communication, May 7, 2021),

> The weak link in current Substance Use Disorder treatment [is] the lack of quality case management. Too often doctors, psychologists, therapists and counselors involved in a patient's care do not coordinate their efforts, fail to follow up, or even to communicate with each other ... family therapists are in the best position to manage the treatment team to assure everyone has input to the overall treatment plan and works toward the same goal.

Cohesion in the treatment process can enhance the recovery process for the family and the addict, leading to a nearly 100 percent success rate *when the FRT protocols are followed*. A fragmented approach does not ensure consistent effort towards the goal of helping addictive/codependent family systems heal, repair, and be restored to optimal development. And the evidence is in: the current approach yields only a 50 percent chance of the addict remaining sober after treatment, and does not address the damage to the family or to others who are in relationship with the addict.

It is finally time to move addiction treatment into the modern era. It is time to integrate modern mental and medical health treatment with the long-established residential rehab movement. It is time to acknowledge that addiction is almost always enabled by well-meaning individuals who need their own support. It is time to understand the need for addiction treatment to comprehensively treat the addict through at least *the first year of continuous sobriety*. This book, *Addiction Therapy and Treatment: A Systems Approach*, describes exactly how this will work. Individuals seeking treatment for addiction should start with a therapist certified in Family Recovery Therapy (FRT). And rehabs seeking interventionists are best served by referring to certified FRT therapists who will work with the addict and the family— the family system— hands on, before and after a residential stay and throughout the initial year of continuous sobriety.

It is my fervent hope, and indeed, the passion that has fueled writing this book, that those invested in good outcomes in treating addiction will grasp the value of the FRT model and adopt it. I hope that the families in need of addiction treatment will seek practitioners who use this model. I hope that community facilities and government agencies will update their approach to incorporate the principles of Family Recovery Therapy. Ultimately, I hope that practitioners involved in addiction treatment at any level will implement the principles of Family Recovery Therapy so that we can finally achieve a high rate of success in treating addictive/codependent family systems.

Appendix A

Erik Erikson's Eight Stages of Psycho-Social Development

In baseball, we need to get to first base before we can move on to second. Psychologist Erik Erikson described the developmental stages we move through in life. We need to master one stage before we can successfully move on to the next. Several factors can delay, disrupt, or otherwise slow or stop our development. Addiction, codependency, living in a dysfunctional home, or other stressors will naturally disrupt our path to optimal health. Getting into recovery provides the basis for slowly uncovering and repairing our deficits and provides us with a process to make up for our losses.

There are many renditions of Erikson's stages. Following is a compilation of several descriptions of Erik Erikson's Eight Stages of Psycho-Social Development adapted from his *Childhood and Society* (1963).

Erik Erikson's Eight Stages of Psycho-Social Stages of Development

Stage 1.
Infancy (Under 2 years) If needs are met, infant develops a sense of basic trust

Age Stages	Psychological Dilemma	Favorable Outcome	Unfavorable Outcome
	Trust vs. Mistrust	Outward signs of healthy growth	Outward signs of unhealthy growth
		Expressions of Trust	Expressions of Mistrust
		1. Shares self and possessions	1. Does not share self or possessions
		2. Good eye contact	2. Poor eye contact
		3. Welcomes touching	3. Loner and unhappy
		4. Lets mother go	4. Unwilling to let mother go
		5. Open, non-suspicious attitude	5. Suspicious, closed, guarded
		6. Invests in relationships	6. Avoids relationships

Appendix A. Erik Erikson's Eight Stages of Psycho-Social Development

Stage 2.

Toddlerhood (2–3 years) Toddler strives to learn independence and self-confidence

Age Stages	Psychological Dilemma	Favorable Outcome	Unfavorable Outcome
	Autonomy vs. Shame and Doubt	Outward signs of healthy growth	Outward signs of unhealthy growth
		Expressions of autonomy	Expressions of shame and doubt
		1. Independent	1. Procrastinates frequently
		2. Not easily led	2. Has trouble working alone
		3. Resists being dominated	3. Needs structure and directions
		4. Able to stand on own two feet	4. Has trouble making decisions
		5. Works well alone or with others	5. Is easily influenced
		6. Assertive when necessary	6. Embarrassed when complimented

Stage 3.

Early childhood (3–6 years) Preschooler learns to initiate tasks and grapples with self-control

Age Stages	Psychological Dilemma	Favorable Outcome	Unfavorable Outcome
	Initiative vs. Guilt	Outward signs of healthy growth	Outward signs of unhealthy growth
		Expressions of initiative	Expressions of guilt
		1. Is a self-starter	1. Gets depressed easily
		2. Accepts challenges	2. Puts self down
		3. Assumes leadership roles	3. Slumped posture
		4. Sets goals—goes after them	4. Poor eye contact
		5. Moves easily, freely with body	5. Has low energy level

Stage 4.

Middle childhood (7–12) Child becomes effective or feels inadequate

Age Stages	Psychological Dilemma	Favorable Outcome	Unfavorable Outcome
	Industry vs. Inferiority	Outward signs of healthy growth	Outward signs of unhealthy growth
		Expressions of Industry	Expressions of inferiority
		1. Wonders how things work	1. Timid, somewhat withdrawn
		2. Finishes what starts	2. Overly obedient
		3. Likes "projects"	3. Procrastinates often
		4. Enjoys learning	4. An observer, not a producer
		5. Likes to experiment	5. Questions own ability

Appendix A. Erik Erikson's Eight Stages of Psycho-Social Development

Stage 5.

Adolescence (13–19 years) Teenager works at developing a sense of self by testing roles, then integrating them to form a cohesive identity

Age Stages	Psychological Dilemma	Favorable Outcome	Unfavorable Outcome
	Identity vs. Role Confusion	Outward signs of healthy growth	Outward signs of unhealthy growth
		Expressions of identity	Expressions of identity confusion
		1. Certain about sex role identity	1. Doubts about sex role identity
		2. Active interest in intimate relations	2. Lacks confidence
		3. Plans for future	3. Overly hostile to authority
		4. Challenges adult authority	4. Overly obedient
		5. Tends to be self-accepting	5. Tends to be self-rejecting

Stage 6.

Early adulthood (20–39 years) Young adult struggles to form close relationships and to gain capacity for intimate love

Age Stages	Psychological Dilemma	Favorable Outcome	Unfavorable Outcome
	Intimacy vs. Isolation	Outward signs of healthy growth	Outward signs of unhealthy growth
		Expressions of Trust	Expressions of Mistrust
		1. Maintains friendships	1. Sabotages relationships
		2. Physical and emotional intimacy	2. Withdraws
		3. Participation in games, groups	3. Avoidance, defensive
		4. Open, willing to interact	4. Self-defeating behavior
		5. Able to make and keep commitments	5. Isolates
			6. Questions job performance

Appendix A. Erik Erikson's Eight Stages of Psycho-Social Development

Stage 7.

Middle Adulthood (40–64 years) Middle-aged person seeks a sense of contributing to the world through, for example, family and work

Age Stages	Psychological Dilemma	Favorable Outcome	Unfavorable Outcome
	Generativity vs. Stagnation	Outward signs of healthy growth	Outward signs of unhealthy growth
		Expressions of Generativity	Expressions of Stagnation
		1. Achieves goals	1. Watching
		2. Confident	2. Complaining, blaming
		3. Productive work	3. Withdraws
		4. Their own person	4. Poor physical health
		5. Willingness to invest in the next generation	5. Fatalist attitude
		6. Willing to risk, explore, produce; has take charge attitude	6. Dissatisfaction with self, job, life, mate

Stage 8.

Late Adulthood (65 years and above) Reflecting on life, the elderly person may experience satisfaction or a sense of failure

Age Stages	Psychological Dilemma	Favorable Outcome	Unfavorable Outcome
	Ego Integrity vs. Despair	Outward signs of healthy growth	Outward signs of unhealthy growth
		Expressions of Integrity	Expressions of Despair and Distrust
		1. Proud, content with self and life	1. Despair
		2. Still actively thinking about the future	2. Deep resentment
		3. Healthy interaction with self	3. Nothing left, uselessness
		4. Self-approving	4. Low self-esteem
		5. Comfortable giving and sharing with others	5. Anger at self, other, world, society
		6. Likes being an example to others	6. Closed to others
		7. Accepts aging process gracefully and death as part of life cycle	7. Complains, irritable
			8. Anger at aging, feels cheated

Appendix B

The Fourteen Principles of Family Recovery Therapy

FRT Principle 1
Addiction is a chronic, relapsing, treatable medical disease with profound mental and physical consequences. Addicts will need long-term, possibly lifelong, recovery support, which can take many forms.

FRT Principle 2
Effective treatment of addiction usually involves treatment of codependents, because codependents enable addiction. Codependency is a chronic relationship pattern that has profound mental and physical consequences and is characterized by an obsessive focus on other people. Codependents may need lifelong recovery support, which can take many forms.

FRT Principle 3
In Family Recovery Therapy (FRT), the client in treatment is the family system that suffers from both addiction and codependency.

FRT Principle 4
During the first year of treatment, the FRT therapist monitors, assesses, and guides the family in an integrated treatment process, which addresses biological, psychological, social, and spiritual recovery.

FRT Principle 5
As the treatment team leader, the FRT therapist guides the family throughout the continuum of care and collaborates with all supportive therapeutic services, which may include other treatment providers, interventionists, treatment programs, physicians, and any other adjunctive services.

FRT Principle 6
The FRT therapist must be well-versed in the 12 Steps and have a thorough understanding and appreciation for the fundamental role that mutual aid programs play in recovery from codependency and addiction.

FRT Principle 7
The FRT therapist, who is a state-licensed medical or mental health

professional, must be knowledgeable and experienced in many paths to growth and recovery. Ideally, the therapist is engaged in a personal recovery practice, whether 12-Step or other, in which capacity, the therapist stands shoulder-to-shoulder with the family members.

FRT Principle 8
Since addiction and the codependency that enables it are chronic conditions, it is recommended that the addict and codependents develop ongoing support beyond the first year of continuous sobriety.

FRT Principle 9
Treatment includes monitoring for co-occurring mental and physical health problems and providing appropriate referrals as needed.

FRT Principle 10
Medically Assisted Treatment may be necessary, if medication is used in the service of recovery and not as a substitute for recovery.

FRT Principle 11
Regular drug testing is a powerful tool and will be used in addiction treatment.

FRT Principle 12
All members of the family seeking treatment must be fully informed of, and understand, the therapeutic goals, as well as understand and agree to the treatment plan, which includes specific recommendations for different stages of treatment.

FRT Principle 13
Optimal recovery is achieved when family members commit to all aspects of the treatment program.

FRT Principle 14
Typically, a member of the enabling subsystem contacts the treatment provider. It is vital that the provider begin to engage the caller in the Family Recovery Therapy treatment model during this first contact.

Appendix C

How AA Works with Professionals

AA and psychotherapy both provide valuable services to help the alcoholic, and AA welcomes collaboration with professionals. Following is an excerpt from AA's publication, *If You Are a Professional, Alcoholics Anonymous Wants to Work with You* (Alcoholics Anonymous World Services, 2018a). The publication is available in its entirety online.

A Resource for the Helping Professional

Professionals who work with alcoholics share a common purpose with Alcoholics Anonymous: to help the alcoholic stop drinking and lead a healthy, productive life.

Alcoholics Anonymous is a nonprofit, self-supporting, entirely independent fellowship—"not allied with any sect, denomination, politics, organization or institution." Yet A.A. is in a position to serve as a resource to you through its policy of "cooperation but not affiliation" with the professional community.

We can serve as a source of personal experience with alcoholism as an ongoing support system for recovering alcoholics.

How the Program Works

A.A.'s primary purpose, as stated in our Preamble, is: "to stay sober and help other alcoholics to achieve sobriety."

The only requirement for A.A. membership is a desire to stop drinking. There are no dues or fees; we are self-supporting through our own contributions. Members share their experiences in recovery from alcoholism on a one-to-one basis, and introduce the newcomer to A.A.'s Twelve Steps of personal recovery and its Twelve Traditions, which sustain the Fellowship itself.

Meetings: At the heart of the program are its meetings, which are conducted autonomously by A.A. groups in cities and towns throughout the world, even in jails, institutions and on military bases. Anyone may attend open meetings of A.A. These usually consist of talks by one or more speakers who share impressions of their past illness and their present recovery in A.A. Some open meetings—to which helping professionals, the media and others are invited—are held for the specific purpose of informing the nonalcoholic (and possibly alcoholic) public about A.A. Closed meeting are for alcoholics only.

Alcoholics recovering in A.A. generally attend several meetings each week.

Anonymity. Anonymity helps the Fellowship to govern itself by principles rather than personalities; by attraction rather than promotion. We openly share our program of recovery, but not the names of the individuals in it.

What A.A. Does NOT Do

A.A. does not: Furnish initial motivation for alcoholics to recover; solicit members; engage in or sponsor research; keep attendance records or case histories; join "counsels" or social agencies (although A.A. members, groups and service offices frequently cooperate with them); follow up or try to control its members; make medical or psychological diagnoses or prognoses; provide detox, rehabilitation or nursing services, hospitalization, drugs, or any medical or psychiatric treatment; offer religious services or host/sponsor retreats; engage in education about alcohol; provide housing, food, clothing, jobs, money or any other welfare or social services; provide domestic or vocational counseling; accept any money for its services or any contributions from non–A.A. sources; provide letters of reference to parole boards, lawyers, court officials, social agencies, employers, etc.

Referrals from Judicial, Health Care, Military, or other Professionals

Today numerous A.A. members come to us from judicial, health care, military or other professionals. Some arrive voluntarily; others do not.

A.A. does not discriminate against any prospective member. Who made the referral to A.A. is not what interests us—it is the problem drinker who elicits our concern.

Proof of attendance at meetings. Sometimes a referral source asks for proof of attendance at A.A. meetings.

- *Groups cooperate in different ways.* There is no set procedure. The nature and extent of any group's involvement in this process is entirely up to the individual group.
- Some groups, with the consent of the prospective member, have an A.A. member acknowledge attendance on a slip that has been furnished by the referral source. The referred person is responsible for returning the proof of attendance.

Singleness of Purpose and Problems Other Than Alcohol

Some professionals refer to alcoholism and drug addiction as "substance abuse" or "chemical dependency." Nonalcoholics are, therefore, sometimes introduced to A.A. and encouraged to attend A.A. meetings. Nonalcoholics may attend open A.A. meetings as observers, but only those with a drinking problem may attend closed meetings.

A.A. Members and Medications

A.A. does not provide medical advice; all medical advice and treatment should come from a qualified health care professional. The suggestions provided in the pamphlet "The A.A. Member—Medications and Other Drugs" may help A.A. members minimize the risk of relapse.

How to Make Referrals to A.A.

Alcoholics Anonymous can be found on the Internet at www.aa.org and in most telephone directories by looking for "Alcoholics Anonymous" or "A.A." (Some professionals ask the person they are referring to call the local A.A. number while still in the office, thus offering an immediate opportunity to reach out for help).

Or you can contact the General Service Office (G.S.O.) of Alcoholics Anonymous for help and information. G.S.O.'s A.A. website, aa.org, can aid in finding local resources. Additionally, online A.A. meetings are available, which members of the military and others often use when they are in places where there are no meetings nearby (Alcoholics Anonymous World Services. [2018a]. https://www.aa.org/assets/en_US/p-46_ifyouareaprofessional.pdf).

APPENDIX D

Dr. Kevin McCauley's Ten Principles of Successful Addiction Treatment

In his CD, *The First Year in Recovery*, addiction physician Dr. Kevin McCauley outlines ten principles essential to a 95 percent success rate of recovery from addiction (2007).

Dr. McCauley worked with addicted commercial and military pilots who were highly motivated to recover and resume flying. His principles form the foundation of the Pilot Recovery Program, also called Return to Flight. McCauley references the FAA-funded substance abuse program for impaired pilots, the Human Intervention and Motivation Study (HIMS), which coordinates identification, treatment, and return to flight for pilots with substance issues (www.himsprogram.com). He notes that not following through on any part of the program lessens the probability of success; that each compromise in adherence to the program's principles can reduce the chance of a successful recovery.

Impaired doctors and nurses achieve an 85 to 95 percent recovery rate in programs that are based on the Pilot Program protocol, and the Pilot Program principles can be applied to other populations with the expectation of high rates of success.

Below, we have summarized Dr. McCauley's ten main principles. Note how closely they relate to the FRT principles. For simplicity and ease of reading, the pronoun, "he," has been used below; the principles apply equally to women and gender-nonconforming individuals in recovery.

McCauley's Ten Principles:

1. *90 Days of Residential Treatment.* It has been demonstrated that both 30 and 60 days of treatment are insufficient to provide a solid foundation for recovery. A full 90 days in a residential program provides a strong base for ongoing recovery.

2. *Seamless Transition into a Sober Living Environment.* McCauley emphasizes that the addict should visit sober living houses—and choose the one he will move into—while still in residential treatment. Upon release from the inpatient facility, the recovering addict should be transported *directly* to the sober living environment, so there is no time during this vulnerable transition for the addict to obtain drugs or alcohol.

Appendix D. McCauley's Principles of Successful Addiction Treatment

3. *Frequent, Non-Random Drug Testing.* Drug testing must continue throughout the first year of recovery and be performed at frequent enough intervals (every two or three days) to detect any time the addict uses his drug of choice. Any lower frequency gives the addict a window in which to use with impunity, which is a disservice to the recovering addict: a clean test enhances motivation for recovery.

4. *Outpatient Treatment Program.* While the addict is residing at a sober living environment after being released from residential care, he needs to continue treatment. This will entail working with a drug addiction counselor and may include individual, family, and/or group therapy.

5. *Relapse Prevention Plan.* A recovering addict may be exposed to old triggers to drink or use, and new situations are likely to arise in which he will have impulses to use again. Very early in outpatient treatment—if this has not been done during the residential stay—it is helpful for an addict, in the presence of his therapist, to draw up a relapse prevention plan that spells out in detail who to call, where to go, and what to do when impulses to use arise. The addict should write out his plan, carry it with him at all times, and rely on it as a valuable recovery tool.

6. *90 AA Meetings in 90 Days.* "90 in 90" means that the addict should attend at least 90 meetings in his first 90 days of being in outpatient treatment. This gives the recovering addict a firm footing in the recovery community of Alcoholics Anonymous. In the environment of AA, the recovering addict can learn sober ways of thinking, behaving, and coping, and observe sober people who are creating sober lives for themselves. AA offers the addict a community in which to develop personal connections, and to feel a sense of belonging, with others who are also in recovery.

7. *Meeting with an Addiction Physician.* There can be medical complications resulting from addiction; a physician versed in the physical effects of addiction, and the physical changes that accompany recovery, will be best able to help the addict understand and manage any medical concerns.

8. *Meeting with an Addiction Psychiatrist.* There may be psychiatric issues that preceded addiction, or that arose during the period of use, or that developed during recovery. A psychiatrist who is knowledgeable about the psychological issues that accompany drug and alcohol dependence can distinguish psychological symptoms that are transitory aspects of recovery from those that may benefit from psychotropic medication. Sometimes an addict needs a period of time as a sober person before a psychiatrist can determine what symptoms are likely to clear up with sobriety.

9. *Return to Work.* Returning to work is an important aspect of becoming fully functional after a lapse into addiction. Furthermore, work helps build self-esteem and offsets the shame that generally accompanies addiction and job loss. Someone in early recovery may benefit from choosing a lower-stress job than

he had had previously, since the goal of working at this phase of recovery is to provide consistency, structure, responsibility, and an opportunity to perform well, rather than to embark on, or resume, a particular career path. For some people in recovery, return to a previous job is appropriate, but for others this is not the case. Determining what constitutes appropriate work for a specific individual is a topic that the recovering person can discuss with a therapist or group leader.

10. *Fun.* The dopamine that has been depleted in addiction needs replenishment. Learning non-drug-using, healthy ways to produce pleasure is essential to rebuilding the natural supplies of dopamine. Without dopamine, recovery will not be appealing; the addict will experience more pain than pleasure, and the option of returning to alcohol or drugs in order to feel good will be compelling.

Appendix E

Addiction/Codependency Family Treatment Agreement

The following are treatment recommendations:

Treatment for the Addict:

1. Addict agrees to stop all substance use, detox, and if appropriate, move into a sober living environment.
2. Individual and Family Therapy.
3. Addict agrees to attend 12-Step meetings, get a sponsor, work the Steps, go to 90 meetings in 90 days, and then continue to go to regular meetings until graduation from the program.
4. Addict agrees to frequent, random drug testing.
5. Addict agrees to get a developmentally appropriate, honorable, entry-level, full-time job.
6. Addict agrees to stay away from "using friends" for 90 days.
7. Addict agrees to go to a detox facility if they relapse.
8. Failure to succeed in this Intensive Outpatient Program (IOP) will result in a referral to a Residential Treatment Program.
9. Referral to other 12-Step programs may be made if the need arises.

Treatment for the Codependents:

1. Individual and Family Therapy.
2. Codependent agrees to attend a minimum of two Al-Anon meetings each week, get a sponsor, and work the 12 Steps.
3. Codependent agrees to remain abstinent from substances during the initial two months of treatment.
4. Referral to other 12-Step programs may be made if the need arises.

Treatment for the Family System:

1. Family Therapy.
2. Family agrees to attend, together, three Al-Anon meetings in the first 90

days of treatment (meeting to be chosen by the FRT therapist). (Arrive 10 minutes early, stay 10 minutes afterward.)

3. Family agrees to attend, together, three AA meetings in the first 90 days of treatment (meeting to be chosen by the FRT therapist). (Arrive 10 minutes early, stay 10 minutes afterward.)

Graduation:

The Intensive Phase ends after all adult family members reach these milestones:

1. Addict: One year of continuous sobriety and completion of the 12 Steps.
2. Codependent: Completion of the 12 Steps.

Signature _____ Date _____

Signature _____ Date _____

Signature (Counselor) _____ Date _____

_____ Copy to client

Appendix F

Additional Resources

For more information about Family Recovery Therapy, please visit www.LarryFritzlan.com where you will find additional resources such as training opportunities and other useful information. The website also provides links to the books listed below, co-written with Avis Rumney, LMFT. Each book, appropriate both for professionals and family members, provides additional case studies tailored to a specific issue related to alcoholism and addiction.

My Addicted Child: A Family Systems Approach That Works (2015)
My Addicted Parent: A Family Systems Approach That Works (2017a)
My Addicted Spouse: A Family Systems Approach That Works (2017b)

The videos listed below offer some additional perspectives on addiction and addiction treatment:

Rehab: Last Week Tonight with John Oliver (HBO)
https://www.youtube.com/watch?v=hWQiXv0sn9Y&t=1021s
(Oliver, 2018)

How Childhood Trauma Leads to Addiction–Gabor Maté
https://www.youtube.com/watch?v=BVg2bfqblGI
(After Skool, 2021)

The Moyers' Journey from Addiction to Recovery
https://www.youtube.com/watch?v=EI86nx4SuB4
(The LBJ Library, 2014)

Everything you think you know about addiction is wrong | Johann Hari
https://www.youtube.com/watch?v=PY9DcIMGxMs
(TED, 2015)

William Cope Moyers on Addiction (The Mary Hanson Show)
https://www.youtube.com/watch?v=WKbO63JQNlg
(Hanson, 2019)

Addiction: A Family's Path to Recovery Bill Moyers, William Moyers and Judith Moyers
https://www.youtube.com/watch?v=QEBWn7RwbEM
(92nd Street Y)

APPENDIX G

Testing Instruments

There are several testing instruments used to assess for addiction. Clinicians may want to use the MAST (Selzer, 1971), or the AUDIT (Babor et al., 2001), as noted on p. 193, both of which are available online. We include here AA's Twelve Questions (Alcoholics Anonymous World Services, 2018b). This publication is designed for individuals to assess their behavior with respect to alcohol. It is *the individual* who needs to answer these questions for themselves, and to decide whether they are an alcoholic. However, other family members can find it informative to review the questions to learn about behaviors that can accompany addiction. Following is AA's publication, *Is AA for You? Twelve Questions Only You Can Answer,* which we have included in its entirety.

Is A.A. for You? Twelve Questions Only You Can Answer

Only you can decide whether you want to give A.A. a try—whether you think it can help you. We who are in A.A. came because we finally gave up trying to control our drinking. We still hated to admit that we could never drink safely. Then we heard from other A.A. members that we were sick. (We thought so for years!) We found out that many people suffered from the same feelings of guilt and loneliness and hopelessness that we did. We found out that we had these feelings because we had the disease of alcoholism.

We decided to try to face up to what alcohol had done to us. Here are some of the questions we tried to answer *honestly*. If we answered YES to four or more questions, we were in deep trouble with our drinking. See how you do. Remember, there is no disgrace in facing up to the fact that you have a problem.

1. Have you ever decided to stop drinking for a week or so, but only lasted for a couple of days?

Most of us in A.A. made all kinds of promises to ourselves and to our families. We could not keep them. Then we came to A.A. A.A. said: *"Just try not to drink today."* (If you do not drink today, you cannot get drunk today.)

2. Do you wish people would mind their own business about your drinking—stop telling you what to do?

In A.A. we do not *tell* anyone to do anything. We just talk about our own drinking, the trouble we got into, and how we stopped. We will be glad to help you, if you want us to.

3. Have you ever switched from one kind of drink to another in the hope that this would keep you from getting drunk?

We tried all kinds of ways. We made our drinks weak. Or just drank beer. Or we did not drink cocktails. Or only drank on weekends. You name it, we tried it. But if we drank *anything* with alcohol in it, we usually got drunk eventually.

4. Have you had to have an eye-opener upon awakening during the past year? Do you need a drink to get started, or to stop shaking?

This is a pretty sure sign that you are not drinking "socially."

5. Do you envy people who can drink without getting into trouble?

At one time or another, most of us have wondered why we were not like most people, who really can take it or leave it.

6. Have you had problems connected with drinking during the past year?

Be honest! Doctors say that if you have a problem with alcohol and keep on drinking, it will get worse—never better. Eventually, you will die, or end up in an institution for the rest of your life. The only hope is to stop drinking.

7. Has your drinking caused trouble at home?

Before we came into A. A., most of us said that it was the people or problems at home that made us drink. We could not see that our drinking just made everything worse. It never solved problems anywhere or anytime.

8. Do you ever try to get "extra" drinks at a party because you do not get enough?

Most of us used to have a "few" before we started out if we thought it was going to be that kind of party. And if drinks were not served fast enough, we would go someplace else to get more.

9. Do you tell yourself you can stop drinking any time you want to, even though you keep getting drunk when you don't mean to?

Many of us kidded ourselves into thinking that we drank because we wanted to. After we came into A.A., we found out that once we started to drink, we couldn't stop.

10. Have you missed days of work or school because of drinking?

Many of us admit now that we "called in sick" lots of times when the truth was that we were hungover or on a drunk.

11. Do you have "blackouts"?

A "blackout" is when we have been drinking hours or days that we cannot remember. When we came to A.A., we found out that this is a pretty sure sign of alcoholic drinking.

12. Have you ever felt that your life would be better if you did not drink?

Many of us started to drink because drinking made life seem better, at least for a while. By the time we got into A.A., we felt trapped. We were drinking to live and living to drink. We were sick and tired of being sick and tired.

What Is Your Score?

Did you answer YES four or more times? If so, you are probably in trouble with alcohol. Why do we say this? Because thousands of people in A.A. have said so for many years. They found out the truth about themselves—the hard way.

But again, only *you* can decide whether you think A.A. is for you. Try to keep an open mind on the subject. If the answer is YES, we will be glad to show you how we stopped drinking ourselves. Just call.

A.A. does not promise to solve your life's problems. But we can show you how we are learning to live without drinking "one day at a time." We stay away from that "first drink." If there is no first one, there cannot be a tenth one. And when we got rid of alcohol, we found that life became much more manageable. (Alcoholics Anonymous World Services, 2018c, https://www.aa.org/assets/en_US/p-3_isaaforyou.pdf)

APPENDIX H

The Cost of Addiction Treatment

The cost of addiction treatment is far less than the cost of *not* treating addiction—costs incurred by individuals, families, government agencies, and costs to society as a whole of untreated addiction are immense. In an ideal world, treating all medical and psychological diseases would constitute a cost-savings approach that benefits society as a whole. The following is from the National Institute of Health:

> Principles of Drug Addiction Treatment: A Research-Based Guide (Third Edition)
> Is drug addiction treatment worth its cost?
>
> Substance abuse costs our Nation over $600 billion annually and treatment can help reduce these costs. Drug addiction treatment has been shown to reduce associated health and social costs by far more than the cost of the treatment itself. Treatment is also much less expensive than its alternatives, such as incarcerating addicted persons. For example, the average cost for 1 full year of methadone maintenance treatment is approximately $4,700 per patient, whereas 1 full year of imprisonment costs approximately $24,000 per person.
>
> According to several conservative estimates, every dollar invested in addiction treatment programs yields a return of between $4 and $7 in reduced drug-related crime, criminal justice costs, and theft. When savings related to healthcare are included, total savings can exceed costs by a ratio of 12 to 1. Major savings to the individual and to society also stem from fewer interpersonal conflicts; greater workplace productivity; and fewer drug-related accidents, including overdoses and deaths. (National Institute on Drug Abuse [NIDA], 2020, June 3.)

As an addiction treatment provider for 25 years, I have conducted my family-based intensive outpatient program as part of my private practice. I have also created and directed a residential treatment program. While much of my work has been "fee for service" (paid directly by the clients), some of it has been paid for or reimbursed by insurance companies.

Unfortunately, getting reimbursement from health insurance companies can be challenging. Insurance companies are corporations that benefit from limiting what they pay for, which can result in failure to pay for needed treatment. At the present time, I only accept clients who are willing to pay for my services out of pocket. I give them a superbill which they can submit to their insurance company for reimbursement. Some clients get most of the fees reimbursed, some get a fraction of the fees reimbursed, and some do not get any reimbursement at all. Each health insurance company has its own regulations about what costs they will cover, and the regulations also vary depending on the individual's particular health plan.

I understand the dilemma families face regarding payment for treatment, and occasionally I offer my services *pro bono* (free of charge). Treatment can be costly. However, I remind my clients that failing to treat addiction early can lead to greater expenses later. Addiction is a chronic disorder. Delayed treatment, and the deterioration of the addict and of the family situation that can occur over time, means that deferred treatment can result in additional expense—not only may treatment be more prolonged and more costly, but there are medical, psychological, legal, and other consequences that far outweigh the cost of treatment. Delaying treatment can also put an addict or a family member's life at risk.

My hope is that addicts and families—not to mention health insurance companies and society at large—will come to understand the progressive nature of addiction and begin treatment as soon as they recognize the possibility of a drug or alcohol problem. A motivated individual can find treatment through low-fee agencies, government programs, and social services agencies such as the Salvation Army, which provides free treatment to those who qualify.

The following are some general guidelines for treatment costs. However, costs do vary in different geographic areas:

- Working with a clinician in private practice: $75 to $300 per session.
- 30-day residential treatment program: $15,000 to $50,000.
- 90-day residential treatment program: $25,000 to $100,000.
- 90-day intensive outpatient program: $10,000 to $15,000.
- Sober living homes: $1,000 a month.
- Upscale sober living homes: $2,000 to $5,000 a month.
- Family Recovery Therapy, as presented in this book, depending on clinician: $12,000 to $25,000 for 12 months.

Insurance reimbursement varies from one insurance company to another, and also varies depending on the geographical area. Some insurance companies reimburse 100 percent of the costs of addiction treatment (once a deductible has been met), and other companies cover only a small percentage of the cost of treatment. Some insurance companies will reimburse some portion of the cost of clinical sessions, but will not cover any drug testing charges. If you want to have some of your costs reimbursed by insurance, it is best to check with your insurance company to find out its specific reimbursement policies.

APPENDIX I

"REQUIEM: My Mother's Unspeakable Illness" by Cynthia Gorney

A daughter tries to redeem a brutal, embarrassing death.

In my mother's hospital room there was a single window, and if you stood before the window you could see the Aerial Bridge. In Minnesota this is a famous bridge, often pictured on postcards, and around the bridge stretched Lake Superior, flat and pearled and vast as the sea. My mother told me over the telephone that she had a view of the lake. I was standing in my kitchen in California and willing my voice not to crack. "You checked into the hospital five days ago without letting any of us know," I said carefully into the telephone, and when she answered me I thought stupidly for a moment: She is drunk in the hospital, how can she be drunk in the hospital? "I don't want you to come," said my mother, thickly, making herself sound jolly. "I wouldn't know what to do with you. I just got tired of feeling sick, my stomach hurt, I was coughing so much. The nurses are nice. I have a view of the lake."

All of this took place in the spring, just a little while ago, and I am writing about it now because I want you to know what happens when someone you love dies of alcoholism.

I am not going to preach, or call in the sociologists, or heave around a lot of numbers and research theories and Alcoholics Anonymous advice. I did that in my own scrabbling way when my mother was alive, and while I did it my mother went on drinking. She drank quietly and discreetly, in the privacy of her pleasantly cluttered home. She was active in her church and traveled internationally and volunteered on committees to help the homeless and care for Latin American refugees; she read prodigiously and wrote in three languages and had friends in such places as Leon, Nicaragua, and Harbin, China. You can see that she was a woman of curiosity and learning and great intelligence. She died in March of cirrhosis of the liver, which is also what kills the men under blankets by the sewer grates.

I want you to know this because if you are like me or like my mother you think you know it, but you don't, not really. You don't know that when an educated lady in her 60s has cirrhosis she will be lying in a hospital bed near the oncology wing, and that when you get off the elevator the nurses will come toward you quickly because they need to prepare you for what you are about to see. You don't know that your first glimpse into the open door of the hospital room will be of skin, the skin of a leg or an arm, you can't tell which because the skin is green and it seems impossible that this could in fact be human skin. There must be makeup involved, or some malfunction of hospital lighting. The nurses are murmuring around you *she looks pretty bad right now* and the body shifts position and you see that it is not bad lighting after all. This is what cirrhosis does to the body. Before it kills you, it turns you ocher green.

I wish somebody had told my mother that before it happened to her.

She was unbearably thirsty and for the first few days, when they thought she might recover, they gave her water only in tiny sips. When my brothers and I arrived she asked us to sneak her some water. I suppose the irony of this quest was not lost on any of us because my mother had never asked us to sneak her alcohol. In our house, the gin and vodka bottles were delivered by the grocery boy and left just as seamlessly in the household garbage, having been emptied in dignified fashion into large glasses with slices of lime. My mother never drove erratically or beat us with hairbrushes or acted like one of the crazy women in the movie star exposes. It was only after she went through a residential treatment program and kept drinking anyway that she began hiding the bottles, putting them under her clothes in the bottom of the suitcase when she came to visit. She never talked about it. When we tried to talk about it she waved her hand and changed the subject, and we sat moving our mouths noiselessly behind the thick glass wall that she had pulled from the air and slammed into the ground between herself and the rest of us. She was able to do this because we were her children and made ourselves too small to beat it down.

In the hospital she wore an eye patch when we arrived, but by the second day the nurses had taken it off and we saw that one eye looked as though it had exploded from inside. Apparently this was not one of the things that hurt her, but a spidery web of blood had spread across the eye and it was difficult to look at her face without staring at the bad eye. Her belly was swollen where the fluids were building up. Her skin was loose around her bones, crepey and soft and green. When I stroked her head, her hair seemed very shiny and black to me, and I remember thinking that this was the only part of her that held what looked like life, the hair on the top of her head.

The doctor was a resident who seemed desperately young, with his unsmiling face and circles under his eyes. He took my brothers and me into a small room with a table and told us the alcohol had turned our mother's liver into something like a piece of leather. He said livers are remarkably resilient and that some people are able to survive with only a portion of the liver left, so that if they had gotten hold of my mother earlier, the doctors might have been able to save her, but that now her liver had ceased any function at all and this was shutting down her kidneys and causing peritonitis, systemic collapse, cardiac exhaustion, various other medical details I was working to follow. The resident said it would take a few days for her to die, perhaps longer, and that if we were able to do it, we might wish to use this time to say goodbye in a way that felt appropriate to us. When we left the room my brothers and I stood with our arms around each other's shoulders and our heads pressed together like a tripod. We had done this in the residential treatment program, which was the only other time, since we were grown, that I had seen my brothers cry.

We called her priest, who was a tough-faced Episcopalian with short black hair and a strong handshake. He told us he was a recovering alcoholic and listened to me without saying anything when I stood in the hallway with my hands jammed into my pockets and said I don't understand, I have never understood, why she couldn't ask for help. She went into the program because she was hallucinating and as soon as she stopped hallucinating, I said to the priest, and the wall came back down and nobody ever busted through again. And the priest said, I know, that is how alcoholism works. The disease keeps you from naming the disease, said my mother's priest; you're so deep inside it that you can't pick up the telephone and pronounce the words: Help me.

The priest described standing in a room at a party, when he was drinking, and seeing that across the room was a man from Alcoholics Anonymous, and the priest just went on standing there, he said, knowing he was sick, knowing this man had a kind of medicine that could help cure him, and being unable to walk toward this man and speak. "That is the disease," the priest said. "I could not do it."

In the afternoon we moved my mother into the hospice, where patients go to die.

There is a lot more I could tell you. Some is about the passages I understand lie before each of us, the last letting go of a hand too tired to squeeze back, and some is about the sound of the breath of a person whose liver is like a piece of leather. In the hospital halls it was possible to hear my mother's breathing two rooms away; when she inhaled there was a small moan and when she exhaled there was a louder moan. I had to walk some distance down the hall, past the oncology wing, to leave the sound of the breaths. At the end of the hall was a room with a curtainless window and a wide view of the lake, and that was when a nurse came to tell me that I needed to go to my mother's room. When she put her hand on my elbow to steady me I knew that my mother had died, and I am telling you this because nobody told it to me: Alcohol killed her, not in the metaphorical way that children of alcoholics talk about in their Emotional Deprivation groups, but precisely and literally and in such a way that for the last three days of her life she had green skin and a bloodied eye and made a terrible noise every time she breathed.

I want someone else to hear this. I want to imagine that in a pleasantly cluttered house somewhere there is a man or a woman who doesn't know, truly doesn't know, and could read about my mother and say, now I do. My mother would have raged at me for shaming her in public, for that is how she would have thought of it. She was a proud woman, and I believe she died frightened and too ashamed to repeat aloud the name of the illness that killed her. I repeat it for her now: Alcoholism. Alcoholism-induced cirrhosis of the liver. Alcoholism-induced peritonitis, followed by renal failure, followed by cardiac arrest. If one person sees these words and picks up a telephone and asks for help, my betrayal will have been worthwhile. (Gorney, 1993, May 2).

Appendix J

From Addiction to Healthy Self

This diagram represents the author's perspective on his progression from addiction to recovery, a process spanning several decades.

The left part of this diagram shows me in the grasp of addiction, unable to clearly process emotions, feelings, and thoughts, or to benefit from education, and bereft of loving relationships or a spiritual connection. The right part of the diagram depicts where I am today. I have developed a healthy self and have the ability to experience emotions and feelings, and to think clearly, and to process my inner world. I have benefited from education. I participate in loving relationships and I experience a spiritual center in my life.

As an addict, I was in a desperate struggle to get my medicine—the substances I craved for relief—and then to do whatever was necessary to "keep it together." Meanwhile, I was gradually losing my capacity to hold things together.

When I was drinking, I was mostly angry, depressed, or anxious. I had little time or inclination to explore my emotions and feelings. My relationships with others mirrored my own retarded development. Most of my peers were substance users. Pursuing education was not a priority. I was caught in a perpetual struggle both internally, and with the world outside my skin. I had little love or joy in my life.

When I got sober, I began the slow process of growth and moving towards

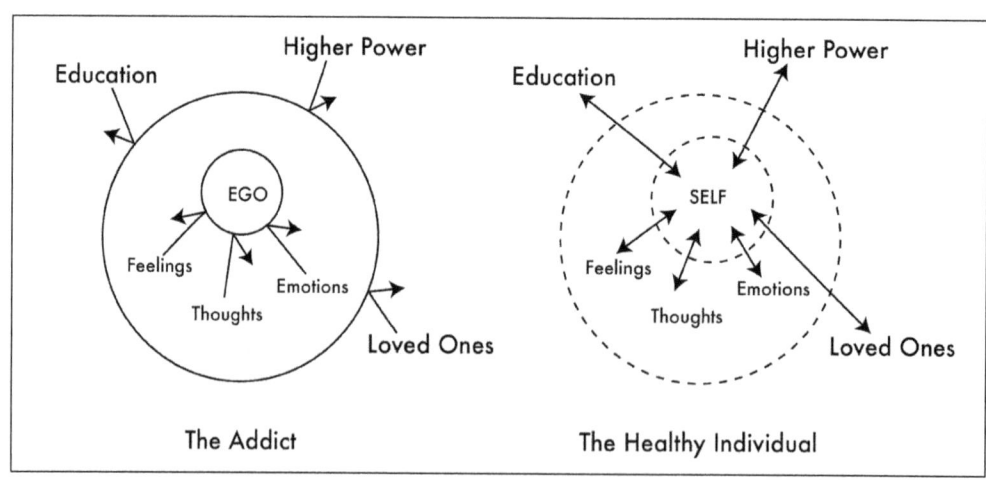

A.1 *Addict vs. Health Person.*

health. With considerable help, I was able to achieve a level of development that I might have reached earlier, had I not succumbed to nearly two decades of active addiction.

I was able to understand that I had a disease that I could not control, that there was a path toward healing, and that I could seek help from many available professionals and resources—medical doctors, psychotherapists, psychologists, support groups, recovery mentors, meditation retreats, spiritual guides, and to connect with several communities of individuals invested in personal growth.

Today, with over four decades of recovery, I can say that I'm good. I have a solid, loving marriage with a wonderful person. I went back to school, got my master's degree, and became a licensed psychotherapist. I have taught courses in graduate school and written a number of books. I discovered that while I have a body, feelings, thoughts, and an ego, I am more than all these parts. I have discovered an experience beyond my body and mind that I call spirituality. I have recovered much of what I lost to addiction, and I am now healthy.

Appendix K

How to Find Social Support Groups

12-Step Social Support Options

To find 12-Step meetings in your area, search online for: Al-Anon and your city, Alcoholics Anonymous and your city, or Co-dependents Anonymous and your city. For additional information about these programs, go to their respective websites which are listed below:

Al-Anon
www.Al-Anon.org

Alcoholics Anonymous
www.AA.org

Co-dependents Anonymous
www.CODA.org

Non–12-Step Social Support Options

Below are listed some non–12-Step recovery organizations:

Celebrate Recovery (Christian 12-Step)
www.celebraterecovery.com

LifeRing Secular Recovery
www.lifering.org

Secular Organizations for Sobriety
www.sossobriety.org

SMART Recovery®
www.smartrecovery.org

Women for Sobriety
www.womenforsobriety.org

Appendix L

Spiritual Experience

After publication of the original version of the Big Book, *Alcoholics Anonymous* (1939), there was confusion and misunderstanding about AA's use of the word "spiritual." In the second edition of the Big Book published in 1955, an appendix entitled "Spiritual Experience" was added to help clarify what AA meant by "spiritual." The subsequent editions of the Big Book also include this appendix.

Below is the appendix, "Spiritual Experience," from the fourth edition of *Alcoholics Anonymous* (2001, pp. 567–568), reprinted in its entirety with permission from AA World Services.

>The terms "spiritual experience" and "spiritual awakening" are used many times in this book which, upon careful reading, shows that the personality change sufficient to bring about recovery from alcoholism has manifested itself among us in many different forms.
>
>Yet it is true that our first printing gave many readers the impression that these personality changes, or religious experiences, must be in the nature of sudden and spectacular upheavals. Happily for everyone, this conclusion is erroneous.
>
>In the first few chapters a number of sudden revolutionary changes are described. Though it was not our intention to create such an impression, many alcoholics have nevertheless concluded that in order to recover they must acquire an immediate and overwhelming "God-consciousness" followed at once by a vast change in feeling and outlook.
>
>Among our rapidly growing membership of thousands of alcoholics such transformations, though frequent, are by no means the rule. Most of our experiences are what the psychologist William James calls the "educational variety" because they develop slowly over a period of time. Quite often friends of the newcomer are aware of the difference long before he is himself. He finally realizes that he has undergone a profound alteration in his reaction to life; that such a change could hardly have been brought about by himself alone. What often takes place in a few months could seldom have been accomplished by years of self discipline. With few exceptions our members find that they have tapped an unsuspected inner resource which they presently identify with their own conception of a Power greater than themselves.

Most of us think this awareness of a Power greater than ourselves is the essence of spiritual experience. Our more religious members call it "God-consciousness."

Most emphatically we wish to say that any alcoholic capable of honestly facing his problems in the light of our experience can recover, provided he does not close his mind to all spiritual concepts. He can only be defeated by an attitude of intolerance or belligerent denial.

We find that no one need have difficulty with the spirituality of the program. *Willingness, honesty and open mindedness are the essentials of recovery. But these are indispensable.*

"There is a principle which is a bar against all information, which is proof against all arguments and which cannot fail to keep a man in everlasting ignorance—that principle is contempt prior to investigation."

—HERBERT SPENCER

References

Ablon, J. (2018, April 30). Al-Anon family groups: Impetus for learning and change through the presentation of alternatives. *The American Journal of Psychotherapy*. https://doi.org/101176/appi.psychotherapy.1974.28.1.30.

After Skool. (2021, January 19). *How childhood trauma leads to addiction-Gabor Maté* [Video]. https://www.youtube.com/watch?v=BVg2bfqblGI

Al-Anon Family Groups. (2018). *Intimacy in alcoholic relationships: A collection of Al-Anon personal stories.*

Al-Anon Family Groups. (n.d.-a). *Detachment.* (Pamphlet 19) Retrieved from https://al-anon.org/pdf/S19.pdf on 2021, May 30.

Al-Anon Family Groups. (n.d.-b). *88% of members say their mental health improved after attending Al-Anon.* Retrieved from https://al-anon.org/blog/members-mental-health-improved-after-attending-al-anon/ on 2021, May 30.

Al-Anon Family Groups. (n.d.-c). *Suggested preamble.* Retrieved from https://al-anon.org/pdf/preamble.pdf on 2021, August 31.

Alcoholics Anonymous. (n.d.). Wikipedia. Retrieved August 31, 2021, from https://en.wikipedia.org/wiki/Alcoholics_Anonymous

Alcoholics Anonymous: The story of how many thousands of men and women have recovered from alcoholism (2nd ed.). (1955). Alcoholics Anonymous World Services, Inc.

Alcoholics Anonymous: The story of how more than one hundred men have recovered from alcoholism. (1939). Works Publishing Company.

Alcoholics Anonymous World Services. (1981). *Twelve steps and twelve traditions.*

Alcoholics Anonymous World Services. (2001). *Alcoholics anonymous* (4th ed.).

Alcoholics Anonymous World Services. (2018a). *If you are a professional, Alcoholics Anonymous wants to work with you.* Retrieved from https://www.aa.org/assets/en_US/p-46_ifyouareaprofessional.pdf on 2021, June 26.

Alcoholics Anonymous World Services. (2018b). *Is A.A. for you: Twelve questions only you can answer.* Retrieved from https://www.aa.org/assets/en_US/p-3_isaaforyou.pdf on 2021, June 25.

Alcoholics Anonymous®. (n.d.-a). *A.A. around the world*. Alcoholics Anonymous®. Retrieved August 24, 2021, from https://www.aa.org/pages/en_us/aa-around-the-world

Alcoholics Anonymous®. (n.d.-b). *Anonymity letter to the media*. Alcoholics Anonymous®. Retrieved August 25, 2021, from https://www.aa.org/pages/en_US/anonymity-letter-to-media

Alcoholics Anonymous®. (n.d.-c). *History and resources*. Alcoholics Anonymous®. Retrieved August 24, 2021, from https://www.aa.org/pages/en_US/history-and-resources

Alcoholics Anonymous®. (n.d.-d). *Members of the clergy ask about Alcoholics Anonymous*. Alcoholics Anonymous®. Retrieved August 25, 2021, from https://www.aa.org/pages/en_US/members-of-the-clergy-ask-about-alcoholics-anonymous

Altarum. (2018, February 13). *Economic toll of opioid crisis in U.S. exceeds $1 trillion since 2001*. Altarum. Retrieved July 8, 2021, from https://altarum.org/news/economic-toll-opioid-crisis-us-exceeded-1-trillion-2001

American Psychiatric Association. (1994). *Diagnostic and statistical manual of mental disorders* (4th ed.).

American Psychiatric Association. (2013). *Diagnostic and statistical manual of mental disorders* (5th ed.). https://doi.org/10.1176/appi.books.9780890425596

American Society of Addiction Medicine. (2011, August 15). *Public policy statement: Definition of addiction*. Retrieved from https://www.asam.org/docs/default-source/public-policy-statements/1definition_of_addiction_long_4-11.pdf?sfvrsn=a8f64512_4 on 2021, June 1.

American Society of Addiction Medicine. (2019). *Definition of addiction*. Retrieved from https://www.asam.org/Quality-Science/definition-of-addiction on 2021, May 30.

Babor, T.F., Higgins-Biddle, J.C., Saunders J.B., & Monteiro, M.G. (2001). *The alcohol use disorders identification test: Guidelines for use in primary care* (2nd ed.). World Health Organization Department of Mental Health and Substance Dependence. Retrieved from https://www.who.int/publications/i/item/audit-the-alcohol-use-disorders-identification-test-guidelines-for-use-in-primary-health-care on 2021, June 19.

Beattie, M. (1986). *Codependent No More.* Hazelden.

Bettinardi-Angres, K., & Angres, D.H. (2010). Understanding the disease of addiction. *Journal of Nursing Regulation, 1*(2), 31–37. https://www.google.com/url?sa=t&rct=j&q=&esrc=s&source=web&cd=&ved=2ahUKEwjGw_b_5sryAhWSHDQIHWkYCF0QFnoECBsQAQ&url=https%3A%2F%2Fwww.ncsbn.org%2FUnderstanding_the_Disease_of_Addiction.pdf&usg=AOvVaw3TNZ9h6gLVR3JjJ8fWAcu9

Bever, L. (2018, January 31). A town of 3,200 was flooded with nearly 21 million pain pills as addiction crisis worsened, lawmakers say. *Washington Post,* Health. https://www.washingtonpost.com/news/to-your-health/wp/2018/01/31/a-town-of-3200-was-flooded-with-21-million-pain-pills-as-addiction-crisis-worsened-lawmakers-say/

Bowen, M. (1961). Family psychotherapy. *American Journal of Orthopsychiatry, 31,* 40–60.

Bowen, M. (1966). The use of family theory in clinical practice. In *Comprehensive Group Psychotherapy, 7,* 345–374.

Bowen, M. (1971). Family therapy and family group therapy. In H. Kaplan & B. Sadock (Eds.), *Comprehensive group psychotherapy* (pp. 384–421). Williams and Wilkins.

Bowen, M. (1974). Alcoholism as viewed through family systems theory and family psychotherapy. *Annals of the New York Academy of Sciences, 233,* 115–122.

Bowen, M. (1978). *Family therapy in clinical practice.* Jason Aronson.

Brown, S. (1985). *Treating the Alcoholic: A Developmental Model of Recovery.* Wiley.

Brown, S. & Lewis, V. (1999). *The alcoholic family in recovery: A developmental model.* The Guilford Press.

Brown, S. (Ed.). (1995). *Treating alcoholism.* Jossey-Bass.

Cadoret, R.J., Cain, C.A., & Grove, W.M. (1980, May). Development of alcoholism in adoptees raised apart from alcoholic biologic relatives. *Arch Gen Psychiatry, 37*(5), 561–563. doi:10.1001/archpsyc.1980.01780180075008.

Cadoret, R.J. (1994). Genetic and environmental contributions to heterogeneity in alcoholism: Findings from the Iowa adoption studies. *Annals of New York Academy of Science, 708,* 59–71.

Cadoret, R.J., Troughton, E., & Gorman, T.W. (1987). Genetic and environmental factors in alcohol abuse and antisocial personality. *Journal of Studies on Alcohol, 48,* 1–8.

Center for Substance Abuse Treatment. (2004). *Substance abuse treatment and family therapy.* Treatment Improvement Protocol (TIP) Series, No. 39. Report No.: (SMA) 04–3957. PMID: 22514845. Substance Abuse and Mental Health Services Administration (US); https://www.ncbi.nlm.nih.gov/books/NBK64269/

Centers for Medicare & Medicaid Services. (n.d.). *The Mental Health Parity and Addiction Equity Act (MHPAEA).* Centers for Medicare & Medicaid Services. Retrieved August 24, 2021, from https://www.cms.gov/CCIIO/Programs-and-Initiatives/Other-Insurance-Protections/mhpaea_factsheet

Cermak, T. (1986). *Diagnosing and treating codependence.* The Johnson Institute.

Chappel, J.N., & DuPont, R.L. (1999). Twelve-step and mutual-help programs for addictive disorders. *Psychiatric Clinics of North America, 22*(2), 425–446.

Compton, W.M., Blanco, C., & Wargo, E.M. (2015). Integrating addiction services into general medicine. *JAMA, 314*(22), 2401–2402.

Dekkers, A., De Ruysscher, C., & Vanderplasschen, W. (2020). Perspectives on addiction recovery: Focus groups with individuals in recovery and family members. *Addiction Research & Theory, 28*(6), 526–536. https://doi.org/10.1080/16066359.2020.1714037

Dennis, M. & Scott, C.K. (2007). Managing addiction as a chronic condition. *Addiction Science and Clinical Practice, 4*(1), 45–55.

Dodes, L. (2002). *The heart of addiction: A new approach to understanding and managing alcoholism and other addictive behaviors.* HarperCollins.

Dube, S.R., Felitti, V.J., Dong, M., Chapman, D.P., Giles, W.H., & Anda R.F. (2003). Childhood abuse, neglect, and household dysfunction and the risk of illicit drug use: The Adverse Childhood Experiences study. *Pediatrics, 111*(3), 564–572. https://doi.org/10.1542/peds.111.3.564

Erikson, E. (1963). *Childhood and society.* Norton.

Erikson, M. (2020, March 11) *Alcoholics Anonymous most effective path to alcohol abstinence.* Stanford Medicine News Center. Retrieved from https://med.stanford.edu/news/all-news/2020/03/alcoholics-anonymous-most-effective-path-to-alcohol-abstinence.html on 2021, May 30.

Erowid (n.d.). *Psychoactive plants and drugs.* Erowid. https://www.erowid.org/psychoactives/psychoactives.shtml

Felitti, V.J., Anda, R.F., Edwards, V., Koss, M.P., Marks, J.S., Nordenberg, D., Spitz, A.M., & Williamson, D.F. (1998, May 1). Relationship of child abuse and household dysfunction to many of the leading causes of death in adults: The adverse childhood experiences (ACE) study. *American Journal of Preventive Medicine, 14* (4), 245–248. https://doi.org/10.1016/S0749-3797(98)00017-8

Fox, M. (1983). *Original blessing: A primer in creation spirituality.* Bear & Company.

Fritzlan, L., & Rumney, A. (2015). *My Addicted Child.* Recovery Works.

Fritzlan, L., & Rumney, A. (2017a). *My Addicted Parent.* Recovery Works.

Fritzlan, L., & Rumney, A. (2017b). *My Addicted Spouse.* Recovery Works.

Galanter, M. (2018). Combining medically assisted treatment and twelve-step programming: A perspective and review. *The American Journal of*

Drug and Alcohol Abuse, 44(2),151–159.https://doi.org/10.1080/00952990.2017.1306747

Goldenberg, I., Stanton, M., & Goldenberg H. (2017). *Family therapy: An overview* (9th ed.). Cengage Learning.

Goldstein, R.Z., & Volkow, N. (2002, October 1). Drug addiction and its underlying neurobiological basis: Neuroimaging evidence for the involvement of the frontal cortex. *The American Journal of Psychiatry*. https://doi.org/10.1176/appi.ajp.159.10.1642

Gorney, C. (1993, May 2). "REQUIEM: My mother's unspeakable illness." *The Boston Sunday Globe*.

Gramlich, J. (2017, October 26). *Nearly half of Americans have a family member or close friend who's been addicted to drugs*. Pew Research Center. http://pewrsr.ch/2gFsr5b

Griffin, R.M. (2014, April 1). *10 health problems related to stress that you can fix*. WebMD. https://www.webmd.com/balance/stress-management/features/10-fixable-stress-related-health-problems

Hanh, T.N. (2006). Chanting from the heart: Buddhist ceremonies and daily practices. Parallax Press.

Hanson, M. (2019, May 4). *William Cope Moyers on Addiction (The Mary Hanson Show)* [Video]. https://www.youtube.com/watch?v=WKbO63JQNlg

Harris, D. (Narrator). (2015, June 24). Meditation 101: A beginner's guide. [Video] YouTube. Retrieved from https://www.youtube.com/watch?v=o-kMJBWk9E0 on 2001, June 18.

Horvath, A.T. (2000). Smart Recovery®: Addiction recovery support from a cognitive-behavioral perspective. *Journal of Rational-Emotive & Cognitive-Behavior Therapy, 18,* 181–191. https://doi.org/10.1023/A:1007831005098
https://www.drugabuse.gov/publications/principles-drug-addiction-treatment-research-based-guide-third-edition/preface

Jarvis, M., Williams, J., Hurford, M., Lindsay D., Lincoln, P., Giles, L., Luongo, P., & Safarian, T. (2017, June). Appropriate use of drug testing in clinical addiction medicine. *Journal of Addiction Medicine, 11*(3), 163–173. https://doi.org/10.1097/ADM.0000000000000323

Johnson, V.E. (1990). *I'll quit tomorrow: A practical guide to alcoholism treatment* (Rev. ed.). HarperSanFrancisco.

Kaij, L., & Rosenthal, D. (1961, September). Alcoholism in twins: Studies on the etiology and sequels of abuse of alcohol. *The Journal of Nervous and Mental Disease, 133*(3), 272.

Karpman, S. (1968). Fairy tales and script drama analysis. *Transactional Analysis Bulletin.* 26 (7): 39–43.

Kilmer, B., Nicosia, N., Heaton, P., & Midgette, G. (2013). Efficacy of frequent monitoring with swift, certain, and modest sanctions for violations: Insights from South Dakota's 24/7 sobriety project. *American Journal of Public Health, 103*(1), 37–43.

Kuhn, T. (1962). *The structure of scientific revolutions*. University of Chicago Press.

Lancer, D. (2017, June 21). Codependency addiction: stages of disease and recovery. *Global Journal of Addiction & Rehabilitation Medicine 2*(2). https://doi.org/10.19080/GJARM.2017.02.555582

La Rosa, J. (2020, February 5) *$42 Billion U.S. Addiction Rehab Industry Poised for Growth, and Challenges*. Marketdata LLC. Retrieved from https://www.marketdataenterprises.com/addiction-rehab-industry-poised-for-growth-and-challenges/ on 2021, April 25.

The LBJ Library. (2014, February 27). *The Moyers' Journey from addiction to recovery* [Video]. https://www.youtube.com/watch?v=EI86nx4SuB4

Leshner, A.I. (1997, October 3). Addiction is a brain disease, and it matters. *Science, 278*(5335), 45–47. https://doi.org/10.1126/science.278.5335.45

Levin, J.D., Culkin, J., & Perrotto. (2001). *Introduction to chemical dependency counseling*. Jason Aronson.

Library of Congress. (2012, June 25–September 29) *Books that shaped America*. Library of Congress Southwest Gallery Exhibition. Retrieved from https://www.loc.gov/exhibits/books-that-shaped-america/1900-to-1950.html on 2021, May 30.

Lyvers, M. (2000). "Loss of control" in alcoholism and drug addiction: A neuroscientific interpretation. *Experimental and Clinical Psychopharmacology, 8*(2), 225–249. https://doi.org/10.1037/1064-1297.8.2.225

Maharaj, N. (1973). *I am that*. Acorn Press.

Maté, G. (2010). *In the realm of hungry ghosts: Close encounters with addiction*. North Atlantic Books.

McCauley, K.T. (2007). *First year: The first year in recovery*. [Audio CD]. The Institute For Addiction Study.

McCrady, B.S., Epstein, E.E., & Kahler, C.W. (2004). Alcoholics Anonymous and relapse prevention as maintenance strategies after conjoint behavioral alcohol treatment for men: 18 month outcomes. *Journal of Consulting and Clinical Psychology, 72*(5), 870–878. https://doi.org/10.1037/0022-006X.72.5.870

McGoldrick, M., Gerson, R., & Petry, S. (2020). *Genograms: Assessment and treatment* (2nd ed.). W.W. Norton & Company.

McLellan, A., Weinstein, R.L., Shen, Q., Kendig, C., & Levine, M. (2005). Improving continuity of care in a public addiction treatment system with clinical case management. *American Journal on Addictions, 14*(5), 426–440.

Mitchell, S.A. (2002) *Can love last?* W.W. Norton and Company.

Moyers, B. (Host). (1998, March 29). The hijacked brain. (Episode 1) [TV Series] *Moyers on addiction: Close to home*. Public Broadcasting Service.

National Institute of Mental Health. (2016, May). Substance use and mental health. Retrieved on 2/20/2021 from https://www.nimh.nih.gov/

health/topics/substance-use-and-mental-health/index.shtml

National Institute on Drug Abuse (NIDA). (2018, January). *Principles of drug addiction treatment: A research-based guide*. https://www.drugabuse.gov/publications/principles-drug-addiction-treatment-research-based-guide-third-edition/preface

National Institute on Drug Abuse (NIDA). (2020, July 10). *Treatment and recovery*. Retrieved from https://www.drugabuse.gov/publications/drugs-brains-behavior-science-addiction/treatment-recovery on 2021, May 30.

National Institute on Drug Abuse (NIDA). (2020, June 3). *Is drug addiction treatment worth its cost?* Retrieved from https://www.drugabuse.gov/publications/principles-drug-addiction-treatment-research-based-guide-third-edition/frequently-asked-questions/drug-addiction-treatment-worth-its-cost on 2021, September 1.

NIDA. 2020, May 29. Preface. Retrieved from https://www.drugabuse.gov/publications/principles-drug-addiction-treatment-research-based-guide-third-edition/preface on 2021, July 7.

92nd Y. (2013, April 18). *Addiction: A Family's path to recovery: Bill Moyers, William Moyers and Judith Moyers* [Video]. https://www.youtube.com/watch?v=QEBWn7RwbEM

Noriega, G. (2004). Codependence: A transgenerational script. *Transactional Analysis Journal, 34*(4), 312–322. https://doi.org/10.1177/036215370403400404

Office of the Surgeon General. (2016). *Facing addiction in America: The Surgeon General's report on alcohol, drugs, and health*. U.S. Department of Health and Human Services.

Oliver, J. (Host). (2018, May 20). *Rehab: Last Week Tonight with John Oliver (HBO)*. [Video]. YouTube. Retrieved from https://www.youtube.com/watch?v=hWQiXv0sn9Y on 2021, May 30.

Redwood Toxicology Laboratory, Inc. (n.d.-c). *Benzodiazepines*. Redwood Toxicology Laboratory, Inc. Retrieved July 8, 2021, from https://www.redwoodtoxicology.com/resources/drug_info/benzodiazepines

Redwood Toxicology Laboratory, Inc. (n.d.-d). *Cocaine*. Redwood Toxicology Laboratory, Inc. Retrieved July 8, 2021, from https://www.redwoodtoxicology.com/resources/drug_info/cocaine

Redwood Toxicology Laboratory, Inc. (n.d.-e). *EtG/EtS alcohol testing*. Redwood Toxicology Laboratory, Inc. Retrieved July 8, 2021, from https://www.redwoodtoxicology.com/services/etg_testing

Redwood Toxicology Laboratory, Inc. (n.d.-f). *Marijuana*. Redwood Toxicology Laboratory, Inc. Retrieved July 8, 2021, from https://www.redwoodtoxicology.com/resources/drug_info/marijuana

Redwood Toxicology Laboratory, Inc. (n.d.-g). *Methadone*. Redwood Toxicology Laboratory, Inc. https://www.redwoodtoxicology.com/resources/drug_info/methadone

Redwood Toxicology Laboratory, Inc. (n.d.-h). *Opiates*. Redwood Toxicology Laboratory, Inc. Retrieved July 8, 2021, from https://www.redwoodtoxicology.com/resources/drug_info/opiates

Redwood Toxicology Laboratory, Inc. (n.d.-i). *Phencyclidine*. Redwood Toxicology Laboratory, Inc. Retrieved July 8, 2021, from https://www.redwoodtoxicology.com/resources/drug_info/phencyclidine

Redwood Toxicology Laboratory, Inc. (n.d.-a). *Amphetamines*. Redwood Toxicology Laboratory, Inc. Retrieved July 8, 2021, from https://www.redwoodtoxicology.com/resources/drug_info/amphetamines

Redwood Toxicology Laboratory, Inc. (n.d.-b). *Barbiturates*. Redwood Toxicology Laboratory, Inc. Retrieved July 8, 2021, from https://www.redwoodtoxicology.com/resources/drug_info/barbiturates

Rogers, C. (1995). *On becoming a person: A therapist's view of psychotherapy*. Houghton Mifflin.

Rotunda, R.J., West, L., & O'Farrell, T.J. (2004). Enabling behavior in a clinical sample of alcohol-dependent clients and their partners. *Journal of Substance Abuse Treatment, 26*(4), 269–276. https://doi.org/10.1016/j.jsat.2004.01.007

Satz, R., Larson, M.J., LaBelle, C., Richardson, J,. & Samet, J. (2008, June). The case for chronic disease management for addiction. *Journal of Addiction Medicine, 2*(2), 55–65. https://doi.org/10.1097/ADM.0b013e318166af74

Selzer, M. (1971). The Michigan alcoholism screening test: The quest for a new diagnostic instrument. *The American Journal of Psychiatry, 127*(12), 1653–1658. https://doi.org/10.1176/ajp.127.12.1653

Staton, M.D., Todd, T.C., & Associates. (1982). *Family therapy of drug abuse and addiction*. Guilford Press.

Substance Abuse and Mental Health Services Administration. (2012, November). *Results from the 2011 National survey on drug use and health: Mental health findings* (NSDUH Series H-44, HHS Publication No. (SMA) 12–4713). Retrieved from https://www.samhsa.gov/data/sites/default/files/2011MHFDT/2k11MHFR/Web/NSDUHmhfr2011.htm on 2021, May 30.

Substance Abuse and Mental Health Services Administration. (2020). *Substance use disorder treatment and family therapy*. Treatment Improvement Protocol (TIP) Series, No. 39. DHHS Publication No. (SMA) 04-3957.

Substance Abuse and Mental Health Services Administration. (2021, March). *What is buprenorphine?* Retrieved from https://www.samhsa.gov/medication-assisted-treatment/medications-counseling-related-conditions/buprenorphine on 2021, May 30.

Sun, F. (2011, August 16). All-time 100 non-fiction books. Time. Retrieved from https://

entertainment.time.com/2011/08/30/all-time-100-best-nonfiction-books/slide/the-big-book-by-alcoholics-anonymous/ on 2021, May 30.

Tartarsky, A. (2002). *Harm reduction psychotherapy: A new treatment for drug and alcohol problems*. Rowman & Littlefield.

TED. (2015, July 9). *Everything you think you know about addiction is wrong: Johann Hari* [Video]. https://www.youtube.com/watch?v=PY9DcIMGxMs

Tiebout, H. (1944). Therapeutic mechanisms of Alcoholics Anonymous. *American Journal of Psychiatry, 100*, 468–473.

Timko, C., & DeBenedetti, A. (2007). A randomized controlled trial of intensive referral to 12-step self-help groups: One year outcomes. *Drug and Alcohol Dependence, 90*(2), 270–279.

Tolle, E. (1999). *The power of now: A guide to spiritual enlightenment*. New World Library.

Twerski, A.J. (1997). *Addictive thinking: Understanding self-deception*. Hazelden.

Wandzilak, K., & Curry, C. (2006). *The lost years: Surviving a Mother and Daughter's Worst Nightmare*. Jeffers Press.

White, W.L. (1998). *Slaying the dragon: The history of addiction treatment and recovery in America*. Chestnut Health Systems/Lighthouse Institute.

World Health Organization. (2018, June 18). *WHO releases new International Classification of Diseases (ICD 11)*. World Health Organization. Retrieved July 8, 2021, from https://www.who.int/news/item/18-06-2018-who-releases-new-international-classification-of-diseases-(icd-11)

Index

ABC Problem Solving Worksheet 259
abstinence 13, 14
abstinence-only social support group 11
addict centered approach 64–65
addicted brain 11, 13
addiction 11; addict, damage to 76; American Society of Addiction Medicine (ASAM) 81–87; behavioral addiction 79; biological basis 17; brain changes 70–72; chronic condition 35–36; clinical overview 67–74; codependent dynamics 75–76; definition 70, 78–79; degrees of abuse 72; *DSM-5* Diagnostic Criteria for Substance Abuse Disorders 79–80; family, damage to 76–77; family disease 74–76; impaired control 79, 80; lack of control 71–72; medical illness 13, 20, 25; mental illness 14–15; neurobiology 82; pharmacological indicators 79, 80; risky use 79, 80; social impairment 79, 80
Addiction/Codependency Family Treatment Agreement 134, 176, 305–306
addiction trained psychiatrists 59
addiction treatment: Affordable Care Act 27; birth 26; cost 311–312; history 16–22; insurance reimbursement 26; new paradigm 12, 13, 22, 24–27, 131, 233, 250; programs 23
addictive/codependent system 18, 27, 42–44, 64
addictive family systems 39
Adverse Childhood Experiences (ACE) 15
aftercare plan 146
Al-Anon 17, 20, 51, 54–55, 56, 266
Alcohol Use Disorders Identification Test (AUDIT) 164, 193
The Alcoholic Family in Recover: A Developmental Model 17, 45, 131, 153, 216
Alcoholics Anonymous 12, 16, 25, 51–53, 252, 259–280
Alcoholics Anonymous 12, 69, 254–256, 264
American Society of Addiction Medicine (ASAM) 11, 13, 17, 20, 67
antidepressants, use of 14
anxiety 14
ASAM *see* American Society of Addiction Medicine (ASAM)
Association of Intervention Specialists (AIS) 244

behavioral addictions 79
behavioral therapy 73
bipolar disorder 14
Bowen, Murray 17, 20, 25–26, 33, 38–39, 131

Bowen's Theory of Family Systems: differentiation of self 109–112, 120–122; emotional cutoff 107, 117–118, 127–128; family projection process 116–117, 126–127; foundation of family recovery therapy 118–120; LO 2—Eight Interlocking Theoretical Concepts 107–108; LO 3 108–109; LO 5 Triangles 112–113; LO 6 117–118; nuclear family emotional system 114–116, 125–126; transgenerational models 107–108; triangles 122–125
brain disease 17, 18
brain disorder of addiction 13
brain imaging techniques 21, 70
Brown, Dr. Stephanie 17, 31, 37, 45, 62, 76, 121–122, 131, 153, 216–230, 256
Buprenorphine 14, 60

Can Love Last 16
case studies: adolescent 207–215; parent 184–206; spouse 159–183; young adult 137–158
Cermak, Timmen 31, 45, 97, 131, 242, 290
Certified Intervention Professional (CIP) 244
character defects 269–270
childhood trauma and substance abuse disorders 15
chronicity 70, 166–167
Cocaine Anonymous 51
Co-Dependents Anonymous 4, 55, 279
codependency 17, 37–40, 44–47, 53–58, 76–77, 121–122
cognitive behavioral therapy 13, 73
compulsive gambling 11
computer gaming 11
consent to the agreement 146
continuum of care 7, 32, 44–46, 89, 93, 102
control (loss of) 70
coordination of treatment, lack of 26
craving 70

Debtors Anonymous 12, 51
denial 61–62
depression 14
desistance theory 72–73
Detachment 54
detox facility 29
Developmental Model of Family Recovery: abstinence stage 217, 224–226; drinking stage 217, 219–222; early recovery stage 217, 219, 226–228; environment 219; family system 216–217, 219; four stages of recovery 219; individual development 217, 219; ongoing recovery 217, 219, 228–230; overview 216;

three domains of change 219; transition stage 217, 218–219, 222–224; trauma of recovery 224–225
differentiation 23
disorder of disconnection 15
Dodes, Dr. Lance 13, 73
Dopamine 68
drug testing: breathalyzers 286–287; frequency 283–284; necessity 281–282; random 285–286; retention rate 283–285; verification 282–283
DSM-5 67, 78–79

Eight Stages of Psycho-Social Development 8, 293–296
Emotional Acre 77
Erikson, Erik 8, 293–296

Facing Addiction in America: The Surgeon General's Report on Alcohol, Drugs, and Health 7, 12, 34–35
family disease 17
family dynamics 18, 20
family-focused therapy 26
family programs 64–65
Family Recovery Therapy (FRT): co-occurring issues, assessment 58–59; codependency 57–58, 63–66; conclusion 289–291; Developmental Model of Family Recovery 216–230; drug testing 60–61; family commitment to treatment 62–63; goals 8; initial contact, engagement of treatment in 63–66; medically assisted treatment 60; mental and physical health problems, monitoring 58–59; mutual aid program, role 49–55; NIDA *Principles of Drug Addiction, versus* 90–106; overview 7; paths to growth and recovery, understanding 55–57; principles 35–67; professional congruity 56–57; social support groups, role 49–55; therapeutic goals, understanding 61–62; treatment recommendations 61–62; 12-step culture, understanding 55–57; Twelve-Step model 49–55
family systems 26, 33, 39–42
family therapist 49
Fellowship and addicts 15–16; *see also* Twelve-Step programs
First Year in Recovery 302–304
fragmented treatment 46–48
Freud, Sigmund 16, 19
FRT Therapist 7, 12, 29, 44–49

Gamblers Anonymous 12, 51
Gamers Anonymous 12
gaming disorder 32–33
genogram 134, 135
Gorney, Cynthia 313–315

harm reduction approaches 13, 73, 240
Harm Reduction Psychotherapy 13
The Heart of Addiction: A New Approach to Understanding and Managing Alcoholism and Other Addictive Behaviors (2002) 73
higher power 54–55
Human Intervention and Motivation Study (HIMS) 148, 302–304

identified patient 30, 64
imaging techniques and addiction 18
in recovery 55–56
In the Realm of Hungry Ghosts: Close Encounters with Addiction 15, 68, 251
ineffective treatment 88–89
informed consent form 135
initial call 134–135
initial sessions with enabling codependents 135–136
integrated treatment process 42–49, 93, 99, 147
Intensive Outpatient Program (IOP) 28, 29, 133
intervention 17, 18, 19, 245
interventionist 29, 47
IP-ing 30

Johnson, Vernon 17, 245
Johnson method 17, 20, 245

Karpman Drama Triangle 161
Kuhn, Thomas 24, 25, 26, 27

letter of accountability 146
Lewis, Dr. Virginia 17, 45, 216
LifeRing Secular Recovery 12, 15, 51, 252, 253, 259, 318
Long Definition of Addiction 11
long-term addiction 11
The Lost Years: Surviving a Mother and Daughter's Worst Nightmare 140

Marijuana Anonymous 51
Maté, Gabor 15, 28, 68
McCauley, Kevin 31, 131, 148, 302–304
medically assisted treatment (M.A.T.) 12, 14, 19, 60
medically defined addiction 11
mental health and addiction 19
Mental Health Parity and Addiction Equity Act of 2008 26, 133
Michigan Alcoholism Screening Test (MAST) 164, 193, 308
Mitchell, Stephen 16
motivational therapy 73
multidimensional family therapy 26
My Addicted Child: Codependency, Enabling, and the Road to Recovery (2015) 75
My Addicted Spouse 159

Naltrexone 14
Narcotics Anonymous 12, 51
Nicotine Anonymous 51
NIDA *Principles of Drug Addiction Treatment* 89–106

Overeaters Anonymous 12, 51

paradigm shifts 25
parentified child 39
peer support, value of 25
personality disorders 14
Pilot Recovery Program 302–304
post-traumatic stress disorder 14
prefrontal cortex 18, 50, 68
presenting problem 134
Principles of Drug Addiction Treatment: A Research-Based Guide 35, 89

problematic substance abusers 73
psychodynamic therapy 13, 73

Recovery Bus 270
Reedy, Brad 1–5, 31, 131
Rehab 133
relapse prevention plan 303
"Requiem: My Mother's Unspeakable Illness" 313–315
residential treatment centers 17, 29, 30, 64–65, 133
resistance to treatment plan 61–63
resources, additional 307
Return to Flight 148, 302–304
Rumney, Avis 75, 159
Rush, Dr. Benjamin 25

Schuckit, Marc 69
Secular Organizations for Recovery 51, 251, 253, 259, 318
self-differentiation 39
Serenity Prayer 37
Sex and Love Addicts Anonymous 12, 51
Silkworth, Dr. William 69
simple abuse 11
SMART Recovery 12, 15, 51, 252, 259, 318
Smith, Dr. Bob 16
sober homes 26–27
Sober Living Environment (SLE) 28, 29, 133, 176
social support groups: Al-Anon 256–257; Alcoholics Anonymous 253–254; availability 252–253; codependents 256–257; foundation to recovery 251–252; non 12 step programs 253–254; role 12, 13, 14, 15, 49–55, 64, 318; secular recovery 258–259; 12-Step programs 259–280
spiritual awakening 276–277, 319–320
Spiritual Experience 319–320
spousified child 39, 221
step-down facility 248
The Structure of Scientific Revolutions 24–25
suboxone 14

Substance Abuse and Mental Health Services Administration (SAMHSA) 26
surprise model interventions 17, 18, 20, 171, 245
systemic interventions 18, 21, 245

Tatarsky, Andrew 13
Ten Principles of Successful Addiction Treatment 302–304
testing instruments 308–310
Tolle, Eckhart 70
transactional analysis 123–124
traumatic developmental deficits 15
Treating the Alcoholic: A Developmental Model of Recovery 17
Treatment Agreement 133, 146, 176
treatment providers: Alcoholics Anonymous 299–301; educational consultants (ECs) 243–244; government agencies 249–250; interventionists 244–245; lawyers, probation officers and courts 242–244; overview 233–236; physicians 236–238; psychiatrists 238–239; psychologists and psychotherapists 239–242; residential treatment center (RTC) clinical directors 245–247; sober living environments (SLEs) 248–249
true addicts 13
12 by 12 51
Twelve Questions 164
12-Step fellowships 12–13, 56–57
Twelve-Step programs 14–16, 19, 318
Twelve Steps and Twelve Traditions 51

unconscious actions 17, 19, 20

Vivitrol 14

Wandazilak, Kristina 270
wilderness program 1, 3, 48, 145
willpower and addiction 18, 23, 25
Wilson, Bill 16, 17, 51, 54, 254
Wilson, Lois 17, 54
Women for Sobriety 12, 51, 318

www.ingramcontent.com/pod-product-compliance
Ingram Content Group UK Ltd.
Pitfield, Milton Keynes, MK11 3LW, UK
UKHW050543150426
5217IPUK00026B/2050